GAS MIXING AND DISTRIBUTION IN THE LUNG

LUNG BIOLOGY IN HEALTH AND DISEASE

Executive Editor: **Claude Lenfant**

Director, National Heart, Lung, and Blood Institute
National Institutes of Health
Bethesda, Maryland

Volume 1 IMMUNOLOGIC AND INFECTIOUS REACTIONS IN THE LUNG, *edited by Charles H. Kirkpatrick and Herbert Y. Reynolds*

Volume 2 THE BIOCHEMICAL BASIS OF PULMONARY FUNCTION, *edited by Ronald G. Crystal*

Volume 3 BIOENGINEERING ASPECTS OF THE LUNG, *edited by John B. West*

Volume 4 METABOLIC FUNCTIONS OF THE LUNG, *edited by Y. S. Bakhle and John R. Vane*

Volume 5 RESPIRATORY DEFENSE MECHANISMS (in two parts), *edited by Joseph D. Brain, Donald F. Proctor, and Lynne M. Reid*

Volume 6 DEVELOPMENT OF THE LUNG, *edited by W. Alan Hodson*

Volume 7 LUNG WATER AND SOLUTE EXCHANGE, *edited by Norman C. Staub*

Volume 8 EXTRAPULMONARY MANIFESTATIONS OF RESPIRATORY DISEASE, *edited by Eugene Debs Robin*

Volume 9 CHRONIC OBSTRUCTIVE PULMONARY DISEASE, *edited by Thomas L. Petty*

Volume 10 PATHOGENESIS AND THERAPY OF LUNG CANCER, *edited by Curtis C. Harris*

Volume 11 GENETIC DETERMINANTS OF PULMONARY DISEASE, *edited by Stephen D. Litwin*

Volume 12 THE LUNG IN THE TRANSITION BETWEEN HEALTH AND DISEASE, *edited by Peter T. Macklem and Solbert Permutt*

Volume 13 EVOLUTION OF RESPIRATORY PROCESSES: A COMPARATIVE APPROACH, *edited by Stephen C. Wood and Claude Lenfant*

Volume 14 PULMONARY VASCULAR DISEASES, *edited by Kenneth M. Moser*

Volume 15 PHYSIOLOGY AND PHARMACOLOGY OF THE AIRWAYS, *edited by Jay A. Nadel*

Volume 16 DIAGNOSTIC TECHNIQUES IN PULMONARY DISEASE (in two parts), *edited by Marvin A. Sackner*

Volume 17 REGULATION OF BREATHING (in two parts), *edited by Thomas F. Hornbein*

Volume 18 OCCUPATIONAL LUNG DISEASES: RESEARCH APPROACHES AND METHODS, *edited by Hans Weill and Margaret Turner-Warwick*

Volume 19 IMMUNOPHARMACOLOGY OF THE LUNG, *edited by Harold H. Newball*

Volume 20 SARCOIDOSIS AND OTHER GRANULOMATOUS DISEASES OF THE LUNG, *edited by Barry L. Fanburg*

Volume 21 SLEEP AND BREATHING, *edited by Nicholas A. Saunders and Colin E. Sullivan*

Volume 22 *PNEUMOCYSTIS CARINII* PNEUMONIA: PATHOGENESIS, DIAGNOSIS, AND TREATMENT, *edited by Lowell S. Young*

Volume 23 PULMONARY NUCLEAR MEDICINE: TECHNIQUES IN DIAGNOSIS OF LUNG DISEASE, *edited by Harold L. Atkins*

Volume 24 ACUTE RESPIRATORY FAILURE, *edited by Warren M. Zapol and Konrad J. Falke*

Volume 25 GAS MIXING AND DISTRIBUTION IN THE LUNG, *edited by Ludwig A. Engel and Manuel Paiva*

Other volumes in preparation

HIGH-FREQUENCY VENTILATION IN INTENSIVE CARE AND DURING SURGERY, *edited by Graziano Carlon and William S. Howland*

PULMONARY DEVELOPMENT: TRANSITION FROM INTRAUTERINE TO EXTRAUTERINE LIFE, *edited by George H. Nelson*

THE THORAX (in two parts), *edited by Charis Roussos and Peter T. Macklem*

CHRONIC OBSTRUCTIVE PULMONARY DISEASE (second edition), *edited by Thomas L. Petty*

THE PLEURA IN HEALTH AND DISEASE, *edited by Jacques Chrétien, Jean Bignon, Albert Hirsch, and Gerard Huchon*

GAS MIXING AND DISTRIBUTION IN THE LUNG

Edited by

Ludwig A. Engel

Thoracic Medicine Unit
Westmead Hospital
Sydney, New South Wales
Australia

Manuel Paiva

Institute of Interdisciplinary Research
and Respiratory Research Unit
Free University of Brussels
Belgium

MARCEL DEKKER, INC. New York • Basel

Library of Congress Cataloging in Publication Data

Main entry under title:

Gas mixing and distribution in the lung.

(Lung biology in health and disease ; v. 25)
Includes bibliographies and indexes.
1. Pulmonary gas exchange. I. Engel, Ludwig A.
II. Paiva, Manuel. III. Series.
[DNLM: 1. Lung--physiology. 2. Pulmonary Gas Exchange.
3. Respiration. W1 LU62 v.25 WF 102 G2465]
QP124.G37 1985 599'.012 85-1662
ISBN 0-8247-7284-9

Marcel Dekker, Inc.
270 Madison Avenue, New York, New York 10016

Current printing (last digit);
10 9 8 7 6 5 4 3 2 1

Printed in the United States of America

CONTRIBUTORS

Terence C. Amis, B.V.Sc., M.R.C.V.S., Ph.D. Assistant Professor, Department of Medicine, School of Veterinary Medicine, University of California at Davis, Davis, California

H. K. Chang, Ph.D.* Professor, Departments of Physiology and Medicine and Biomedical Engineering Unit, McGill University, Montreal, Quebec, Canada

Jeffrey M. Drazen, M.D. Associate Professor, Department of Medicine, Harvard Medical School, and Brigham and Women's Hospital, Boston, Massachusetts

Ludwig A. Engel, M.B.B.S., Ph.D., F.R.A.C.P. Head, Thoracic Medicine Unit, Westmead Hospital, Sydney, New South Wales, Australia

Keith Horsfield, D.Sc., Ph.D., M.D., F.R.C.P. Deputy Medical Director, The Midhurst Medical Research Institute, Midhurst, West Sussex, England

J. M. B. Hughes, M.A., D.M., F.R.C.P. Senior Lecturer, Respiratory Division, Department of Medicine, Royal Postgraduate Medical School, and Consultant Physician, Hammersmith Hospital, London, England

Roger D. Kamm, Ph.D. Associate Professor, Department of Mechanical Engineering, Massachusetts Institute of Technology, Cambridge, Massachusetts

Manuel Paiva, Ph.D. Senior Research Scientist, Institute of Interdisciplinary Research and Respiratory Research Unit, Free University of Brussels, Brussels, Belgium

---

Present affiliation:
*Professor, Department of Biomedical Engineering and Department of Physiology and Biophysics, University of Southern California, Los Angeles, California

Johannes Piiper, M.D. Director, Abteilung Physiologie, Max-Planck-Institut für experimentelle Medizin, Göttingen, Federal Republic of Germany

Peter Scheid, M.D. Professor, Institut für Physiologie, Ruhr-Universität, Bochum, Federal Republic of Germany

Arthur S. Slutsky, M.A.Sc., M.D.* Assistant Professor, Department of Medicine, Harvard Medical School, Boston, and Staff Physician, West Roxbury Veterans Administration Medical Center, West Roxbury, Massachusetts

James S. Ultman, Ph.D. Professor, Department of Chemical Engineering and the Bioengineering Program, The Pennsylvania State University, University Park, Pennsylvania

---

Present affiliation:
*Associate Professor, Department of Medicine, University of Toronto, and Mount Sinai Hospital, Toronto, Ontario, Canada

PREFACE

Ever since Hooke's classical demonstration in 1667 that it is the flow of fresh gas into the lungs, rather than their movement, that is essential for sustaining life, the study of the way inspired gases are distributed and mix in the lung has been a source of great interest to life scientists. The more recent observation that, in many respiratory disorders, ventilation distribution and gas mixing are impaired early in the course of the disorder adds a pragmatic component to the need to understand this process in both health and disease.

It is appropriate that this volume should be edited by a physician and a physicist who not only share an interest in the subject but have collaborated in their research for nearly a decade. This collaboration illustrates the multidisciplinary approach that has been applied to the investigation of gas mixing in the lung for many years and is reflected in the varied professional backgrounds of the contributors to this volume.

The flow of gases and their transport to the lung periphery have attracted the attention of both mechanical and chemical engineers who have specialized knowledge of fluid dynamics and mass transport. Chapter 3 offers a comprehensive description of the dispersion of gases in conducting airways during transport between mouth and alveoli. When tidal volumes are smaller than the anatomical dead space, the various mechanisms for axial dispersion can sustain adequate alveolar ventilation and gas exchange at high frequencies of ventilation. This relatively new and developing subject is dealt with in Chapter 4. The topographical or regional distribution of ventilation is largely determined by respiratory mechanics and is covered in Chapter 5. In this field, radioactive gas isotopes have been of fundamental importance in advancing our knowledge. Improvements in the nature of the isotopes and the imaging facilities continue to make this an interesting area.

Because of the large increase in the number of airways in the terminal generations of the bronchial tree, most of the lung volume is contained within units distal to the terminal bronchioles, i.e., the acini. Indeed, this is where most of the gas mixing takes place. The physical processes involved encompass fundamental phenomena such as molecular diffusion and convection, as well as various types of interaction between them. Basic principles of molecular diffusion, the most important mechanism of gas mixing, are reviewed in Chapter 1. Surprisingly, although gas distribution is probably very sensitive to lung anatomy, detailed information on acinar structure is very limited. Yet the geometrical boundaries within which gas transport takes place are the starting point for any accurate quantitative description. What is known and how lung anatomy influences gas mixing and its distribution are discussed in Chapter 2.

Currently, there is no available technique for measuring gas concentrations within the lung acinus. Consequently, most of the experimental data, reviewed in Chapter 7, consist of inferences drawn from measurements made on gases expired from whole lungs or sampled within relatively large conducting airways. Partly for this reason there has been substantial use made of mathematical modeling to understand gas mixing within the lung. Indeed, during the past decade, sophisticated computer simulations of gas transport in the lung periphery have constituted the most exciting steps toward a better understanding of this subject. This theoretical approach beginning with a pedagogical exposition is given in Chapter 6.

Finally, in Chapter 8, instructive comparisons are made between gas-exchanging organs in mammalian and nonmammalian vertebrates, providing a broad framework within which to understand the structure and function of the human lung.

This volume offers a synthesis of most aspects of gas mixing and ventilation distribution in the lung. It provides the theoretical basis as well as an up-to-date account of experimental findings in this field, not available in any other single publication. We hope that the contents will help to clarify some difficult and often confusing aspects of gas mixing and its study using mathematical models. In addition, the volume will hopefully serve as a valuable reference source for both experimental and theoretical information useful to clinicians, physiologists, and investigators in a wide variety of disciplines.

Ludwig A. Engel
Manuel Paiva

INTRODUCTION

Ever since Grehant's publication of "Recherches physiques sur la respiration de l'homme" in 1864, the matter of gas distribution in the lungs has been a topic of great interest and creative research. The beginning of the 20th century brought a realization of the importance of this problem. It is Arthur Keith who must be credited for this realization when, at a meeting of the Medical Society of the London Hospital in 1903, he asked the question: "Why does phthisis attack the apex of the lung?"

For nearly 80 years, an incredible amount of research has been directed to the study of the magnitude and the mechanisms of uneven gas distribution in the lungs in health and in disease. The greatest names in respiratory physiology have been associated with this research, which at the time was responsible for unrelenting scientific debates. Over the years, opposing sides developed around the questions "Stratified inhomogeneity in the alveolar ducts without regional inhomogeneity?" or "Regional inhomogeneity without stratified inhomogeneity in the alveolar ducts?" The fathers of modern respiratory physiology, Haldane, Priestly, Krogh, Lindhard, Meakins, Barcroft, Hasselbach, and Rohrer, among others, were all directly or indirectly involved in these debates. Today the study of gas distribution in the lungs is just as important and popular as it was decades ago, but at last the consensus seems to be that both interregional and intraacinar inhomogeneities are responsible.

During the last 20 years, remarkable techniques and innovative approaches have been developed and used to study gas distribution unevenness. Advances in anatomy, modeling, and computation have shed tremendous light on this problem. Even the recognition that observations in species other than mammalian can make extremely important contributions has been a landmark in our current understanding.

For years Manuel Paiva and Ludwig Engel have been interested in gas distribution. Their contributions have been essential to what we know today. It was, therefore, a great asset to the series of monographs "Lung Biology in Health and Disease" when they agreed to edit this volume. As those who are familiar with the series will recognize, it is one of the shortest monographs. Yet it stands out by virtue of some remarkable characteristics: The editors have assembled a truly international group of authors, all leaders in their field. Although small, this volume is both broad and comprehensive. To have seen this volume develop has been a rewarding experience to me, and I am confident that its readers will be informed and challenged by its content.

Claude Lenfant, M.D.
Bethesda, Maryland

CONTENTS

1

General Concepts of Molecular Diffusion

H. K. CHANG*

McGill University
Montreal, Quebec, Canada

I. Introduction

The earliest investigators in diffusion were motivated primarily by their desire to understand the processes of biological transport. They studied diffusion of liquids, especially across membranes. In the early part of the nineteenth century, physicists and chemists who attempted to unravel the mystery of atomic and molecular forces also became interested in diffusion, principally in the gaseous state. Among this group was Thomas Graham (1805-1869). Using a glass tube with a dense stucco plug at one end and submerged in water at the other end, Graham measured the rate of flux of various gases through the stucco plug. Because the flux of the experimental gas does not equal the flux of air, the water level in the tube will either rise or fall during diffusion. Graham correctly saw that this change in water level would lead to a pressure gradient which would in turn alter diffusion. To overcome this, he continually adjusted the tube position so that the water level stayed constant. His experimental results then consisted of a volume change reflecting the diffusional property of each gas originally held in the tube. Graham showed that this volume change was inversely propor-

**Present affiliation:* University of Southern California, Los Angeles, California.

tional to the square root of the density of the gas. "Graham's law" (Graham, 1833) was thus stated: "The diffusion or spontaneous intermixture of two gases in contact is affected by an interchange of position of infinitely minute volumes, being, in the case of each gas, inversely proportional to the square root of the density of the gas. . . ."

It should be noted that Graham's experiments involved a moving frame of reference for measuring the diffusion fluxes. What was kept constant was the pressure gradient across the stucco plug, not the number of molecules exchanged between air and the experimental gas. This feature of Graham's experiments has caused considerable confusion among later workers. Furthermore, the inverse square-root relationship was specifically derived with air as the second gas in the diffusion process. When applied to other situations, Graham's law as it is known to today's respiratory physiologists may lead to erroneous results.

Taking an analogy from the heat conduction law, which states that the flux of heat is directly proportional to the temperature gradient that causes it, Fick (1855) suggested that "the diffusion of the dissolved material" and "the spreading of warmth in a conductor" were both "left to the influence of molecular forces basic to the same law." Hence he postulated that the concentration gradient of a substance and the resulting diffusional flux are linearly related. Namely,

$$J_z = -\mathcal{D}\frac{dc}{dz} \tag{1}$$

where J_z is the mass flux and dc/dz is the concentration gradient, both in the z direction. The proportionality constant $\mathcal{D}$ is known as the diffusion coefficient.

Fourier's law of heat conduction, Fick's law of diffusion, and Newton's law of viscosity, which states that the shear stress in a flowing fluid is directly proportional to the local velocity gradient, all describe *macroscopic* phenomena. These phenomenological laws, which have similar forms, do not themselves give any insight into the reasons for the behavior they describe. As was correctly foreseen by Fick, there is indeed a molecular or *microscopic* basis which links these macroscopic phenomena. This link was to be found in the kinetic theory of gases, initially developed by Rudolf Clausius (1822-1888) and James Maxwell (1831-1879).

In this chapter we shall be concerned mainly with the application of the macroscopic, phenomenological laws, namely, the determination of diffusion coefficients and the prediction of diffusional fluxes. Before setting out to do that, however, it is useful to examine the general nature of gaseous diffusion and the microscopic basis of molecular diffusion.

II. General Description of Gaseous Diffusion

When a gas mixture contains two or more different kinds of molecules whose spatial distribution is nonuniform, a process called *diffusion* occurs continuously in such a way as to diminish the nonuniformity of composition. The kinetic theory of gases offers an explanation of this phenomenon.

The molecules in the gaseous state are in constant thermal motion due to their thermal energy. They collide with each other, rebound, then collide again. The motion and collisions are purely random. In homogeneous mixtures, if one considers an imaginary plane fixed in space, the net number of molecules that move across the plane over a sufficiently long time should be zero for molecules of the same kind. In nonhomogeneous mixtures, as a consequence of the thermal motion, more molecules of a given kind travel from regions rich in that kind to regions of scarcity than travel in the opposite direction. The process tends to smooth out the original nonuniform distribution. Obviously, the net movement of each kind of molecule is likely to be in the direction in which its density increases most rapidly, where *density* means the number of molecules of the same kind per unit volume.

The description above applies to a general mixture of any number of different kinds of molecules (i.e., gas species). For convenience of discussion, the following refers to binary mixtures, those containing only two kinds of gas molecules. Since each kind of molecule moves according to its own density gradient, the rate of diffusion of the two constituents, in general, will not be equal. For different kinds of molecules having widely different velocities of thermal motion, the difference in diffusion rates may be very large. If nothing more than the thermal motion processes were involved in the phenomenon of diffusion, a greater number of the faster-moving molecules would be transferred in one direction than of the other in the opposite direction. The gas mixture as a whole would thus move bodily toward one side. Indeed, this was what Graham (1833) discovered in his glass-tube experiments.

The phenomenon of bodily motion caused by diffusion requires that for a quantitative description of the diffusion process, the frame of reference be appropriately defined. The most commonly used frame of reference is the *molar* frame of reference, which moves with the molar average velocity (i.e., the net difference among the rates of diffusion in molar units in a mixture). Therefore, when the net flux with respect to the molar frame of reference is zero, the diffusion is called *equimolar.* The general free diffusion with respect to a stationary frame of reference is *nonequimolar.*

III. Physical Basis of Molecular Diffusion

The number of molecules per mole of a substance (Avogadro's number) has been determined to be 6.023×10^{23}. From this number one can calculate that in 1 cm^3 of an ideal gas under standard conditions (STPD) there are 2.688×10^{19} molecules. The average distance of molecular separation at atmospheric pressure will be approximately the cube root of the inverse of this number, or 3.34×10^{-7} cm. The molecular diameter for a simple inorganic gas is in the range of $2\text{-}5 \times 10^{-8}$ cm (see Table 1). Thus for the common gases the average distance of molecular separation is approximately 10 times the molecular diameter.

At ordinary conditions of temperature and pressure, gas molecules have speeds of the order of 10^4 cm/sec (see Table 1). In contrast, actual diffusion velocities are much less, about 1 cm/sec. This great decrease in apparent molecular speed occurs because diffusion is dominated by collisions which deflect the molecules along tortuous paths. The collisions in turn are controlled by the forces of interaction between the molecules. By the formulas of kinetic theory, knowledge of these fundamental intermolecular forces can lead to predictions of the gaseous diffusion coefficients. The task of the kinetic theory of gases, then, is to construct a hypothetical model for the interaction between gas molecules, describe the molecular velocities and molecular collisions in a rational manner, and derive mathematically the transport coefficients and other macroscopic quantities.

The common hypotheses of all kinetic theories are that matter is composed of small discrete units known as the *molecules,* that all molecules of a given substance are alike, and that the three states of matter differ essentially in the arrangement and state of motion of the molecules. In the kinetic theory of gases, it is further assumed that all molecules are monoatomic and all molecular collisions are binary, involving only two molecules. Three body collisions are assumed to occur with only negligible frequency. Except at very low temperatures, pressures of less than 100 atm are low enough to ensure the validity of this hypothesis.

The discovery of wavelike subatomic particles in modern physics has made the original hypotheses of the kinetic theory appear rather crude. Nevertheless, this theory is very useful in explaining the aggregate behavior of a large number of molecules. As a demonstration of the power of the kinetic theory of gases and to give a crude physical explanation to the phenomenological laws, a very simple theory will be presented here.

In this simplified theory it is assumed that gas molecules are rigid, nonattracting spheres, all traveling with the same speed and only in the coordinate directions (x, y, z). It is also assumed that the total number of mole-

Table 1 Molecular Constants of Some Gases

Gas	Average velocity at 20°C (cm/sec × 10^2)	Mean free path at 75 cmHg (cm × 10^{-6})	Collision frequency at 20°C (sec^{-1} × 10^6)	Molecular diameter[a] (cm × 10^{-8})
Air	453	–	–	–
Argon (Ar)	395	9.88	4000	2.94
Carbon monoxide (CO)	471	9.73	5100	3.12
Carbon dioxide (CO_2)	376	6.15	6120	3.23
Helium (He)	1252	27.45	4540	2.65
Krypton (Kr)	272	–	–	3.69
Neon (Ne)	557	–	–	2.66
Nitrogen (N_2)	471	9.29	5070	3.15
Nitrous oxide (N_2O)	392	6.10	–	4.66
Oxygen (O_2)	440	9.93	4430	2.92
Water vapor (H_2O)	587	–	–	2.88
Xenon (Xe)	218	–	–	4.02

[a]Computed from van der Waals equation.
Source: Compiled from various sources.

cules is large in a small volume and that the conservation laws of classical mechanics apply.

Let the diameter of the gas molecules be d. Imagine two molecules A and B. When the centers of these two molecules are at a distance d, collision occurs. Thus each molecule has a "collision sphere" of radius d. A collision occurs whenever the center of another molecule comes within this sphere. If there are n molecules per unit volume and if equal numbers of molecules are traveling in each coordinate direction, there will be n/6 molecules moving in the +x direction, and these molecules will collide with those traveling in the -x direction at a rate $(n/6)\pi d^2(2u)$, where πd^2 is the cross-sectional area of the collision sphere of each molecule and 2u is the relative velocity at which two molecules approach each other. The molecules moving in the +x direction will collide with those moving in the +y, -y, +z, and -z directions at a right angle and at a rate $(n/6)\pi d^2(\sqrt{2}u)$, where $\sqrt{2}u$ is the relative velocity between the colliding molecules. There being no collision with molecules moving in the same direction, the molecules moving in the +x direction will experience

$$\Gamma = \frac{n}{6}\pi d^2(2u) + 4\left[\frac{n}{6}\pi d^2(\sqrt{2}u)\right] = 1.276n\pi^2 u \tag{2}$$

collisions per unit time.

An important quantity in kinetic theory is the average distance that a molecule travels between collisions. This is called the *mean free path.* The average number of collisions experienced by one molecule in unit time is given in Eq. (2). In this time the molecule has traveled a distance u. The mean free path is therefore u/λ, or

$$\lambda = \frac{1}{\xi n\pi d^2} \tag{3}$$

where $\xi = 1.276$ in the present case, but for a slightly improved derivation in which the molecules are allowed to move in all directions, $\xi = \sqrt{2}$ or 1.414. Although Eq. (3) is based on an ultrasimplified theory, it is qualitatively correct and yields results that are within the range of the best available data (see Table 1).

Consider now the net flux of molecules in the +z direction through plane 0, as shown in Figure 1. Let the number density of molecules in plane O be n_0. Molecules approaching O from below have suffered their last collision at a distance λ below plane O. That is, they have come from plane A and have the number density n_A, characteristic of that location. Similarly, molecules arriving at plane O from above have come from plane B, and possess the number density n_B, characteristic of that plane. As an ap-

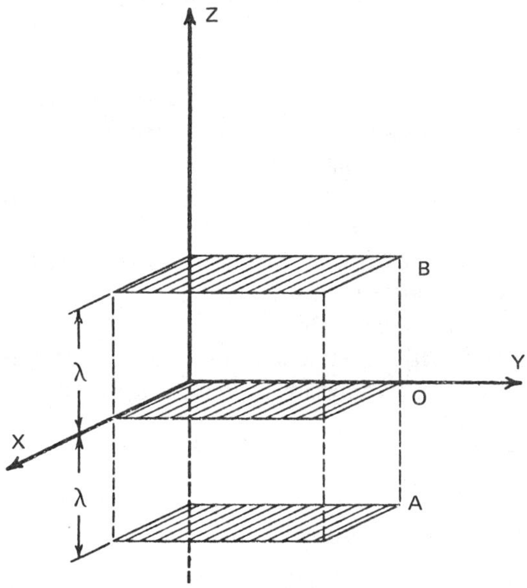

Figure 1 Sketch of molecular flux through plane O in the z direction.

proximation we may assume a constant gradient of density dn/dz over distances of the order of magnitude of the mean free path and write

$$n_A = n_0 - \lambda \frac{dn}{dz} \qquad n_B = n_0 + \lambda \frac{dn}{dz} \tag{4}$$

The number of molecules passing through plane O from below is (1/6) $n_A u$ and from above, $-(1/6)n_B u$. Hence the net flux (flow of molecules per unit area)

$$J_z = -\frac{1}{6}(n_B - n_A)u = -\frac{1}{3}u\lambda\frac{dn}{dz} \tag{5}$$

Comparing Eq. (5) with Fick's law as given in Eq. (1), we obtain the coefficient of self-diffusion of this kind of molecule:

$$\mathcal{D} = \frac{1}{3}u\lambda \tag{6}$$

Thus the proportionality constant in Fick's phenomenological law is given a microscopic interpretation from this simple theory. The diffusion coefficient increases when the molecules move faster or the mean free path increases.

IV. Phenomenological Laws of Molecular Diffusion

A. Steady Diffusion: Fick's First Law

As given in Eq. (1), Fick's law describes the relationship between the diffusional flux and the concentration gradient in steady-state diffusion. This law, sometimes also called Fick's first law (as opposed to Fick's second law, to be discussed later), relates a concentration c, a spatial coordinate z, a flux J_z, and a dimensional proportionality constant $\mathcal{D}$. To give a precise meaning to Fick's first law of diffusion, these quantities must be clearly defined and their dimensions must be consistent.

Since diffusion in a multicomponent system will be discussed in a later section, the definitions that follow are not merely suitable for a binary mixture but apply equally to a mixture containing n species. We shall define a consistent set of concentration, velocity, and flux.

Molar Concentration

$$c_i = \frac{\text{moles of the ith species (in g-moles)}}{\text{volume of mixture (in cm}^3\text{)}}$$

Thus the total *molar concentration* of the mixture is $c = \sum_{i=1}^{n} c_i$ (in g-moles/cm^3), and the *molar fraction* is $x_i = c_i/c$.

Molar Average Velocity

In an n-component system, each species moves at a different velocity. We designate the diffusion velocity of species i with respect to a stationary coordinate system by v_i, which should not be mistaken as the velocity of an individual molecule but should be regarded as the average of the velocities of all the molecules of species i in the mixture. We define

$$v = \frac{\sum_{i=1}^{n} c_i v_i}{\sum_{i=1}^{n} c_i} = \frac{1}{c}\sum_{i=1}^{n} c_i v_i = \sum_{i=1}^{n} x_i v_i \tag{7}$$

Molar average velocity (v) is the velocity of the "centroid of molar concentration" of the system. Thus the quantity $v_i - v$ is the diffusion velocity of species i with respect to the centroid of molar concentration.

Molar Fluxes

For a pure substance, ρv, the density times the velocity, gives the mass flux. In an n-component system, the molar flux may be defined as the flux with respect to the centroid of molar concentration:

$$J_i = c_i(v_i - v)$$

$$= c_i v_i - \frac{c_i}{c}\sum_{j=1}^{n} c_j v_j = N_i - x_i \sum_{j=1}^{n} N_j \tag{8}$$

From this result it can be seen that the molar diffusion flux J_i is the difference between the molar flux N_i with respect to a stationary coordinate system and the rate of the bodily transport of species i due to the local molar flux of the mixture. Summation of Eq. (8) from i = 1 to i = n gives

$$\sum_{i=1}^{n} J_i = 0 \tag{9}$$

which shows that the sum of *molar diffusion fluxes* relative to the molar velocity is zero in any mixture.

In Eq. (1) the concentration gradient is given as dc/dz. This is assuming in fact that the concentration gradient is only along the z axis of a certain coordinate system. In general, the concentration gradients along different axes of a coordinate system are different. To generalize the concept of "gradient" we use the vector operator ∇, which is independent of, and therefore may be represented in, any given coordinate system. Thus, in the cylindrical system,

$$\nabla c = \frac{\partial c}{\partial r}\hat{r} + \frac{1}{r}\frac{\partial c}{\partial \theta}\hat{\theta} + \frac{\partial c}{\partial z}\hat{z} \tag{10}$$

where $\hat{r}$, $\hat{\theta}$, and $\hat{z}$ are unit vectors in the r, θ, and z directions, respectively.

For a binary mixture containing species A and B, Fick's first law may be written in terms of the fluxes as follows:

$$J_A = -\mathcal{D}_{AB}\nabla c_A = -c\,\mathcal{D}_{AB}\nabla x_A \qquad J_B = -\mathcal{D}_{BA}\nabla c_B = c\,\mathcal{D}_{BA}\nabla x_B \tag{11}$$

$$N_A = x_A(N_A + N_B) - c\,\mathcal{D}_{AB}\nabla x_A \qquad N_B = x_B(N_A + N_B) - c\,\mathcal{D}_{BA}\nabla x_B \tag{12}$$

J_A and J_B are relative to the molar average velocity, and N_A and N_B are relative to stationary coordinates. These four fluxes are vectors having a component in the direction of each coordinate axis. The negative signs in Eqs. (11) and (12) indicate that the fluxes are positive in the direction of decreasing or negative gradients. Equation (11) is the more common form of Fick's first law; Eq. (12) shows that the diffusion flux N_A relative to stationary coordinates is the resultant of two vectors, the vector $x_A(N_A + N_B)$, which is the molar flux of A resulting from the bulk motion of the fluid mixture, and the vector $J_A = -c \mathscr{D}_{AB} \nabla x_A$, which is the molar flux of A resulting from the diffusion superimposed on the bulk flow.

From Eq. (9), it is clear that

$$J_A = -J_B \tag{13}$$

From Eqs. (11), (12), and (13), it is also clear that $N_A \neq -N_B$. Using the relation $x_A + x_B = 1$ and applying Eq. (13) to (11), it can be easily shown that

$$\mathscr{D}_{AB} = \mathscr{D}_{BA} \tag{14}$$

Thus diffusion in a binary mixture is characterized by a single diffusion coefficient.

B. Binary Diffusion Coefficient

Diffusion coefficients of binary mixtures of dilute gases have been comprehensively compiled, critically evaluated, and correlated by new semiempirical expressions (Marrero and Mason, 1972). They are strongly dependent on the molecular weights of the individual gases, and are in general independent of the composition of the mixture. They increase with increasing temperature and vary inversely with pressure. Table 2 gives the experimentally obtained diffusion coefficients at 1 atm of some common gas pairs.

Binary diffusion coefficients of nonpolar gases may be predicted within about 5% using the formula derived from the Chapman-Enskog theory (Chapman and Cowling, 1970; Bird et al., 1960):

$$\mathscr{D}_{AB} = 0.001858 \frac{T^{3/2}}{p\sigma_{AB}{}^2 \Omega_{\mathscr{D},AB}} \left(\frac{1}{M_A} + \frac{1}{M_B} \right)^{1/2} \tag{15}$$

where T is ambient temperature in °K; p is ambient pressure in atm; M_A and M_B are molecular weights of gases A and B, respectively; σ_{AB} is the Lennard-Jones force constant for the binary mixture in Å (10^{-8} cm); and $\Omega_{\mathscr{D},AB}$ is a dimensionless quantity pertaining to molecular collision. The Lennard-Jones potential for a binary gas mixture may be approximated by

$$\phi_{AB}(r) = 4\epsilon_{AB} \left[\left(\frac{\sigma_{AB}}{r} \right)^{12} - \left(\frac{\sigma_{AB}}{r} \right)^{6} \right] \tag{16}$$

where ϵ_{AB} and σ_{AB} are molecular force constants. The numerical values of the quantities Ω, ϵ, and σ may be found in the work of Hirschfelder et al. (1954) and in other, more recent publications. Usually for nonpolar, nonreacting molecule pairs, the force constants in Eq. (16) may be estimated satisfactorily by combining the Lennard-Jones parameters of gas species A and B, namely,

Table 2 Experimental Values of Binary Diffusion Coefficients of Some Gas Pairs[a]

Gas pair	(cm^2/sec)	T (°C)	Gas pair	(cm^2/sec)	T (°C)	Gas pair	(cm^2/sec)	T (°C)
Air-Ar	0.192	22	CO-O_2	0.211	27	Kr-Kr	0.101	35
Air-CO_2	0.139	0				Kr-Ne	0.233	0
Air-He	0.708	20	CO_2-CO_2	0.125	40	Kr-N_2	0.159	35
Air-Kr	0.134	0	CO_2-He	0.605	20	Kr-Xe	0.0725	18
Air-O_2	0.178	0	CO_2-Kr	0.109	20			
Air-H_2O	0.260	25	CO_2-Ne	0.267	22	Ne-Ne	0.484	20
			CO_2-N_2	0.167	25	Ne-N_2	0.315	20
Ar-Ar	0.178	2	CO_2-N_2O	0.128	40	Ne-Xe	0.208	18
Ar-CO_2	0.133	3	CO_2-O_2	0.153	20			
Ar-He	0.729	25	CO_2-H_2O	0.198	34	N_2-N_2	0.188	0
Ar-Kr	0.128	15				N_2-O_2	0.208	27
Ar-Ne	0.309	20	He-Kr	0.616	18	N_2-SF_6	0.1	20
Ar-N_2	0.189	20	He-Ne	1.01	20	N_2-H_2O	0.256	34
Ar-SF_6	0.05	20	He-N_2	0.687	25			
Ar-Xe	0.107	18	He-O_2	0.703	20	N_2O-O_2	0.096	0
			He-SF_6	0.4	20			
CO-CO	0.323	100	He-H_2O	0.902	34	O_2-O_2	0.232	25
CO-N_2	0.207	27	He-Xe	0.518	20	O_2-H_2O	0.282	35

[a]Experimental conditions: pressure at 1 atm; temperature as specified.
Source: Taken from various sources.

$$\sigma_{AB} = \frac{1}{2}(\sigma_A + \sigma_B) \tag{17}$$

$$\epsilon_{AB} = \sqrt{\epsilon_A \epsilon_B} \tag{18}$$

As an example of the use of the Chapman-Enskog formula, the diffusion coefficient of the Ar-O_2 pair at 37°C and 1 atm is computed:

$$M_{Ar} = 39.9 \qquad M_{O_2} = 32.0$$

$$\sigma_{Ar} = 3.542 \text{ Å} \qquad \sigma_{O_2} = 3.468 \text{ Å}$$

$$\frac{\epsilon_{Ar}}{k} = 93\text{K} \qquad \frac{\epsilon_{O_2}}{k} = 107\text{K}$$

$$\sigma_{Ar\text{-}O_2} = \frac{1}{2}(3.542 + 3.467) = 3.505 \qquad \text{[from Eq. (17)]}$$

$$\frac{\epsilon_{Ar\text{-}O_2}}{k} = (93 \times 107)^{1/2} = 99.9 \qquad \text{[from Eq. (18)]}$$

$$T = 310\text{K} \qquad \frac{kT}{\epsilon_{Ar\text{-}O_2}} = \frac{310}{99.8} = 3.11$$

$$\Omega_{\mathcal{D},Ar\text{-}O_2}(3.11) = 0.9406$$

$$\mathcal{D}_{Ar\text{-}O_2} = \frac{(1.858 \times 10^{-3})(310)^{1.5}(1/39.9 + 1/32.0)^{0.5}}{(1)(3.505)^2(0.9406)} = 0.2083 \text{ cm}^2/\text{sec}$$

[from Eq. (15)]

Based on Chapman-Enskog theory the mutual diffusion coefficients of 11 gases at 37°C and 1 atm have been calculated and are tabulated in a symmetric matrix form in Table 3. They compare very favorably with the experimental values given in Table 2.

Since considerable effort is needed to apply Eq. (15), it may be tempting to use a simpler formula such as Graham's law when only the relative diffusivity between two gases is desired. It must be borne in mind, however, that the latter is less reliable than the former. In general, Graham's law tends to underestimate the difference between the diffusivities of two gases. For example, since the density of Argon is 10 times that of helium, Graham's law predicts that He should diffuse $\sqrt{10}$ or 3.16 times faster than argon in a given medium. The Chapman-Enskog theory yields that the dif-

Table 3 Binary Diffusion Coefficients (cm^2/sec) at 37°C and 1 atm Computed from Chapman-Enskog Theory

	He	H_2O	Ne	CO	N_2	Air	O_2	Ar	CO_2	N_2O	SF_6
He	1.7790										
H_2O	0.9059	0.2039									
Ne	1.1301	0.4038	0.5439								
CO	0.7506	0.2261	0.3394	0.2163							
N_2	0.7407	0.2315	0.3363	0.2164	0.2162						
Air	0.7538	0.2313	0.3399	0.2172	0.2171	0.2180					
O_2	0.7907	0.2285	0.3491	0.2184	0.2187	0.2195	0.2204				
Ar	0.7715	0.2219	0.3319	0.2073	0.2073	0.2079	0.2083	0.1957			
CO_2	0.6345	0.1602	0.2678	0.1647	0.1663	0.1660	0.1640	0.1545	0.1191		
N_2O	0.6467	0.1584	0.2713	0.1650	0.1669	0.1665	0.1641	0.1548	0.1183	0.1173	
SF_6	0.4349	0.0992	0.1686	0.1031	0.1047	0.1037	0.1001	0.0921	0.0707	0.0698	0.0366

fusivities of the He-air pair and the Ar-air pair differ by a ratio of 3.63 (Table 3); the experimental values at 20°C form a ratio of 3.7 (Table 2). Thus Eq. (15) gives a 2% error and Graham's law underestimates the diffusivity ratio by 15%.

There are many improved versions or variations of the formula given in Eq. (15). These have been discussed in detail by Reid et al. (1977) and Marrero and Mason (1972).

C. Unsteady Diffusion: Fick's Second Law

In a steady-state phenomenon, no parameter of the physical phenomenon varies with time. When unsteady or transient diffusion occurs, time must be featured as a variable in the governing equation. Thus Fick's first law, which contains no time variable, cannot be used alone. It must be combined with the principle of conservation of mass to form the unsteady diffusion equation.

To derive such an equation, consider a segment of length dz of a trumpet-shaped container whose cross-sectional area at axial position z is A(z), as shown in Figure 2. The principle of conservation of mass can be stated as follows:

$$\begin{bmatrix}\text{Rate of accu-}\\\text{mulation of a}\\\text{given substance}\\\text{in the infinitesi-}\\\text{mal segment}\\\text{considered}\end{bmatrix} = \begin{bmatrix}\text{rate at which this}\\\text{substance is}\\\text{brought into the}\\\text{segment}\end{bmatrix} - \begin{bmatrix}\text{rate at which this}\\\text{substance is re-}\\\text{moved from the}\\\text{segment}\end{bmatrix} + \begin{bmatrix}\text{rate at which}\\\text{this substance}\\\text{is produced in}\\\text{the segment by}\\\text{chemical or bio-}\\\text{logical reactions}\end{bmatrix}$$

Assuming a linear variation of cross-sectional area in the infinitesimal segment between z and z + dz, and designating the molar concentration of the substance considered in the infinitesimal volume by c, one can write the left-hand side of the preceding equation as

$$\frac{\partial}{\partial t}\left\{[A + (A + dA)]\,\frac{dz}{2}\,c\right\} = \frac{\partial c}{\partial t}\,\frac{dA\,dz}{2} \approx \frac{\partial c}{\partial t}\,A\,dz \tag{19}$$

where the partial derivative $\partial/\partial t$ is used because c varies both with time t and with axial position z. If there are no chemical reactions in the container and if we assume that diffusion occurs only in the z direction (i.e., diffusion is instantaneous in the direction perpendicular to z), we can write the right-hand side of the equation for the conservation principle as

$$AN_z - (A + dA)(N_z + dN_z) = -N_z\,dA - A\,dN_z - dA\,dN_z \simeq -N_z\,dA - A\,dN_z \tag{20}$$

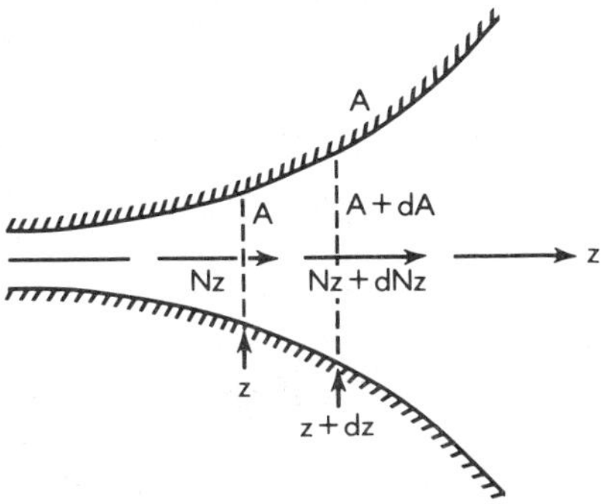

Figure 2 Axisymmetric container with variable cross-sectional area. Diffusion takes place in this container; N is molar flux with respect to a stationary frame of reference.

where N_z is the molar flux in the z direction relative to the stationary coordinate axis, z. Equating Eqs. (19) and (20), we have

$$\frac{\partial c}{\partial t} A\ dz = -N_z\ dA - A\ dn_z \tag{21}$$

which is a general statement of unsteady-state one-dimensional mass transfer.

If there is no bulk flow through the container, from Eqs. (11) and (12), $J_z = N_z = -\mathcal{D}(\partial c/\partial z)$. Therefore, Eq. (21) becomes

$$\frac{\partial c}{\partial t} A\ dz = -\left(-\mathcal{D}\frac{\partial c}{\partial z}\right) dA - A\ d\left(-\mathcal{D}\frac{\partial c}{\partial z}\right) \tag{23}$$

Recalling that $\mathcal{D}$ is a constant and dividing Eq. (22) by A dz, we obtain

$$\frac{\partial c}{\partial t} = \mathcal{D}\frac{\partial^2 c}{\partial z^2} + \frac{\mathcal{D}}{A}\frac{dA}{dz}\frac{\partial c}{\partial z} \tag{23}$$

which is the equation of the one-dimensional diffusion process in an axisymmetric container. In the limiting case in which the container becomes a cylinder, namely when $dA/dz = 0$, we have

$$\frac{\partial c}{\partial t} = \mathcal{D}\frac{\partial^2 c}{\partial z^2} \tag{24}$$

Equation (24) is the simplest form of diffusion equation and is also called Fick's second law of diffusion.

When diffusion occurs in all directions of a coordinate system, a three-dimensional equation may be derived by applying Fick's first law [Eq. (12)] to a general statement of conservation of mass which may be derived in a manner similar to that in which Eq. (21) is derived.

D. Multicomponent Diffusion

Exceptions to Fick's law of diffusion have been discovered frequently and continually since its formulation. The most important exceptions have to do with multicomponent systems in which more than two species are involved in the diffusion process. Under such circumstances the diffusion coefficient defined in Fick's law is often not constant but dependent on the composition of the mixture.

As an illustration of the multicomponent effect, Figure 3 shows two connected tubes as used by Arnold and Toor (1967): one containing 50% methane and 50% argon, the other containing 50% hydrogen and 50% argon. As the partition between the two tubes is removed, although initially there is no gradient of the argon concentration, a transient diffusion flux of argon from the methane side toward the hydrogen side will be observed. This is because hydrogen diffuses faster than methane, and as hydrogen molecules accumulate on the methane side, a pressure gradient is created, causing all species on the methane side, including argon, to move to the hydrogen side.

A transient pressure gradient is an inherent feature of a closed system such as the apparatus shown in Figure 3. The effect of the pressure gradient is to enhance the motion of the slower component and suppress the motion of the faster component, making the net flux with respect to stationary coordinates equal. When a multicomponent mixture is contained in a closed system, the equimolar condition states that

$$\sum_{i=1}^{n} N_i = 0 \tag{25}$$

Since there are n components involved, the flux of each species becomes a function of the fluxes of the other species.

In an attempt to explore the implications of multicomponent diffusion in the lung, Chang et al. (1975) made a model study of ternary equimolar diffusion. Although this model study is highly idealized, it has served to point out the possible effects of multicomponent diffusion in the alveolar spaces (Chang, 1980) and other biological systems (Erasmus and Rahn, 1976). Physiologists who deal with multicomponent gas mixtures therefore should be well aware of such possible effects.

The transport phenomenon of multicomponent diffusion is quite com-

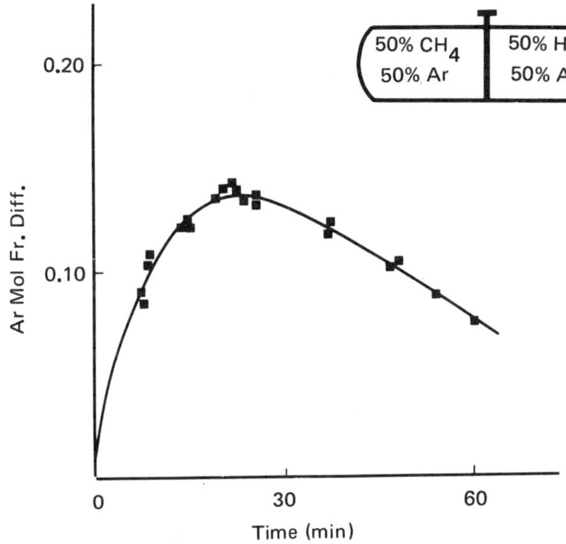

Figure 3 Diffusion of argon in a system of hydrogen-methane-argon. Although there is initially no gradient in argon concentration, argon will move transiently from the methane side toward the hydrogen side. (Based on experiments performed by Arnold and Toor, 1967.)

plex and often defies intuition; theoretically, it is much less well understood than is binary diffusion. Nevertheless, the total knowledge about multicomponent diffusion has to date permitted a fair understanding of this phenomenon and has provided some practical means to predict the pertinent qualities in a multicomponent system. By necessity, the treatment of this subject in the present chapter will be brief and confined to ideal gas mixtures.

For an ideal gas mixture of constant temperature and pressure, the steady-state flux equations, known as the Stefan-Maxwell equations, have the form

$$\frac{p}{RT} \nabla x_i = \sum_{\substack{j=1 \\ j \neq i}}^{n} \frac{1}{\mathcal{D}_{ij}} (x_i N_j - x_j N_i) \tag{26}$$

where p is pressure of the mixture in atm, T is temperature in K, R is the ideal gas constant in cm^3 atm/(1K g-mole), N_j N_i are molar fluxes in g-mole/cm^2 sec with respect to a stationary frame of reference, and $\mathcal{D}_{ij}$ is the binary diffusion coefficient of the i-j gas pair in cm^2/sec. Stefan-Maxwell equations make it evident that the fluxes in a multicomponent mixture are the resultant of coupled actions of the binary gas pairs. Since the total pressure is constant and $\Sigma x_i = 1$, there are only n - 1 independent equations in Eq. (26).

An alternative form of the multicomponent flux equations has been derived by Onsager (1945) from the laws of thermodynamics. These equations have the appearance of a generalized Fick's law:

$$J_i = -\frac{p}{RT} \sum_{j=1}^{n-1} D_{ij} \nabla x_j \tag{27}$$

where J_i is the molar flux of the ith species with respect to the molar average velocity as already defined, and the D_{ij} are the multicomponent diffusion coefficients, which are not constant but dependent on the composition of the mixture. It is clear from Eq. (27) that the flux of any component depends on the concentration gradients of all the components in the mixture. Since the net sum of all fluxes J_i as well as concentration gradients ∇x_i must be zero (i.e., $\Sigma J_i = 0$ and $\Sigma \nabla x_i = 0$), there are only n - 1 independent equations in Eq. (27). The solution methods of Eq. (26) or (27) have been developed by Toor (1964a,b); they are beyond the scope of the present chapter.

E. Effective Diffusion Coefficients

As the solution of Eq. (26) or (27) is rather difficult, it is often advantageous to take the alternative approach of finding the effective diffusion coefficients and applying the binary form of Fick's law to obtain the diffusion fluxes. The effective diffusion coefficient is usually a function of the binary diffusion coefficients and local or boundary concentrations. With this coefficient, one may relate the flux of a certain species to its own concentration gradient,

$$J_i = -cD'_{im} \nabla x_i \tag{28}$$

where D'_{im} denotes the effective diffusion coefficient of the ith species.

Many forms of effective diffusion coefficients have been proposed and used (Cussler, 1976). Perhaps the simplest formula has been proposed by Wilke (1950), who considered the effective diffusion coefficient of a single gas (species 1) with respect to a multicomponent mixture of stagnant gases. He obtained

$$D'_1 = \frac{1 - x_1}{x_2/\mathcal{D}_{12} + x_3/\mathcal{D}_{13} + \cdots x_n/\mathcal{D}_{1n}} \tag{29}$$

Table 4 Effective Diffusion Coefficients for O_2 (D'_{O_2}) and CO_2 (D'_{CO_2}) in Diffusion Between the Inspired Gas[a] and the Alveolar Gas[b]

Mixture	Diffusing gas	Measured at 742 mmHg and 37°C[c] (cm^2/sec)	Computed for 742 mmHg and 37°C[d] (cm^2/sec)	Computed for 713 mmHg and 37°C[e] (cm^2/sec)
O_2-H_2 vs.	O_2	0.549	0.773	—
O_2-CO_2-H_2	CO_2	0.415	0.439	—
O_2-He vs.	O_2	—	0.620	0.530
O_2-CO_2-He	CO_2	—	0.440	0.438
O_2-N_2 vs.	O_2	0.240	0.251	0.240
O_2-CO_2-N_2	CO_2	0.173	0.179	0.177
O_2-SF_6 vs.	O_2	0.107	0.101	0.143
O_2-CO_2-SF_6	CO_2	0.090	0.084	0.096

[a] 21% O_2 + 79% y; y = H_2, He, N_2, or SF_6.
[b] 14% O_2 + 6% CO_2 + 80% y; y = H_2, He, N_2, or SF_6.
[c] By Worth and Piiper (1978b).
[d] From Wilke's equation (1950).
[e] By Chang and Farhi (1980).

where $x_1, x_2, \ldots, x_n$ are the molar fractions. Equation (29) was tested experimentally and was found to be very satisfactory (Fairbanks and Wilke, 1950).

The effective diffusion coefficients offer a simple way to handle a complex problem and are preferred by a number of biologist-investigators who have studied multicomponent diffusion (Chang, 1980; Erasmus and Rahn, 1976; Worth and Piiper, 1978a,b). For ternary gas mixtures similar to the inspired gas and the alveolar gas, Worth and Piiper (1978b) have made in vitro measurements, while Chang and Farhi (1980) have computed the effective diffusion coefficients based on the nonequimolar theory (Tai and Chang, 1979). The two sets of values are compared with the values computed using Eq. (29) and are given in Table 4. The agreement among the three sets of values is good. When diffusion fluxes of O_2 and CO_2 in the alveolar space are computed from Fick's first law, the values in Table 4 should be used as the diffusion coefficients.

V. Summary

The process of diffusion is fundamental to the maintenance of life in all organisms. In respiratory physiology, diffusion in the gas phase plays an important role in the delivery of oxygen to, and removal of carbon dioxide from, the sites of gas exchange. This is even more evident in extreme conditions such as diving and hibernation.

The macroscopic phenomenon of gaseous diffusion can be explained from a microscopic point of view using the kinetic theory of gases. In particular, it can be used to predict accurately the binary diffusion coefficients for nonpolar, nonreacting gas pairs.

Ordinary binary diffusion is well understood and Fick's first law is a phenomenological description of steady-state diffusion caused by a concentration gradient. Mass also can be transported because of temperature or pressure gradients, but such occurrences are virtually nonexistent in organisms and are therefore not discussed.

For the proper application of Fick's law, concentration as well as flux must be appropriately defined. The common definition for concentration is the molar concentration (c). Fluxes may be described as molar flux; a certain frame of reference must be specified for a proper measurement of flux. Unsteady-state binary diffusion is characterized by the diffusion equation, the solution of which yields concentration values in the entire space domain of diffusion at all instants of time, from which fluxes and concentration profiles may be established.

Diffusion in multicomponent mixtures often does not obey Fick's law.

Since gas mixtures in the respiratory tract always contain more than two gases, the effects of multicomponent diffusion must be properly accounted for. A practical way to handle this is to use effective diffusion coefficients and to apply Fick's law or the unsteady-state diffusion equation. For alveolar gas mixtures, values of effective diffusion coefficients for O_2 and CO_2 are given.

References

Arnold, K. R., and Toor, H. L. (1967). Unsteady diffusion in ternary gas mixtures. *AIChE J.*, **13**:909-914.

Bird, R. B., Stewart, W. E., and Lightfoot, E. N. (1960). *Transport Phenomena.* New York, Wiley.

Chang, H. K. (1980). Multicomponent diffusion in the lung. *Fed. Proc.*, **39**:2759-2764.

Chang, H. K., and Farhi, L. E. (1980). Ternary diffusion and effective diffusion coefficients in alveolar spaces. *Respir. Physiol.*, **40**:269-279.

Chang, H. K., Tai, R. C., and Farhi, L. E. (1975). Some implications of ternary diffusion in the lung. *Respir. Physiol.*, **23**:109-120.

Chapman, S., and Cowling, T. G. (1970). *The Mathematical Theory of Non-uniform Gases,* 3rd ed. New York, Cambridge University Press.

Cussler, E. L. (1976). *Multicomponent Diffusion.* Amsterdam, Elsevier.

Erasmus, D., and Rahn, H. (1976). Effects of ambient pressures, He and SF_6 on O_2 and CO_2 transport in the avian egg. *Respir. Physiol.*, **27**: 53-64.

Fairbanks, D. F., and Wilke, C. R. (1950). Diffusion coefficients in multicomponent gas mixtures. *Ind. Eng. Chem.*, **42**:471-475.

Fick, A. E. (1855). Uber Diffusion. *Pogg. Ann.*, **94**:59.

Graham, T. (1833). On the law of the diffusion of gases. *Phil. Mag.*, **2**: 175-190, 269-276, 351-358.

Hirschfelder, J. O., Curtiss, C. F., and Bird, R. B. (1954). *The Molecular Theory of Gases and Liquids.* New York, Wiley.

Marrero, T. R., and Mason, E. A. (1972). Gaseous diffusion coefficients. *J. Phys. Chem. Ref. Data,* **1**(3):1-119.

Onsager, L. (1945). Theories and problems of liquid diffusion. *Ann. N.Y. Acad. Sci.*, **46**:241-265.

Reid, R. C., Prausnitz, J. M., and Sherwood, T. S. (1977). *The Properties of Gases and Liquids,* 3rd ed. New York, McGraw-Hill.

Tai, R. C., and Chang, H. K. (1979). A mathematical study of non-equimolar ternary gas diffusion. *Bull. Math. Biol.*, **41**:591-606.

Toor, H. L. (1964a). Solution of the linearized equations of multicomponent mass transfer: I. *AIChE J.*, **10**:448-455.

Toor, H. L. (1964b). Solution of the linearized equations of multicomponent mass transfer: II. Matrix methods. *AIChE J.*, **10**:460-465.

Wilke, C. R. (1950). Diffusional properties of multicomponent gases. *Chem. Eng. Prog.*, **46**:95-104.

Worth, H., and Piiper, J. (1978a). Diffusion of helium, carbon monoxide and sulfur hexafluoride in gas mixtures similar to alveolar gas. *Respir. Physiol.*, **32**:155-166.

Worth, H., and Piiper, J. (1978b). Model experiments on diffusional equilibration of oxygen and carbon dioxide between inspired and alveolar gas. *Respir. Physiol.*, **35**:1-7.

2

Anatomical Factors Influencing Gas Mixing and Distribution

KEITH HORSFIELD

The Midhurst Medical Research Institute
Midhurst, West Sussex, England

I. Introduction

The evolution of animals capable of surviving on dry land necessitated the development of an internal gas exchange membrane housed in the lungs, from which excessive water loss could be avoided. Air enters the lung and is distributed therein by convective flow in a system of branching tubes, the conducting airways. Because they end blindly, convective flow cannot take inspired oxygen all the way up to the gas exchange membrane, so the last part of its journey must be completed by molecular diffusion. The frog's lung has poorly developed intrapulmonary conducting airways, whereas in reptiles such as the crocodile they are well developed. Because the conducting airways bring gas nearer to the gas exchange membrane in reptiles, the diffusion distance is less and the lung works more effectively. Thus the development of intrapulmonary conducting airways may be seen as a means of reducing the diffusion distance in the gas phase. The lungs cannot be completely emptied (diving mammals are an interesting exception) and so contain some residual gas at the end of expiration. Inspired fresh gas has to mix with the residual gas by molecular diffusion, in order to transport oxygen to, and carbon dioxide from, the gas exchange membrane. This mixing process will be dealt with in subsequent chapters. Fresh gas present in the conducting airways at the end of inspiration cannot take part in gas exchange (in fact, a small quantity may pass through the walls of small airways) so that this part of the inspirate is wasted. Another consequence of airways being a cul-de-sac is that ventilatory flow must be reciprocating, taking the same route out by which it came in. This can be compared with gills in fish, where the flow of water is unidirectional, and birds, which have a different arrangement described in Chapter 8. Alveolar gas remaining in the conducting airways at the end of expiration, the dead space gas, has to be reinspired. In the process it may be unevenly distributed, due to factors discussed later, resulting in small inequalities of dilution of the inspired fresh gas which follows into the acini. The residual gas in the lungs has the function of smoothing out and damping down the changes in gas concentration that would occur if the lungs were emptied with each breath. Thus arterial blood has a relatively constant PO_2 and PCO_2, although variations in phase with respiration can be detected.

II. The Conducting Airways

A. The Central Airways

The trachea divides into right and left main bronchi, which in turn give rise to five lobar bronchi, an upper and a lower on each side, and a middle one on the right only. The lobar bronchi divide into about 20 bronchopulmonary segment bronchi. Variations of the pattern are common, but that most frequently found is shown in Figure 1. Values for diameter, length, and branching angles for these airways from three lungs are given in Table 1.

B. Classification of Branches

In order to describe the 50,000 or so branches of the conducting airways, some method of classification is required. The three most commonly used methods are those described by Weibel, Horsfield, and Strahler, respectively. In Weibel's (1963) well-known and much used symmetrical model A the branches are classified by generation, starting with the trachea as zero, and increasing by 1 at each bifurcation in a centrifugal direction (Fig. 2A). Generations can also usefully be employed with asymmetrical trees (Fig. 2B). In the method described by Horsfield (Horsfield, 1967; Horsfield and Cumming, 1968a) peripheral branches are labeled order 1, and ordering proceeds centripetally increasing by 1 at each bifurcation. When unlike branches meet, the numbering is continued from the higher of the two branches (Fig. 3A). The method of Strahler (1953, 1957) proceeds in two stages. In the first, periph-

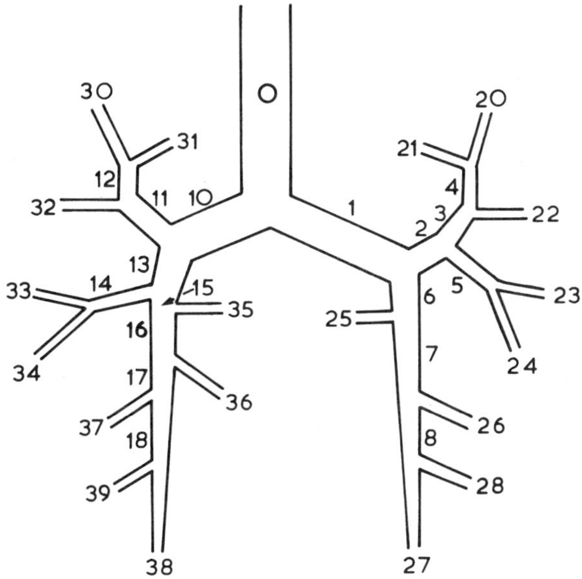

Figure 1 Central airways of the human lung. For identification of bronchi and their dimensions, see Table 3.

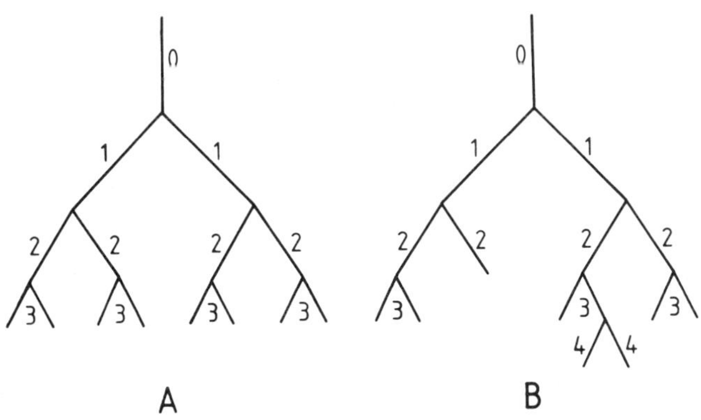

Figure 2 Generations in (A) a symmetrical tree and (B) an asymmetrical tree.

Table 1 Diameters, Lengths, and Branching Angles of the Upper Airways of Three Human Lungs[a]

Branch number	Name	Diameter (mm)			Length (mm)			Branching angle (°)		
		HC	HM2	HM3	HC	HM2	HM3	HC	HM2	HM3
0	Trachea	16.0	20.1	23.5	–	120.0	139.0	–	–	–
Left lung										
1	Left main	12.0	17.5	14.5	50.0	30.9	68.0	73	25	20
2	Upper lobe	7.5	10.3	10.0	16.0	14.5	21.0	48	35	35
3	Upper lobe	7.3	8.8	9.6	1.0	11.8	3.0	65	15	0
4	Apicoposterior	5.0	6.5	8.1	9.0	14.5	6.3	28	20	0
5	Lingula	5.5	7.9	7.2	11.0	9.8	17.0	25	45	60
6	Lower lobe	8.0	11.5	10.5	11.0	14.2	15.5	44	25	20
7	?	6.5	9.9	8.0	18.0	15.3	14.0	28	10	0
8	?	7.0	8.9	8.1	4.5	9.8	4.6	17	5	30
20	Upper apical	5.3	6.1	6.4	13.5	10.2	19.5	14	25	45
21	Upper posterior	–	–	–	–	–	–	–	–	–
22	Upper anterior	–	–	–	–	–	–	–	–	–
23	Lingular superior	3.5	5.5	5.4	11.5	17.5	12.5	28	25	15
24	Lingular inferior	3.5	6.4	5.6	7.5	11.0	24.0	8	25	20
25	Lower apical	5.5	8.2	6.2	8.5	11.2	10.5	70	85	75
26	Lower anterior	5.0	7.1	8.0	11.5	14.2	16.5	36	45	35
27	Lower posterior	5.5	9.5	5.8	7.5	5.0	15.5	33	30	20
28	Lower lateral	5.0	9.1	5.6	8.5	13.0	13.0	31	30	15

Right lung										
10	Right main	11.1	17.5	18.5	22.0	30.9	42.0	35	25	25
11	Upper lobe	7.3	10.2	10.0	15.6	12.2	22.5	63	60	55
12	Apicoposterior	8.5	8.3	7.7	6.4	6.9	6.9	18	10	30
13	Right main	8.9	13.3	14.2	26.0	30.2	27.5	15	15	15
14	Middle lobe	5.2	7.2	7.4	21.0	22.7	21.5	61	25	25
15	Lower lobe	6.4	10.1	11.2	8.0	8.8	12.5	14	5	0
16	?	6.0	9.0	10.5	8.4	11.4	7.9	8	5	5
17	?	6.2	8.0	10.5	14.8	10.0	9.5	0	0	5
18	?	—	—	—	—	—	—	—	—	—
30	Upper apical	4.0	6.5	5.6	2.0	16.1	8.5	40	35	30
31	Upper posterior	4.0	7.1	6.8	13.4	9.4	13.5	10	30	15
32	Upper anterior	5.5	6.9	7.4	17.0	9.1	7.5	33	45	35
33	Middle medial	4.0	5.7	5.8	10.0	11.4	12.0	35	15	25
34	Middle lateral	4.4	6.7	7.0	9.6	15.4	14.5	18	20	5
35	Lower apical	4.4	7.0	5.1	6.2	10.4	14.0	54	40	50
36	Lower medial	3.2	6.0	7.0	6.2	23.0	14.5	58	35	25
37	Lower anterior	4.8	5.5	6.3	6.8	17.0	15.0	35	50	20
38	Lower posterior	5.8	9.0	6.8	10.6	7.5	19.5	31	0	15
39	Lower lateral	—	—	—	—	—	—	—	—	—

[a]Branch numbers are shown in Fig. 2. Numbers 20-39 are bronchopulmonary segments. Branches 3, 8, 12, 15, and 18 may be very short, giving the appearance of trichotomy. HC, lung described by Horsfield and Cumming (1968a). HM2, lung HM-2-72, and HM3, lung HM-3-73, described by Raabe et al. (1976). Additional data from Horsfield et al., 1971. Information not available for branches 18, 21, 22, and 39, owing to a variation in pattern in lung HC and difficulty in identifying data in lungs HM2 and HM3.

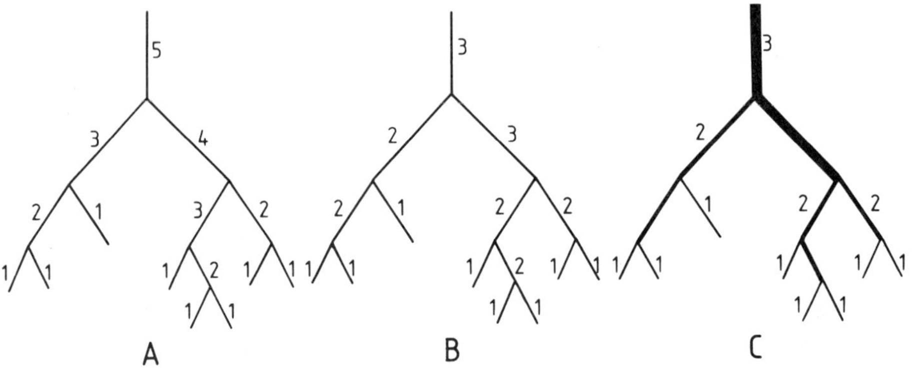

Figure 3 (A) Orders as described by Horsfield. (B, C) Orders as described by Strahler: (B) stage 1; (C) stage 2. (See the text.)

eral branches are designated order 1, increasing by one only at those bifurcations where two like branches meet (Fig. 3B). In the second stage, contiguous branches of the same order are joined to constitute just one branch (Fig. 3C). By comparing Figure 3A and C it will be seen that an asymmetrical tree has fewer branches and fewer orders by Strahler's method than it has by Horsfield's method. As we shall see later, the diameter of a branch is related to the flow it carries, so that in asymmetrical trees the daughter branches at a bifurcation are commonly of unequal diameter. Classification of the branches of asymmetrical trees by generations results in dissimilar branches being grouped together, and is therefore not very satisfactory from a functional point of view. Strahler orders are the best for grouping like branches together, although even with this method there is considerable variation within an order.

C. Numbers of Branches

In a dichotomously branching tree, whether it is symmetrical or asymmetrical the total number of branches N is given by $N = 2E - 1$, where E is the number of terminal branches (order 1). For example, in Figure 2A and B, $N = 2 \times 8 - 1 = 15$. The conducting airways end at the terminal bronchioles, each of which by definition supplies an acinus, so an estimate of their number allows the total number of conducting airways to be calculated. Weibel's model has 65,536 terminal bronchioles, and hence 131,071 conducting airways. This estimate was not based on a direct count, but on the number of symmetrical dichotomous divisions required to give 13.8×10^6 alveolar ducts

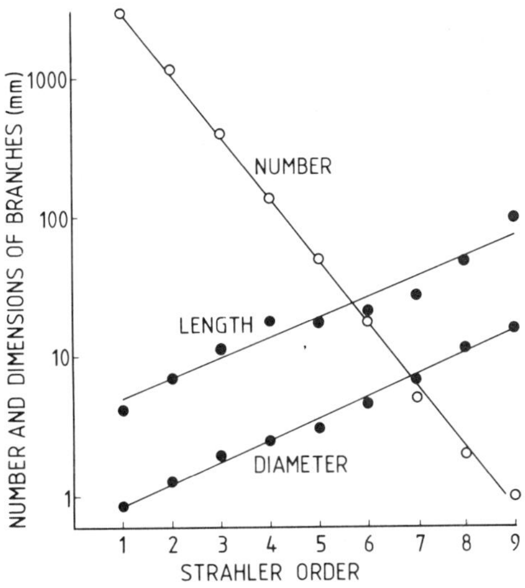

Figure 4 Number, mean diameter, and mean length of branches in each Strahler order of a human bronchial tree cast. The straight lines are drawn from the regression equations.

in four successive generations (Weibel, 1963). Most workers in this field would now consider these numbers to be in error for three reasons: (1) because branching is asymmetrical both in the conducting airways and within the acinus; (2) the number of generations of ducts is very variable between pathways, and on average exceeds four; and (3) the total number of ducts was underestimated for technical reasons (Hansen and Ampaya, 1974). Other estimates of the number of terminal bronchioles include 11,911 (Rohrer, 1915), 54,000 (Findeison, 1935), 27,992 (Horsfield and Cumming, 1968a), and from 16,000 to 26,000 (Thurlbeck and Wang, 1974; Hansen and Ampaya, 1975). These estimates average about 25,000, giving approximately 50,000 conducting airways. This total may be divided up into the numbers present in each order and these plotted on a logarithmic scale against order (Fig. 4). When this is done a linear plot is obtained, which demonstrates a constant proportional increase in numbers with decreasing order. The constant factor is the branching ratio, Rb, and it is defined as the antilog of the absolute value of the slope of the line of best fit by least-squares regression. Table 2 gives values of Rb obtained from three lungs, and Table 3 gives data for human airways based on Horsefield orders.

Table 2 Morphometric Parameters Obtained from Measurements of Airway Casts[a]

Animal	Rb	Rd	Rℓ
Human	2.805	1.427	1.402
Dog 1	3.609	1.692	1.675
Dog 2	3.468	1.562	1.662
Dog 3	3.445	1.480	1.560
Dog 4	3.261	1.495	1.596
Dog 5	3.379	1.558	1.624
Dog 6	3.057	1.516	1.704
Sheep 1	3.533	1.666	1.508
Sheep 2	3.565	1.712	1.387
Human HM-2-72	2.508	1.351	1.333
Human HM-3-73	2.735	1.452	1.464
Dog DM-2-72	3.583	1.530	1.692
Dog DM-5-72	3.040	1.509	1.528
Rat	3.314	1.532	1.820
Hamster	3.258	1.502	1.915

[a]The table is in two sections: the upper section based on data obtained by Horsfield and co-workers, and the lower section based on data obtained by Raabe et al. (1976).
Rb, branching ratio; Rd, diameter ratio; Rℓ, length ratio.
Source: Adapted from Horsfield and Thurlbeck (1981a).

D. Dimensions of Airways

From a tracheal diameter of 15 to 20 mm the airways decrease in diameter and length with decreasing order. The mean diameter and mean length of branches in each order can be plotted on a logarithmic scale against order and linear plots obtained, especially with Strahler orders (Fig. 4). Thus mean diameter and length each increase by a constant factor with order, these factors being the diameter ratio Rd and the length ratio Rℓ. They are the antilogs of the slopes of their respective regression lines on order. Table 2 gives values based on Strahler orders. Data for dimensions of human airways based on Horsefield orders are given in Table 3.

Table 3 Morphometric Data Obtained from a Human Airway Cast[a]

Horsfield order	Number	Diameter (mm)	Length (mm)	Number of acini	Percentage of tracheal flow
28	1	16.0	100.0	25,000	100.0000
27	1	11.1	22.0	13,797	55.1886
26	2	10.5	38.0	9,927	39.7069
25	2	7.0	12.0	7,142	28.5669
24	2	7.0	9.7	5,138	20.5527
23	3	6.7	11.3	3,697	14.7865
22	6	5.9	11.3	2,660	10.6381
21	8	5.4	9.7	1,913	7.6538
20	12	4.3	10.8	1,377	5.5064
19	14	3.5	9.5	990	3.9618
18	20	3.5	8.6	713	2.8503
17	30	3.1	9.9	513	2.0505
16	37	2.9	8.0	369	1.4752
15	46	2.8	9.2	306	1.2222
14	64	2.7	8.2	191	0.7636
13	85	2.5	8.1	137	0.5493
12	114	2.4	7.7	99	0.3952
11	158	2.2	6.4	71	0.2844
10	221	2.0	6.3	51	0.2045
9	341	1.8	5.2	37	0.1474
8	499	1.6	4.8	26	0.1058
7	760	1.3	4.2	19	0.0764
6	1,104	1.1	3.6	14	0.0549
5	1,675	0.95	3.1	10	0.0393
4	2,843	0.76	2.5	7	0.0286
3	5,651	0.64	1.1	4	0.0143
2	11,300	0.56	1.3	2	0.0071
1	25,000	0.51	1.1	1	0.0036
	49,999				

[a]The trachea is order 28. Terminal bronchioles are defined as order 1, the number of which was estimated to average 25,000 (see the text). Each terminal bronchiole supplies one acinus. Percentage of tracheal flow was calculated assuming that each acinus receives equal flow.

Source: Adapted from Horsfield (1981).

E. Flow in Airways

In general, it is obvious that larger airways carry a greater flow than that carried by small ones. For example, flow in the trachea is greater than flow in either main bronchus, both of which are smaller than the trachea. The flow that occurs in an airway during life is dependent on many factors, but here we are concerned only with the volume of lung distal to the airway. If the lung were to expand evenly and synchronously all over (we know that it does not), flow down an airway would be proportional to the volume of lung is supplies. If all the acini were similar, the volume of lung would be proportional to the number of acini supplied. Hence a count of the number of acini supplied by an airway gives a first-order approximation of the flow through it. Table 3 gives these data for the human airways, and Table 4 for lungs, lobes, and bronchopulmonary segments.

F. Bifurcations

The dynamics of flow and diffusion in long straight tubes is relatively well understood and can be analyzed both experimentally and methematically. In the conducting airways, however, there are 25,000 bifurcations, giving rise to 50,000 branches. The length of a branch between bifurcations averages about three times its diameter, so that findings based on long straight tubes are not necessarily applicable to the airways. Bifurcations have profound effects on flow which differ markedly between inspiration and expiration, and these will be dealt with in Chapter 3. Successive bifurcations are frequently found to lie in planes at right angles to each other, an arrangement that reduces the unequal distribution of flow caused by successive bifurcations in the same plane (Snyder et al., 1981). Both of the daughter branches arising at a bifurcation diverge from the line of the parent. Usually, the daughter branches differ in diameter, but occasionally they are equal, in which case their branching angles are approximately equal.

Where a daughter branch arises at a bifurcation, its lateral wall commonly curves away from the parent branch before extablishing its new line of direction. The degree of curvature is quite variable in the larger branches, and rather less in the smaller. It can be expressed as the ratio r/d, where r is the radius of curvature and d the diameter of the daughter branch. It ranges from 0.5 to 18 in the larger and medium airways, to below 1.5 in the smaller (Horsfield et al., 1971). A structure similar to the carina between right and left main bronchi forms a flow divider at the meeting of the medial walls of the daughter branches. When sectioned in the plane of the bifurcation the free edge of the flow divider is curved, with a radius r (Fig. 5). The ratio r/d varies from zero for a very sharp edge to 1.0 for a blunt one. When sectioned at right angles to the plane of the bifurcation

Table 4 Terminal Bronchioles in Segments, Lobes, and Lungs as a Percentage of the Total[a]

Structure		Name	Branch numbers	Percent of terminal bronchioles
Bronchopulmonary segments	Left	upper apical	20	7.19
		upper anterior	21 + 22	7.05
		lingula upper	23	3.64
		lingula lower	24	2.91
		lower apical	25	5.07
		lower anterior	26	6.84
		lower posterior	27	8.01
		lower lateral	28	4.70
	Right	upper apical	30	7.93
		upper posterior	31	3.25
		upper anterior	32	9.72
		middle medial	33	4.50
		middle lateral	34	4.48
		lower apical	35	7.11
		lower median	36	3.43
		lower anterior	37	7.14
		lower posterior	38	7.03
Lobes	Left	upper		20.79
		lower		24.62
	Right	upper		20.90
		middle		8.98
		lower		24.71
Lungs	Left			45.41
	Right			54.59

[a]In this bronchial tree there was no separate left upper posterior segment nor right lower lateral segment, these areas being supplied from adjacent segmental branches. Branch numbers are shown in Fig. 2.

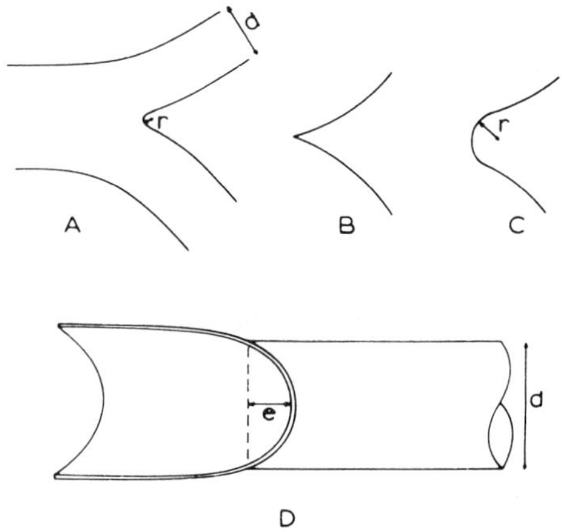

Figure 5 (A) Section of a bronchial bifurcation showing radius of curvature r of flow divider, and diameter d of daughter branch; (B) sharp flow divider; (C) blunt flow divider; (D) section of a bifurcation through parent branch at right angles to section in (A) (see arrow in Fig. 6). e, Depth of chord of flow divider. (From Horsfield et al., 1971.)

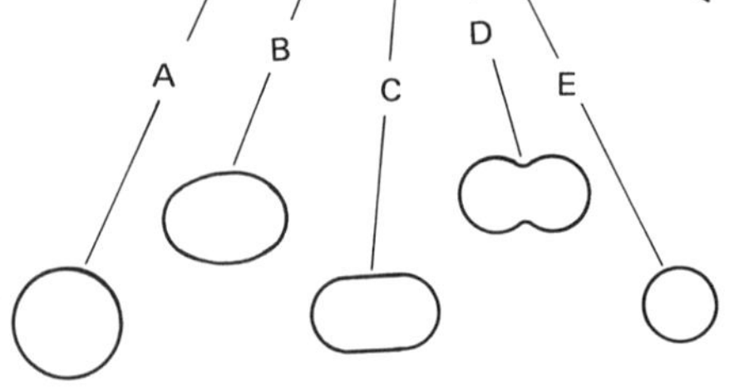

Figure 6 Section of a bronchial bifurcation to show changes in shape over transitional zone T. Arrow shows direction of section in Figure 5D. A to E are cross sections. (A) Parent branch of circular section; (B) section becomes elliptical; (C) section flattens; (D) flow divider indents sections; (E) circular section of daughter branch. (From Horsfield et al., 1971.)

the flow divider has a crescentic shape, and e, the depth of the chord, is less than or equal to d (Fig. 5D). While most intrapulmonary bronchi are circular in section, the shape changes at bifurcations to allow for the development of the daughter branches (Fig. 6). First the section becomes elliptical, with the long axis in the plane of the bifurcation, then flattened, with lateral curvature similar to that of the daughter branches. The cross-sectional area is now about equal to that of the two daughter branches taken together. Next, the ends of the crescent of the flow divider indent the section, and finally, two daughters of circular section are formed.

G. Asymmetry

The lung with its gas exchange membrane is a three-dimensional structure, and the airways supplying it form a three-dimensional tree. A symmetrical dichotomously branching tree supplying space-filling "solid" geometric forms can only be of very limited extent (Suwa, 1981), so if the 25,000 acini are taken to be space filling, it follows that the bronchial tree must be asymmetrical.

That this is so is evident from inspection of a bronchial tree cast. This asymmetry is a priori likely to affect the way in which gas molecules are transported, both by convective flow and molecular diffusion and by the interaction of these two processes. Asymmetry can be expressed in different ways, on the basis of the tree as a whole or at individual bifurcations. From a cast of the airways the number of generations down each pathway can be counted and the result expression as a frequency distribution. Figure 7 shows the distribution of generations down to lobular branches, which ranges from 8 to 25. A lobular branch is here defined as the first branch down any pathway the diameter of which is equal to or less than 0.7 mm. From the lobular branch to the end of the respiratory bronchioles a range of from two to seven generations was found in a sample of lobules (Horsfield and Cumming, 1968a), giving a total range of 10 to 32 generations down to distal respiratory bronchioles. It seems probably that the extremes of the range would be even greater than this if an entire airway system could be studied.

As a molecule of gas traverses the bronchial tree the minimum path it takes is equal to the sum of the lengths of the individual branches along that pathway. With asymmetry these path lengths will vary, their distribution being similar in shape to that shown in Figure 7. The shortest path from the carina to a lobular branch is 8 cm and the longest 22 cm, so that as with generations, there is about a threefold range.

A more general measure of asymmetry is the branching ratio. Both Horsfield and Strahler orders give Rb = 2.0 for symmetrical trees such as Weibel's model, but as asymmetry increases, Rb (Strahler) increases while

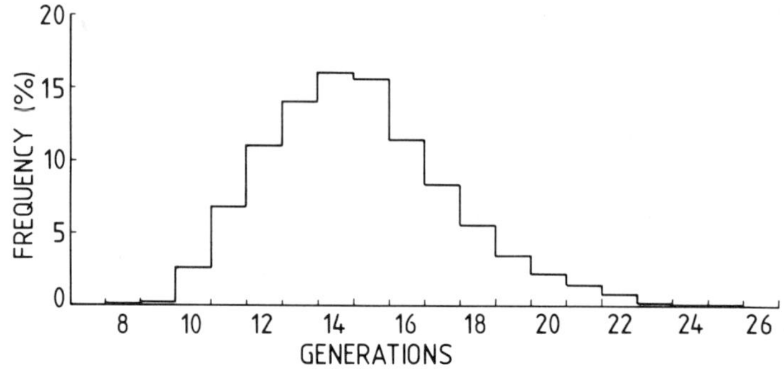

Figure 7 Distribution of generations from carina to lobular branches (0.7 mm diameter) in a human bronchial tree cast. (Adapted from Horsfield and Cumming, 1968a.)

Rb (Horsfield) decreases. In the human bronchial tree the values found were 2.8 and 1.38, respectively, on the same cast. As Table 2 shows, the more asymmetrical lungs of animals have higher values of Rb (Strahler).

At individual bifurcations asymmetry is manifest by differing diameters of the daughter branches and their branching angles. Let D_1 be the diameter of the parent branch, D_2 the diameter of the larger (major) daughter branch, and D_3 the diameter of the smaller (minor) daughter branch. The ratio D_3/D_2 is the symmetry ratio, and its distribution in a sample of bifurcations is shown in Figure 8. Figure 9 shows the reciprocal of the symmetry ratio, D_2/D_3, in relation to the diameter of the parent branch. Values for the symmetry ratio range from about 0.3 to 1.0. Lower values are not found in human airways, in contrast to the pulmonary arteries, where values of 0.1 or less may be seen. The ratios D_2/D_1 and D_3/D_1 are shown in Figure 8 and it will be noted that values of 1.0 and greater are sometimes found. Figure 9 shows these ratios in relation to the diameter of the parent branch. An important consequence of the diameters at a bifurcation is the change in cross-sectional area. Although the daughter diameters are usually less than that of the parent, the summed cross-sectional area usually increases. The ratio $D_1^2/(D_2^2 + D_3^2)$ expresses this, and Figure 8 shows the distribution of values from a sample of bifurcations. A few are greater than 1.0, which says that cross-sectional area decreases distally at these bifurcations.

The branching angle is that made by the center line of the daughter branch with the continuation beyond the bifurcation of the center line of the parent; it is usually less than 90°. The distribution found in a sample of bifurcations is shown in Figure 10. Mean branching angles for major and

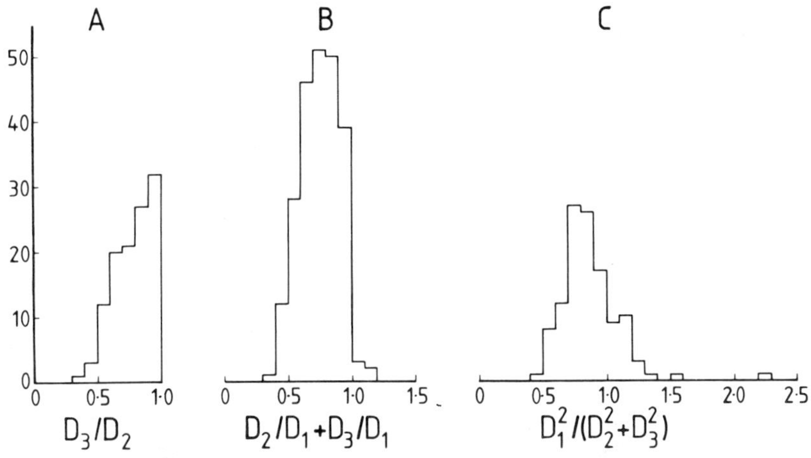

Figure 8 Distributions of ratios of diameters in a sample of 116 bifurcations, from a cast of a human bronchial tree. D_1, Diameter of parent branch; D_2, diameter of major daughter branch; D_3, diameter of minor daughter branch. (A) Symmetry ratio: (B) daughter/parent ratios; (C) area ratio. (See the test.) (Adapted from Horsfield and Cumming, 1967.)

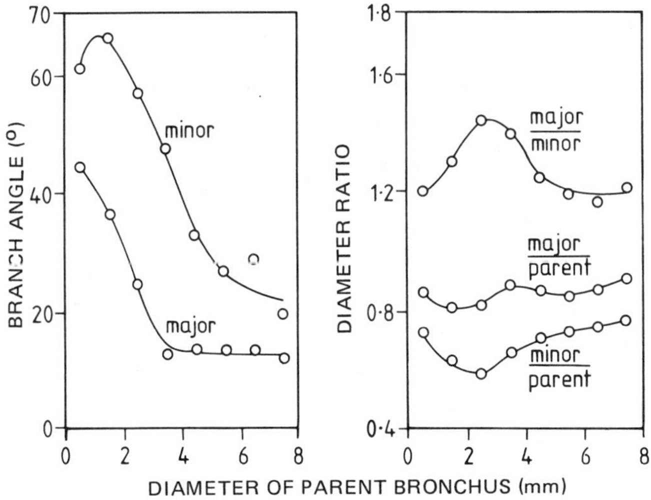

Figure 9 Left panel: Mean branching angles of major and minor daughter branches related to parent branch diameter. Right panel: Diameter ratios of major and minor daughter branches and their parent branch, related to parent branch diameter. Data from two human bronchial tree casts. (Redrawn from Phalen et al., 1978. Courtesy of *The Anatomical Record,* a Wistar Press Publication.)

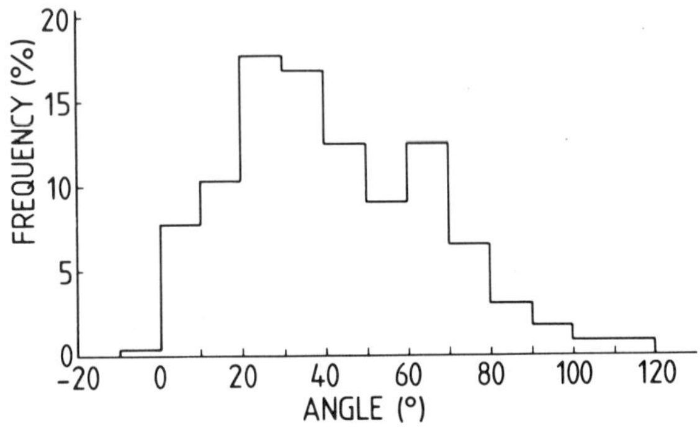

Figure 10 Distribution of branching angles in a sample of 116 bifurcations in a human bronchial tree cast. (Adapted from Horsfield and Cumming, 1967.)

minor branches are shown in relation to parent diameter in Figure 9. It may be seen that the mean angle for the minor branch is consistently greater than that for the major branch. Mean branching angles related to Strahler order in four mammalian species are shown in Figures 11 and 12.

H. Relationship Between Diameter and Flow

An hypothesis which has attracted considerable interest is that the diameters of the airways are adapted and adjusted to minimize some function. An illustration of this is that if airway diameters were increased, resistance to flow, and hence the work of breathing, would be decreased, but dead space and the metabolic cost of the airways themselves would be increased. An optimum diameter might exist at which the total cost to the animal would be minimized. Murray (1926) believed that minimum power dissipation is the main determinant, and assuming laminar flow, he showed that $f = kr^3$, where f = flow, r is the radius of the vessel, and k is a constant. Although this idea was developed for blood vessels, the concept can nevertheless be applied directly to the airways. Uylings (1977) extended the concept to include transitional and turbulent flow regimes by employing a constant j related to relative roughness of the tube wall and Reynold's number. He stated that

$$f = kr^{(j+2)/(j-2)} \qquad (1)$$

The value of j ranges from 4 for laminar flow to 5 for turbulent, so that $f = kr^3$ for laminar flow (as Murray) and $f = kr^{2.333}$ for turbulent. Another way of looking at this is as follows. The relation of flow to the number of

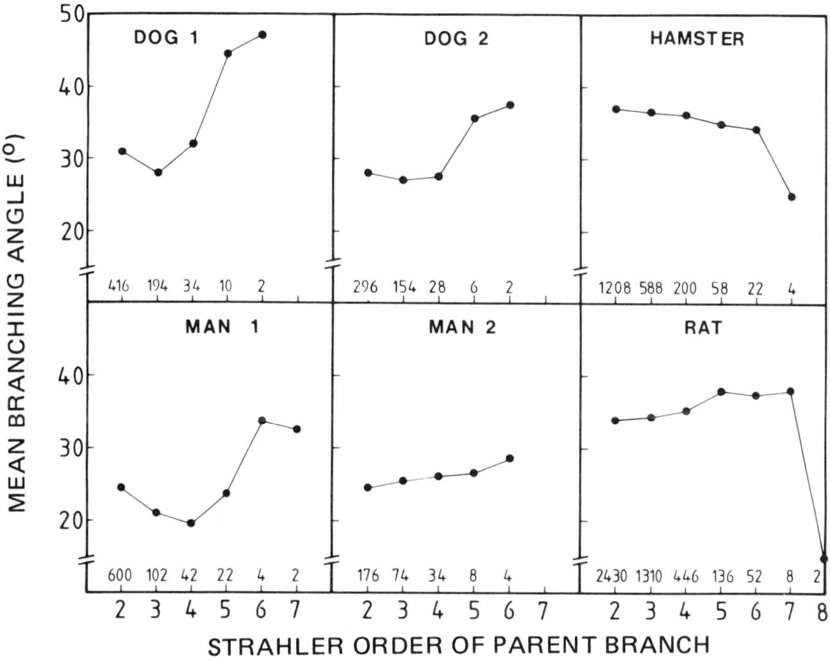

Figure 11 Mean angles of branching in the bronchial tree of four species related to Strahler order of the parent branch. The numbers in the panels are the sample size for each order. (From Thurlbeck and Horsfield, 1980.)

terminal branches supplied has already been discussed in Section II.E. Since both log number of branches and log mean diameter of branches are linearly related to order (Fig. 4), they should be related to each other. Substituting flow for number of branches, we expect that

$$\log f = x \log r \tag{2}$$

Taking antilogs gives us

$$f = kr^x \tag{3}$$

where the exponent x is to be determined (Roy and Woldenberg, 1982). An overall value for x may be calculated from morphometric data (Horsfield and Thurlbeck, 1981b). It is given by

$$x = \frac{\log Rb}{\log Rd} \tag{4}$$

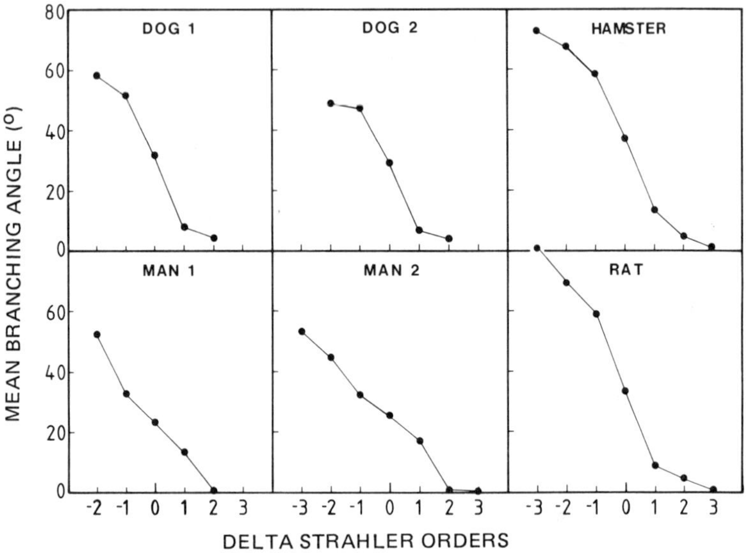

Figure 12 Mean angles of branching in the bronchial tree of four species related to delta Strahler orders, the difference in order between the two daughter branches. When delta = 0, the bifurcation is symmetrical with respect to order. Increasing absolute values of delta define increasing asymmetry, with positive values referring to the major daughter and negative values referring to the minor daughter branch. It can be seen that as asymmetry increases, the major branch angle decreases and the minor branch angle increases.

As an example from a cast of the human bronchial tree, Rb = 2.805 and Rd = 1.427, so

$$x = \frac{\log 2.805}{\log 1.427} = 2.9 \tag{5}$$

This is close to the value calculated for laminar flow. Thus it appears that the radius of an airway is fine-tuned to the flow it carries, and this matching could easily be achieved during growth. At a bifurcation $f_1 = kr_1{}^x$, $f_2 = kr_2{}^x$, and $f_3 = kr_3{}^x$, where the subscripts 1, 2, and 3 refer to parent, major daughter, and minor daughter branches, respectively. Since the flow into a bifurcation equals the flow out,

$$kr_1{}^x = kr_2{}^x + kr_3{}^x \tag{6}$$

$$1 = \frac{r_2}{r_1}^x + \frac{r_3}{r_1}^x \qquad (7)$$

There is only one positive solution for x, so that if r_1, r_2, and r_3 are known, and $r_0 > r_1 \geqslant r_2$, x for a single bifurcation can be determined by an iterative calculation. The value of x thus calculated shows considerable variation between bifurcations, but with a median value in the range 2.333-3.0 (Horsfield and Thurlbeck, 1981b).

Other authors have used different starting points to calculate an optimal value of Rd. These include minimum volume (Kamiya and Togawa, 1972), minimum resistance (Cohn, 1955; Horsfield and Cumming, 1967; Rashevsky, 1973; Weibel, 1963), and minimum entropy production (Wilson, 1967). Each of these authors assumed symmetrical dichotomy, and hence Rb = 2.0, although this was not explicitly stated. They found that $r_1/r_2 = 2^{1/3}$ (note that r_1/r_2 = Rd). By substituting the variable Rb into their equations a more general result can be obtained, namely $Rd = Rb^{1/3}$ instead of $Rd = 2^{1/3}$. Taking logs yields

$$\log Rd = \frac{1}{3} \times \log Rb \qquad (8)$$

$$\frac{\log Rb}{\log Rd} = 3 \qquad (9)$$

and from Eqs. (4) and (9),

$$x = 3 \qquad (10)$$

This result is not surprising because laminar flow was also assumed by each of the authors cited above.

The concept of minimum entropy production which has been applied to rivers (Leopold and Langbein, 1962) has been applied to the pulmonary airways (Horsfield, 1977). It suggests that for minimal entropy production the pressure drop in each order should be equal. Assuming laminar flow once again, this occurs when $Rb \times R\ell/Rd^4 = 1$, and given that $Rb = Rd^3$, then $Rd = R\ell$. These are the theoretical equations that apply for both minimal entropy production and minimum resistance together. Values from one human airway cast are very close to these. Thus Rb = 2.805, $Rb^{1/3}$ = 1.410, Rd = 1.427, and $R\ell$ = 1.402.

I. Species Differences

There are three main types of bronchial tree among the mammals commonly studied in respiratory physiology. The first is that of humans; the second is

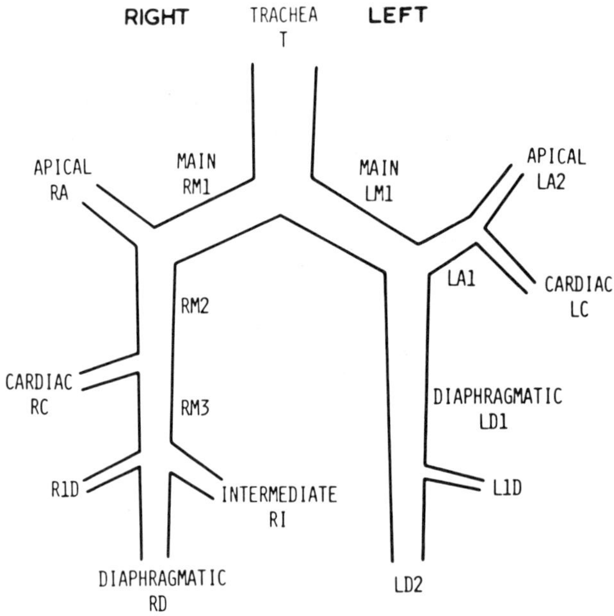

Figure 13 Central airways of the dog's lung. (See Table 5 for dimensions and branching angles.)

exemplified by the dog, and includes cats and rabbits; the third is exemplified by the pig and includes other ungulates such as the sheep.

The dog's lung has seven lobes, an apical, cardiac, and diaphragmatic on each side, and in addition an intermediate lobe on the right. Figure 13 shows the branching pattern of the major airways, and Table 5 gives their dimensions and branching angles. In the ungulates the right apical lobe bronchus arises direct from the trachea, but otherwise the pattern is similar to that in the dog. In both of these groups the axial pattern is well developed, but especially so in ungulates. The main bronchus in a lobe, or even in a lung, runs with very little change of course at bifurcations, producing a branching pattern resembling a pine tree. This contrasts with the more dichotomous pattern seen in humans, which resembles an oak tree. Table 2 gives morphometric parameters for the airways of various species, the higher values of Rb in animals, and especially in sheep, reflecting their more asymmetrical branching.

Table 5 Mean Diameters, Lengths, and Branching Angles of the Upper Airways of 15 Dogs[a]

Branch	$D/W^{1/3}$ (mm/kg^3)	$L/W^{1/3}$ (mm/kg^3)	Branching angle (°)
T	7.10	–	–
LM1	5.04	8.07	46
LA1	3.37	4.70	54
LA2	2.90	3.84	48
LC	2.30	3.33	25
LD1	4.80	3.23	22
L1D	1.79	–	56
LD2	3.73	3.91	13
RM1	6.02	4.71	36
RA	3.79	4.08	73
RM2	5.71	3.40	18
RC	2.85	6.65	62
RM3	5.56	4.36	19
RI	2.66	5.36	41
R1D	1.55	–	18
RD	4.46	5.06	29

[a]The identification of the branches is shown in Fig. 13. D, diameter; L, length; W, body weight. Dimensions are normalized for body weight.
Source: Adapted from Woldehiwot and Horsfield (1978).

III. The Acinus

A. Structure of the Acinus

Each terminal bronchiole supplies a segment of lung called an acinus, the structure of which is summarized in Table 6 and Figure 14. At the smoothly rounded part of the pleural surface it is commonly pyramidal in shape, but on sharper edges, and inside the lung where other structures also occupy space, the shape may be markedly irregular and asymmetrical. The anatomy of the acinar airways is not well understood, despite numerous studies employing various techniques. Variations in terminology over the years have compounded the difficulties. The description given below is based on the work of Hansen and Ampaya (1975), Hansen et al. (1975), and Parker et al. (1971). Both groups reconstructed part of an acinus from serial sections,

Table 6 Numbers and Dimensions of Structures in a Human Acinus[a]

Generation	Structure	Number in acinus	Diameter (mm)	Length (mm)	Sacs on RB and AD	Alveoli on RB, AD, and sacs	Mean number of alveoli	
							Per sac	Per RB or AD
1	Terminal bronchiole	1	0.55	1.20	0	5	—	5.0
2	Respiratory bronchiole 1	2	0.47	0.97	4	32	3.5	9.0
3	Respiratory bronchiole 2	4	0.47	0.97	16	96	3.5	10.0
4	Respiratory bronchiole 3	8	0.49	0.88	24	119	2.4	7.7
5	Alveolar duct 1	19	0.50	0.66	74	373	3.0	8.2
6	Alveolar duct 2	45	0.49	0.51	186	678	2.6	4.3
7	Alveolar duct 3	108	0.51	0.58	405	1542	2.6	4.6
8	Alveolar duct 4	254	0.40	0.43	627	2812	2.9	3.8
9	Alveolar duct 5	374	0.38	0.41	1020	4516	3.4	2.9
10	Alveolar duct 6	366	0.30	0.30	1135	6420	4.0	4.0
11	Alveolar duct 7	146	0.27	0.28	498	2191	3.7	2.3
12	Alveolar duct 8	58	0.24	0.22	274	973	2.8	3.7

[a]RB, respiratory bronchiole; AD, alveolar duct; sac, alveolar sac. Alveolar sacs not taken as a separate generation.
Source: Horsfield (1981). Data from Hansen and Ampaya (1975) and Hansen et al. (1975).

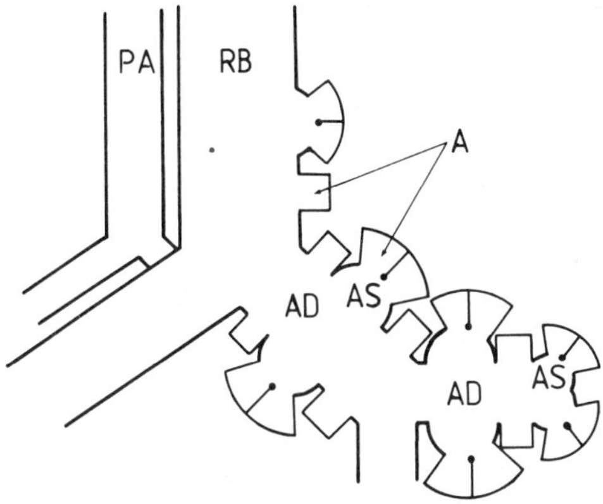

Figure 14 Diagrammatic representation of the structures in a human pulmonary acinus. PA, Pulmonary artery; RB, respiratory bronchiole; AD, alveolar duct; AS, alveolar sac; A, alveolus. Alveolar sacs arise laterally from RBs and ADs, and also form the terminations of the ADs. Alveoli arise from ASs and directly from RBs and ADs. ADs are almost completely surrounded by openings into alveoli, ASs, and other Ads. The pulmonary artery runs adjacent to the RB on the side free from alveoli. (Data from Hansen and Ampaya, 1975; Hansen et al., 1975; Parker et al., 1971.)

making a positive (hollow) enlarged model with sheets of polyurethane foam. They were then able to follow the various pathways through the model. Although the description of Hansen and co-workers is the most complete account so far of the asymmetrical structure of the acinus, the technique used is very difficult in practice, with major problems in deciding where a given structure starts and finishes. Furthermore, no group has ever studied one complete acinus by the method of serial sections, so the data are incomplete. Because of these problems, the following description is tentative and subject to revision as more data become available. Readers interested in previous studies should refer to these directly (Boyden, 1971; Miller, 1947; Ogawa, 1920; Pump, 1964, 1969; Weibel, 1963, Willson, 1922).

The terminal bronchiole most commonly gives rise to three generations of dichotomously branching respiratory bronchioles, although pathways are sometimes seen which terminate in less than three generations. Respiratory bronchioles are tubular structures that give rise laterally to a few alveolar sacs and alveoli. They are lined with cuboidal bronchial epithelium, which is flattened around the mouths of the alveoli. From two to nine generations of alveolar ducts arise from the respiratory bronchioles, branching by dichotomy, trichotomy, or polychotomy with marked variations both within and between acini. An alveolar duct is surrounded by the openings of the other ducts, sacs, and alveoli which spring from it. Their walls consist almost entirely of the margins of these openings, which are lined with flattened epithelium only. Because their lengths and diameters are approximately equal, they are either barrel-shaped or form irregular polyhedra. Alveolar sacs have a similar structure to the ducts, but are hemispherical or saucer-shaped. They average 260 μm in diameter at the orifice, and 180 μm deep. Sacs arise from the sides of respiratory bronchioles and ducts, and also form the terminal division of the ducts distally, although less than half their total number are formed in this way. They give rise to alveoli only, about three or four per sac on average. In expanded lungs alveolar walls are flat, and alveoli form complex polyhedra of varied form. They have one opening averaging 200 μm in diameter, and are of about the same depth, but show wide variations in size. Alveoli arise from the walls of respiratory bronchioles, alveolar ducts, and alveolar sacs. Approximately equal numbers of alveoli arise from respiratory bronchioles and ducts directly or via sacs, but in absolute numbers there are many more peripherally because of the increasing number of structures. In previous descriptions where the total number of ducts was less, more alveoli were attributed to each duct.

B. Number of Acinar Structures

In an acinus there are 2 + 4 + 8 = 14 respiratory bronchioles when these branch by symmetrical dichotomy, giving about 350,000 in the lungs. The total number of alveolar ducts was estimated by Weibel (1963) to be 13.8×10^6, by Parker et al. (1971) to be 23×10^6, and by Hansen and Ampaya (1975) to be 31.5×10^6. The lower value is probably an underestimate for technical reasons (Hansen and Ampaya, 1974), so the number can be put between 25 and 30×10^6. Alveolar sacs were estimated by Hansen and Ampaya (1975) to number 98×10^6 or 4263 acinus. Estimates of alveolar numbers range from 2×10^8 to 6×10^8 (Angus and Thurlbeck, 1972); Dunnill, 1962; Hansen and Ampaya, 1975; Weibel, 1963). Mean alveolar size is relatively constant, the larger numbers being found in lungs from taller subjects.

C. Collateral Ventilation

Although the terminal branches of the airways end blindly, communications between parallel structures are well recognized. The part they play in normal respiration is unknown, but they are probably of considerable importance in diseases in which airway blockage occurs. In this case collateral communications could offer alternative routes for inspired air to reach those alveoli whose supplying bronchiole has been blocked. Three types of collateral com-

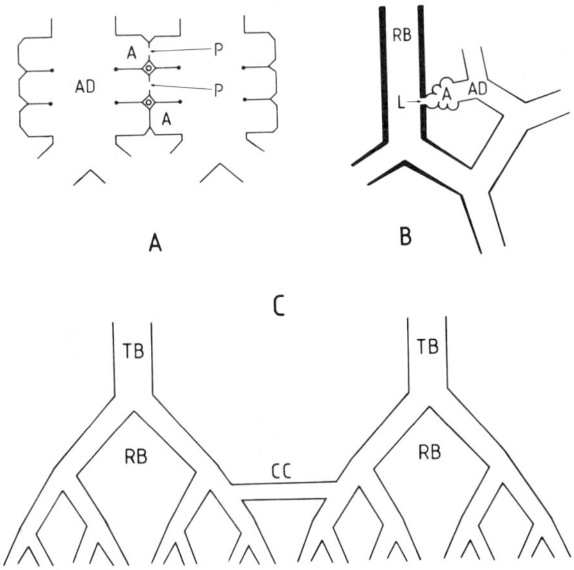

Figure 15 Possible routes of collateral ventilation: (A) interalveolar pores; (B) canal of Lambert; (C) interbronchiolar channels. A, Alveoli; AD, alveolar duct; CC, interbronchiolar channel; L, canal of Lambert; P, interalveolar pore; RB, respiratory bronchiole; TB, terminal bronchiole. (See the text.)

munication have been described: interalveolar pores, the canals of Lambert, and interbronchiolar channels.

1. Interalveolar communications, or pores of Kohn (Fig. 15A), are holes in alveolar septae situated within the interstices of the capillary network (Loosli, 1937; Macklin, 1935). They can be found in most species, range from 3 to 15 μm in diameter, and according to Martin (1966) average about eight per "alveolus" in the dog. (From his paper, he seems to mean eight per alveolar wall.) They have the form of a simple orifice, tube, or hourglass, are present at birth, and increase in size and number with age. In the dog, where interlobar septae are poorly developed, interalveolar pores could, at least potentially, allow movement of gas between all alveoli in a lobe. Whether these pores are in fact patent during life is not known, but it seems likely that they are normally covered by a film of alveolar surfactant. Even if they are patent, Menkes and Traystman (1977) have calculated that the behavior of resistance to collateral flow with changing lung volume is more likely to be due to flow via larger accessary airways than through the pores.

2. The canals of Lambert (Lambert, 1955; Duguid and Lambert, 1964) are tubular passages about 30 μm in diameter which pass from the lumen of a respiratory bronchiole, through its wall, to join an adjacent alveolus. Such alveoli mainly, and probably entirely, arise from structures distal to the respiratory bronchiole concerned, which have turned back to become adjacent to it. Thus any collateral ventilation going through the canal would be within the one acinus (Fig. 15B). Although the canals are "fairly numerous" (Duguid and Lambert, 1964), they are not large and it seems unlikely that they constitute an important route for collateral ventilation.

3. Interbronchiolar channels (Fig. 15C) from 60 to 200 μm in diameter were described in the dog by Martin (1963, 1966) and have since been demonstrated in human lungs (Andersen and Jespersen, 1980; Henderson et al., 1968-1969; Raskin and Herman, 1975). Numerous experiments have demonstrated convective flow through such channels, most simply by blocking one branch in a lobe and then inflating the whole lobe via another bronchus. This phenomenon occurs most readily in dog lungs, which have poorly developed interlobular septae; less readily in human lungs, which have partially developed septae; and least in pig lungs, in which the lobules are completely separated by septae. Although collateral channels are much less frequent at septae, they do sometimes cross them (Raskin and Herman, 1975). These communications have been described as short tubes (Henderson et al., 1968-1969; Raskin and Herman, 1975) and as respiratory bronchioles (Anderson and Jespersen, 1980; Martin, 1966). Their diameters have been demonstrated histologically, by casting and by the passage of graded polystyrene spheres. They join respiratory bronchioles of adjacent acini and probably also permit respiratory bronchiole-alveolar duct and duct-duct communication. In normal lungs they are the most important route for collateral ventilation. Numerous studies have been made of the physiology of flow through collateral channels; this topic has been reviewed by Menkes and Traystman (1977). The finding that resistance to flow was greater in the upper and middle lobes than in the lower (Menkes and Traystman, 1977) received anatomical confirmation when Andersen and Jespersen (1980) found that collateral channels are more numerous in the lower lobes.

4. Collateral channels constitute a reserve mechanism for ventilating a segment of lung whose supplying bronchus has been blocked. To a degree they are self-regulating, because if the airways are patent, ventilation of adjacent acini by the normal route would prevent the development of a pressure difference between them, and hence no convective flow would occur in the collaterals. If the airway to one acinus becomes blocked, a pressure difference would develop between the two acini on inspiration, causing convective flow from the acinus with the patent bronchus to that with the blocked bronchus. In addition to this, the patency of collateral channels to flow is

regulated by PO_2 and PCO_2 in the lungs, expecially PCO_2 (Traystman et al., 1976; Traystman et al., 1978). When PCO_2 rises, indicating reduced alveolar ventilation, the channels open up, and the resistance to flow through them falls. This regulation is probably mediated locally and may respond to both airway and small vessel PCO_2.

IV. Airway Cross-Sectional Area

Although for the most part the diameter of a daughter branch is less than that of its parent, the summed cross-sectional area of the two daughter branches is usually greater than that of its parents. Thus, passing down the airways, the summed cross-sectional area of successive generations increases. This is not true of the first three or four generations, however, down which cross-sectional area actually decreases slightly. Within the acinus cross-sectional area increases rapidly in successive generations. These features are most easily illustrated by Weibel's model, which has the well-known trumpet or thumbtack shape. This is conceptually helpful, as it is obvious that the velocity of convective flow diminishes down the airways, while mass transfer by diffusion, which is proportional to cross-sectional area, increases. These are the conditions in which the stationary interface of concentration forms (Cumming et al., 1971; Paiva, 1973), as will be described in Chapter 6. Although the thumbtack model is conceptually helpful, it is anatomically inaccurate. The asymmetry of the conducting airways, shown in Figure 7, and of the acinus, shown in Table 6, imply a wide range of generations and path lengths to the terminal alveolar sac. As a result, the shape of the cross-sectional area-length plot is in fact better likened to that of an onion with a pointed end (Horsfield, 1978).

V. Asymmetry and Function

Asymmetry of the airways is now recognized as being an important factor in the way gas is distributed by convection and diffusion, and their interaction, as will be described in Chapter 6. The time taken for a molecule of gas to traverse the conducting airways is the transit time, and this has a distribution similar to that of path length and generations. Its calculation has been described elsewhere (Horsfield and Cumming, 1968a,b). Acini supplied by longer bronchial paths inspire dead-space gas in the first part of inspiration for a longer time, and therefore receive more dead-space gas as a proportion of their tidal volume. On expiration, alveolar gas reaches the mouth distributed in both time and volume, and this contributes to the sigmoid shape of phase II of the single-breath nitrogen test. From one airways cast its distribution in volume due to anatomical asymmetry was calculated to be 169 ml (Horsfield and Cumming, 1968b). The range of this distribution may of course be increased by functional factors, such as regional differences in ventilation, asynchronous emptying, or by pathological changes in disease.

VI. Diseased Lungs

A. Lung Parenchyma

A number of disease processes may affect alveoli and connective tissue, either locally or generally. Fibrosis, often accompanied by shrinkage and loss of elasticity, results in diminished flow to the affected parts. When the disease is widespread, the more severely affected parts have the lower flow. Fibrosis may also reduce the lumen of small airways, going on to complete obliteration, with obvious effects on flow. Air-filled cysts, especially valved ones, may gradually increase in size, collapsing nearby lung tissue and decreasing or preventing flow to it. In emphysema the patchy loss of elastic tissue probably results in different parts of the lungs having different pressure-volume curves. At end expiration different parts of the lung will be at different points on these curves, so that on inspiration they expand differently, causing unequal distribution of inspired gas. In general, fibrosis reduces lung volume whereas panacinar emphysema increases it, so that the lung volume at which inspiration starts may differ considerably from normal. Two mechanisms may then contribute to a change in the distribution of inspired gas: first, the regional expansion of the chest wall may be different at different volumes, and second, the pressure-volume curves and the starting points on them will be different.

B. Dilatation of the Alveolar Ducts

Duct dilatation occurs as part of normal aging, but this process shades almost imperceptibly into emphysema, so that it is difficult to say where one ends and the other starts (Fig. 16a). The resulting increase in the cross-sectional area of the airways at this level may affect the mixing of gases by diffusion.

C. Emphysema and Chronic Obstructive Lung Disease

These conditions have much in common and for simplicity will be grouped together. When following a pathway down a cast of normal airways a progressive decrease in diameter may be noted. In airways disease the diameter is much more irregular (Linhartova et al., 1974; Scott and Steiner, 1975). An alternating increase and decrease may be seen, or there may be localized narrowing which can be severe enough to be called a stenosis (Fig. 16b).

Dilatations may be present, either in the form of cysts (Fig. 16c) or as bronchiectasis. Sometimes, probably associated with loss of elastic tissue, the airways may become corkscrew-shaped (Fig. 16d).

An increase in the number of alveolar pores in emphysema was noted by Kohn (1893) and it is possible that the destruction of alveolar walls in panacinar emphysema starts with an enlargement of the pores. Evenually, alveolar walls are lost, leaving abnormally large air spaces of various sizes and distribution. In centrilobular emphysema (Leopold and Gough, 1957) there is a dilatation of first- and second-generation respiratory bronchioles (Fig. 17a), followed by a breaking down of the tissues between them to form an abnormal space (Fig. 17b). These should be compared with the normal structures shown in Figure 17d (Horsfield et al., 1966). The apices of the acini are at the center of the lobule (like the sharp ends of slices of a round cake), so that the process comes to affect the center of the lobule first. Alevolar ducts and alveoli distal to the centrilobular space are relatively normal, although later they too may be affected. Thus in centrilobular emphysema there is an in-series dilatation at the level of the respiratory bronchioles, a critical point because this is where the stationary interface will normally become established. The form of the interface will be altered to a major degree, and the dilatation will act as a dilution chamber, interfering with the transport of O_2 and CO_2. It has been calculated that if the dilatations of centrilobular emphysema are widely and evenly distributed and affect 10-20% of the lung volume, retention of CO_2 and an increased slope of the single-breath nitrogen test would result (Horsfield et al., 1973). This should be contrasted with panacinar emphysema involving 10-20% of the lung, which would have minimal effect. In addition to the dilatation, stenosis of bronchioles has been described in centrilobular emphysema, including the entry bronchioles to the emphysematous spaces (Bignon et al., 1969, 1970; Depierre et al., 1972). This would diminish flow into the acinus and further raise the P_{CO_2}.

In panacinar emphysema all of the acinus is affected, eventually resulting in a large, irregular dilatation with gross loss of alveolar walls (Fig. 17c). Gas mixing in such a structure must be slower than in a normal acinus, and the stationary interface, if it exists at all, would be at the entry bronchiole. The breakdown of alveolar walls between adjacent acini increases the possibilities for collateral ventilation (Hogg et al., 1969). Thus although airways may be partially or completely occluded from one cause or another in panacinar emphysema, collateral channels may be able to maintain ventilation in the affected parts of the lung. Airways may be affected in emphysema by loss of elastic recoil, reducing the forces holding them open, and by loss of cartilage and connective tissue, which makes their walls floppy and more liable to collapse on expiration.

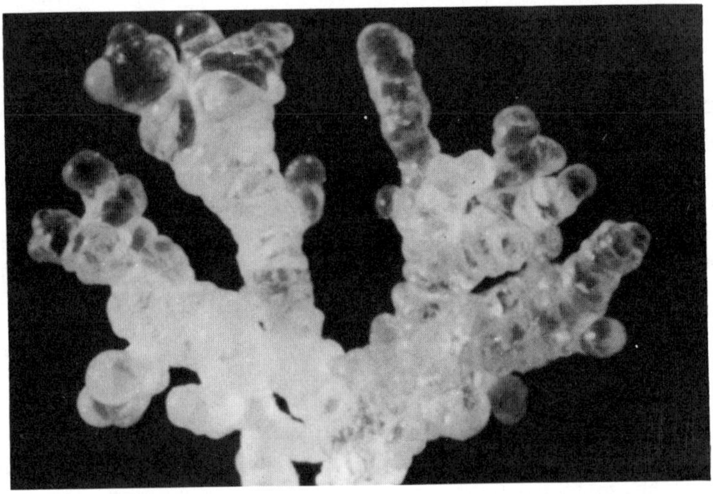

(a)

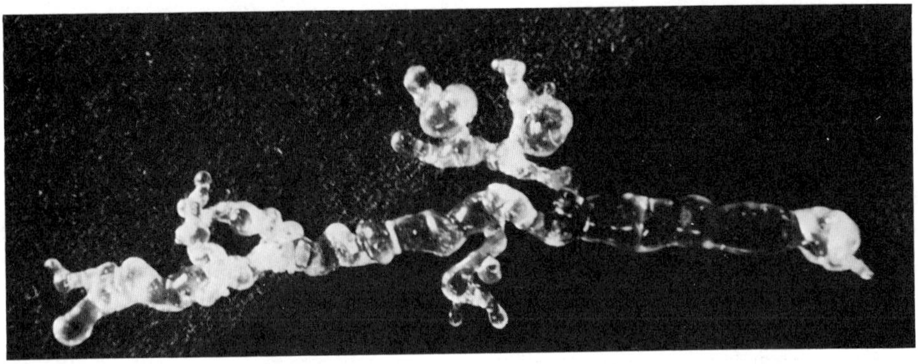

(b)

Figure 16 Airway casts: (a) dilatation of alveolar ducts; (b) airways in chronic obstructive lung disease (COLD) showing varying diameter, focal narrowing, and dilatations; (c) dilated airways in honeycomb lung; (d) corkscrew airway in COLD.

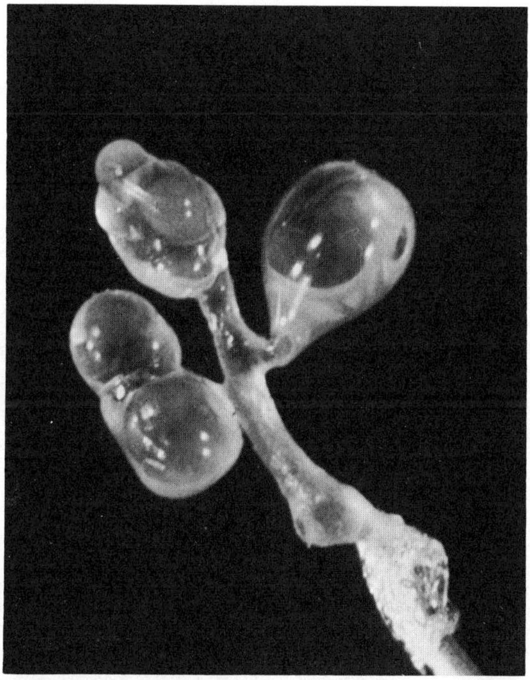

(c)

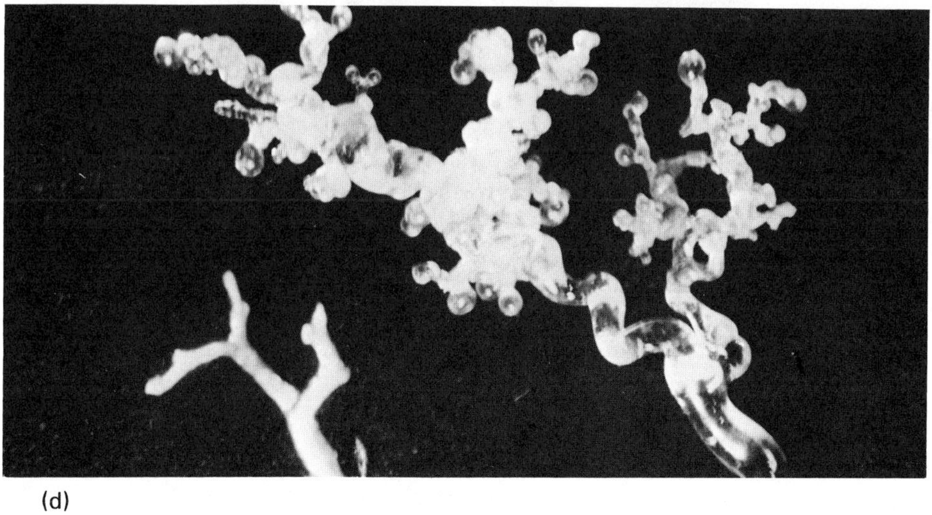

(d)

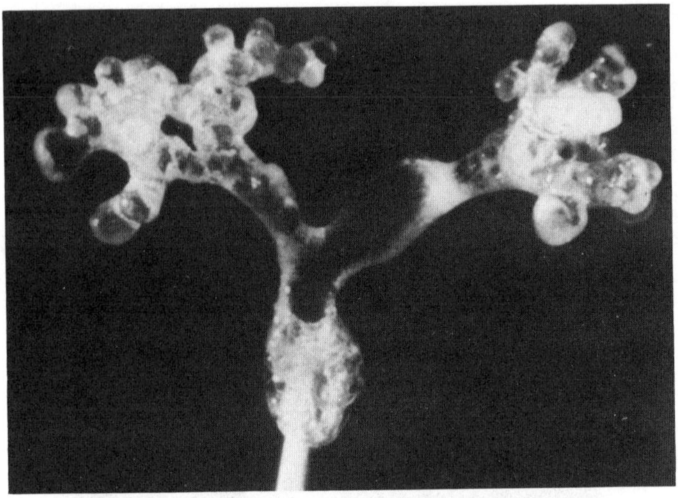

(a)

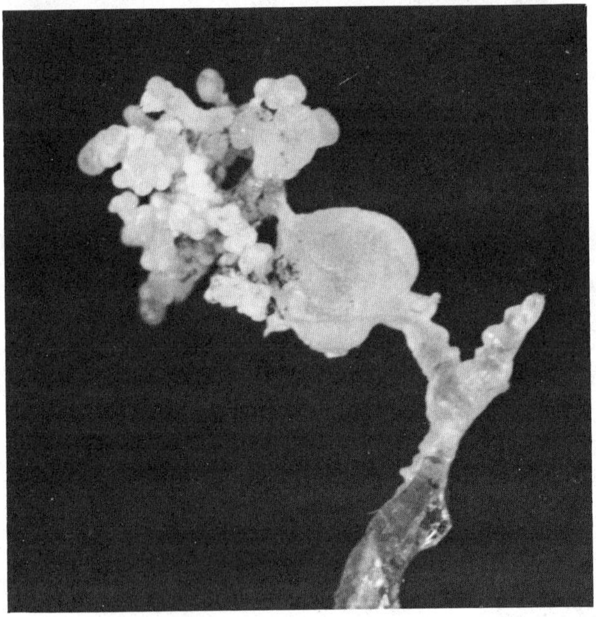

(b)

Figure 17 Airway casts: (a) dilated respiratory bronchiole in early centrilobular emphysema; (b) dilatation of centrilobular emphysema, with alveolar ducts and alveoli distal to it; (c) panacinar emphysema, with total destruction of the acinus; (d) normal acinus, partly pruned, for comparison.

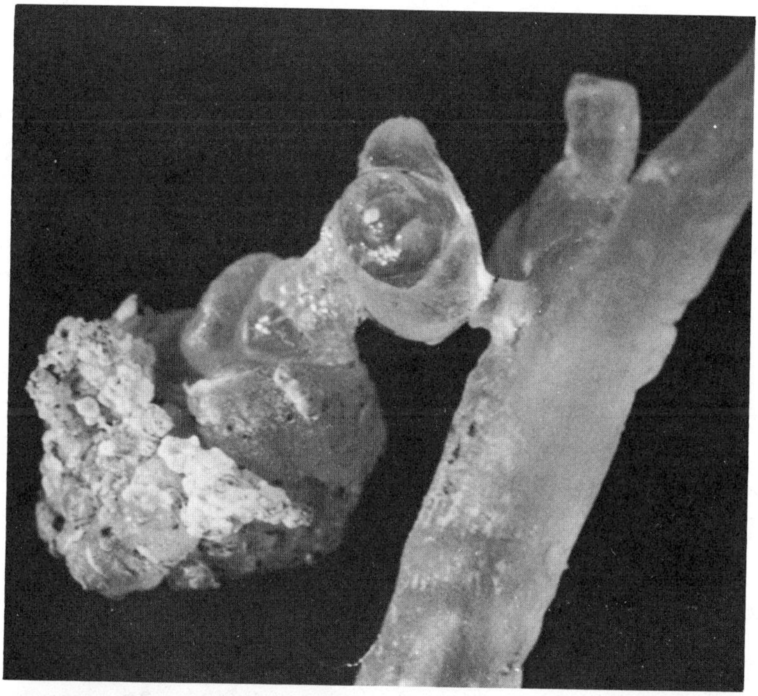

(c)

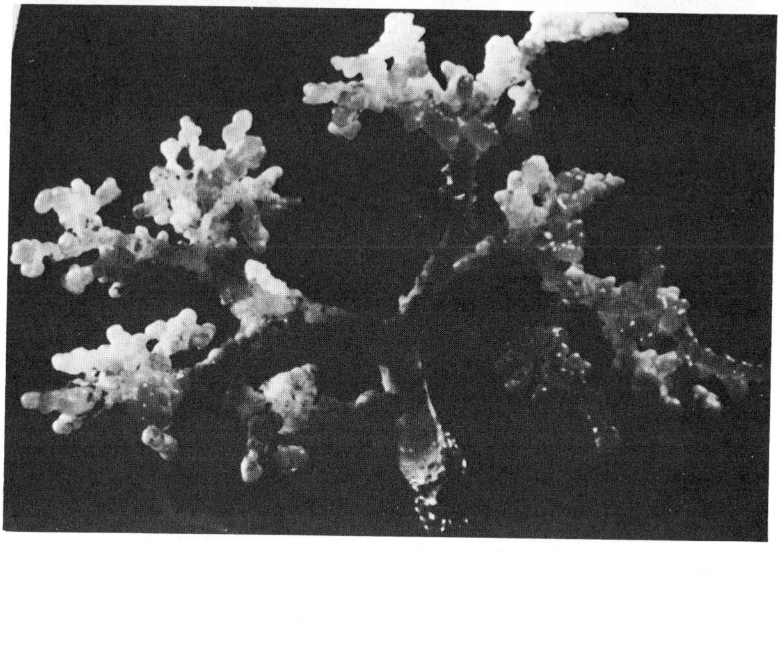

(d)

D. Asthma

Partial or complete blockage of small airways occurs in asthma, due to any combination of bronchoconstriction, edema of the mucosa, and mucus in the lumen. Again, collateral ventilation may be very important in maintaining ventilation to the affected acini, while contributing to the incompleteness of gas mixing and V/Q abnormalities (Brown et al., 1969). Depending on circumstances, total convective flow by all routes to these acini may be normal or reduced, but even if normal, gas mixing along the abnormal route will be impaired. This will result in an increased slope on the single-breath test for nitrogen (Hogg et al., 1972) and a reduced gas mixing efficiency (Cumming and Guyatt, 1981).

E. Pulmonary Edema

Airways and blood vessels enter the lung at the hilum and run into the lung in a tunnel of fibrous tissue, the peribronchial sheath. Between the sheath and the bronchial wall is a potential space, the peribronchial space, which is traversed by some loose connective tissue. This space extends about as far down as the cartilage in the bronchial walls, approximately to 2-mm-diameter airways. Beyond this the airways are attached directly to the lung parenchyma. The elastic recoil of the lung is normally transmitted across the peribronchial space to the bronchial wall, in much the same way as it is transmitted across the potential pleural space, helping to keep the airway open

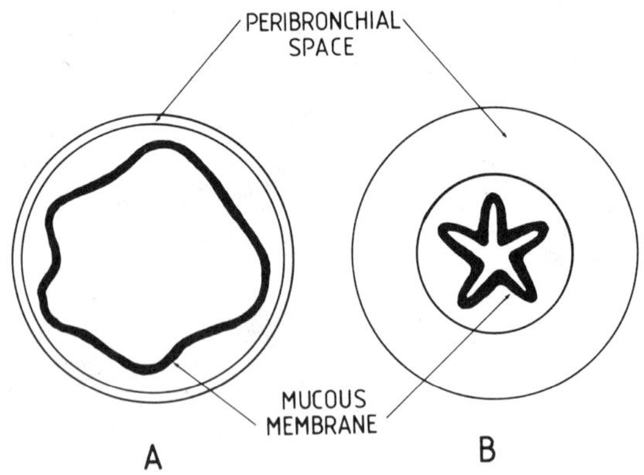

Figure 18 Diagrams of bronchial cross sections: (A) normal, with potential peribronchial space; (B) edema fluid in peribronchial space causing decreased bronchial diameter, folding of the mucosa, and marked narrowing of the airway.

(Fig. 18A). When the lungs become edematous, fluid gathers in the peribronchial space, and at a later stage in the lumen of the airways. The bronchus becomes isolated from the recoil pressure and its diameter decreases, producing folding of the mucous membrane into the lumen (Fig. 18B). This may become completely occluded, especially if fluid is present. If fluid accumulates in the distal respiratory bronchioles, alveolar ducts, and alveoli (i.e., distal to the stationary interface), diffusive mixing will be adversely affected.

References

Andersen, J. B., and Jespersen, W. (1980). Demonstration of intersegmental respiratory bronchioles in normal human lungs. *Eur. J. Respir. Dis.*, **61**: 337-341.

Angus, G. E., and Thurlbeck, W. M. (1972). Number of alveoli in the human lung. *J. Appl. Physiol.*, **32**:483-485.

Bignon, J., Khoury, F., Even, P., André, J., and Brouet, G. (1969). Morphometric study in chronic obstructive bronchopulmonary disease. Pathologic, clinical and physiologic correlations. *Am. Rev. Respir. Dis.*, **99**:669-695.

Bignon, J., Andre-Bougaran, J., and Brouet, G. (1970). Parenchymal, bronchiolar, and bronchial measurements in centrilobular emphysema. Relation to weight of right ventricle. *Thorax*, **25**:556-567.

Boyden, E. A. (1971). The structure of the pulmonary acinus in a child of six years and eight months. *Am. J. Anat.*, **132**:275-300.

Brown, R., Woolcock, A. J., Vincent, N. J., and Macklem, P. T. (1969). Physiological effects of experimental airway obstruction with beads. *J. Appl. Physiol.*, **27**:328-335.

Cohn, D. L. (1955). Optimal systems: II. The vascular system. *Bull. Math. Biol.*, **17**:219-227.

Cumming, G., and Guyatt, A. R. (1981). Alveolar gas mixing efficiency in the human lung. *Clin. Sci.*, **62**:541-547.

Cumming, G., Horsfield, K., and Preston, S. B. (1971). Diffusion equilibrium in the lungs examined by nodal analysis. *Respir. Physiol.*, **12**: 329-345.

DePierre, A., Bignon, J., Lebeau, A., and Brouet, G. (1972). Quantitative study of parenchyma and small conductive airways in chronic nonspecific lung disease. *Chest*, **62**:699-708.

Duguid, J. B., and Lambert, M. W. (1964). The pathogenesis of coal miners' pneumoconiosis. *J. Pathol. Bacteriol.*, **88**:389-403.

Dunnill, M. S. (1962). Postnatal growth of the lung. *Thorax*, **17**:329-333.

Findeisen, W. (1935). Uber das Absetzen kleiner, in dur Luft suspendierter Teilchen in der menschlichen Lunge bei der Atmung. *Arch. Ges. Physiol.,* **236**:367-379.

Hansen, J. E., and Ampaya, E. P. (1974). Lung morphometry: a fallacy in the use of the counting principle. *J. Appl. Physiol.,* **37**:951-954.

Hansen, J. E., and Ampaya, E. P. (1975). Human air space shapes, sizes, area, and volumes. *J. Appl. Physiol.,* **38**:990-995.

Hansen, J. E., Ampaya, E. P., Bryant, G. H., and Navin, J. J. (1975). Branching pattern of airways and air spaces of a single human terminal bronchiole. *J. Appl. Physiol.,* **38**:983-989.

Hendersen, R., Horsfield, K., and Cumming, G. (1968-1969). Intersegmental collateral ventilation in the human lung. *Respir. Physiol.,* **6**:128-134.

Hogg, J. C., Macklem, P. T., and Thurlbeck, W. M. (1969). The resistance of collateral channels in excised human lungs. *J. Clin. Invest.,* **48**:421-431.

Hogg, W., Brunton, J., Kryger, M., Brown, R., and Macklem, P. (1972). Gas diffusion across collateral channels. *J. Appl. Physiol.,* **33**:568-575.

Horsfield, K. (1967). Morphology of the Human Bronchial Tree. M.D. thesis, University of Birmingham, Birmingham, England.

Horsfield, K. (1977). Morphology of branching trees related to entropy. *Respir. Physiol.,* **29**:179-184.

Horsfield, K. (1978). Quantitative morphology and structure: functional correlations in the lung. In *The Lung.* International Academy of Pathology Monograph 19. Edited by W. M. Thurlbeck and M. R. Abell. Baltimore, Williams & Wilkins, pp. 151-159.

Horsfield, K. (1981). The structure of the tracheo-bronchial tree. In *Scientific Foundations of Respiratory Medicine.* Edited by J. G. Scadding and G. Cumming. London, William Heinemann.

Horsfield, K., and Cumming, G. (1967). Angles of branching and diameters of branches in the human bronchial tree. *Bull. Math. Biophys.,* **29**:245-259.

Horsfield, K., and Cumming, G. (1968a). Morphology of the bronchial tree in man. *J. Appl. Physiol.,* **24**:373-383.

Horsfield, K., and Cumming, G. (1968b). Functional consequences of airway morphology. *J. Appl. Physiol.,* **24**:384-390.

Horsfield, K., and Thurlbeck, A. (1981a). Volume of the conducting airways calculated from morphometric parameters. *Bull. Math. Biol.,* **43**:101-109.

Horsfield, K., and Thurlbeck, A. (1981b). Relation between diameter and flow in branches of the bronchial tree. *Bull. Math. Biol.,* **43**:681-691.

Horsfield, K., Cumming, G., and Hicken, P. (1966). A morphologic study of airway disease using bronchial casts. *Am. Rev. Respir. Dis.*, **93**: 900-906.

Horsfield, K., Dart, G., Olson, D. E., Filley, G. F., and Cumming, G. (1971). Models of the human bronchial tree. *J. Appl. Physiol.*, **31**:207-217.

Horsfield, K., Barer, D. H., and Cumming, G. (1973). Centrilobular emphysema studied with a mathematical model. *J. Appl. Physiol.*, **31**:386-391.

Kamiya, A., and Togawa, A. (1972). Optimal branching structure of the vascular tree. *Bull. Math. Biophys.*, **34**:431-438.

Kohn, H. N. (1893). Zur Histologie des indurirenden fibrosen Pneumonie. *Muench. Med. Wochschr.*, **40**:42-45.

Lambert, M. W. (1955). Accessory bronchiole-alveolar communications. *J. Pathol. Bacteriol.*, **70**:311-314.

Leopold, J. G., and Gough, J. (1957). The centrilobular form of hypertrophic emphysema and its relation to chronic bronchitis. *Thorax*, **12**: 219-235.

Leopold, L. B., and Langbein, W. B. (1962). The concept of entropy in landscape evolution. *Geological Survey Professional Paper 500-A.* Washington, D.C., U.S. Government Printing Office, pp. A1-A20.

Linhartova, A., Anderson, A. E., and Foraker, A. G. (1974). Topology of nonrespiratory bronchioles of normal and emphysematous lungs. *Hum. Pathol.*, **5**:729-735.

Loosli, C. G. (1937). Interalveolar communications in normal and in pathological mammalian lungs. *Arch. Pathol.*, **24**:743-762.

Macklin, C. C. (1935). Pulmonic alveolar vents. *J. Anat.*, **69**:188-192.

Martin, H. B. (1963). The effect of ageing on the alveolar pores of Kohn in the dog. *Am. Rev. Respir. Dis.* **88**:773-784.

Martin, H. B. (1966). Respiratory bronchioles as the pathway for collateral ventilation. *J. Appl. Physiol.*, **21**:1443-1447.

Menkes, H. A., and Traystman, R. J. (1977). Collateral ventilation. *Am. Rev. Respir. Dis.*, **116**:287-309.

Miller, W. S. (1947). *The Lung,* 2nd ed. Springfield, Ill., Charles C Thomas.

Murray, C. D. (1926). The physiological principle of minimal work: I. The vascular system and the cost of blood volume. *Proc. Natl. Acad. Sci. USA*, **12**:207-214.

Ogawa, C. (1920). The finer ramifications of the human lung. *Am. J. Anat.*, **27**:315-332.

Paiva, M. (1973). Gas transport in the human lung. *J. Appl. Physiol.*, **35**: 401-410.

Parker, H., Horsfield, K., and Cumming, G. (1971). Morphology of the distal airways of the human lung. *J. Appl. Physiol.*, **31**:386-391.

Phalen, R. F., Yeh, H. C., Schum, G. M., and Raabe, O. G. (1978). Application of an idealized model to morphometry of the mammalian tracheobronchial tree. *Anat. Rec.,* **190**:167-176.

Pump, K. K. (1964). The morphology of the finer branches of the human lung. *Dis. Chest,* **46**:379-398.

Pump, K. K. (1969). Morphology of the acinus of the human lung. *Dis. Chest,* **56**:126-134.

Raabe, O. G., Yeh, H. C., Schum, G. M., and Phalen, R. F. (1976). *Tracheobronchial Geometry–Human, Dog, Rat, Hamster,* Albuquerque, N. Mex., Lovelace Foundation for Medical Education and Research.

Rashevsky, N. (1973). The principle of adequate design. In *Foundations of Mathematical Biology,* Vol. III. Edited by R. Rosen. New York, Academic Press, pp. 143-175.

Raskin, S. P., and Herman, P. G. (1975). Interacinar pathways in the human lung. *Am. Rev. Respir. Dis.,* **111**:489-495.

Rohrer, F. (1915). Der Stromungswiderstand in der menschlichen Atemwegen und der Einfluss der unregelmassigen Verzweigung des Bronchialsystems auf der Atmungsverlauf in vershiedenen Lungenbezinken. *Arch. Gesamte Physiol.,* **162**:225-229.

Roy, A. G., and Woldenberg, M. J. (1982). A generalization of optimal models of arterial branching. *Bull. Math. Biol.,* **44**:349-360.

Scott, K. M. W., and Steiner, G. M. (1975). Postmortem assessment of chronic airways obstruction by tantalum bronchography. *Thorax,* **30**:405-414.

Snyder, B., Dantzker, D. R., and Jaeger, M. J. (1981). Flow partitioning in symmetric cascades of branches. *J. Appl. Physiol.,* **51**:598-606.

Strahler, A. N. (1953). Revision of Horton's quantitative factors in erosional terrain. *Trans. Am. Geophys. Union,* **34**:345.

Strahler, A. N. (1957). Quantitative analysis of watershed geomorphology. *Trans. Am. Geophys. Union,* **38**:913-920.

Suwa, N. (1981). Supracellular structural principle and geometry of blood vessels. *Virchows Arch. (Pathol. Anat.),* **390**:161-179.

Thurlbeck, A., and Horsfield, K. (1980). Branching angles in the bronchial tree related to orders of branching. *Respir. Physiol.,* **41**:173-181.

Thurlbeck, W. M., and Wang, N. S. (1974). The structure of the lungs. In *MTP International Reviews of Science: Respiration Physiology,* Series 1, Vol. 2. London, Butterworth, p. 4.

Traystman, R. J., Batra, G. K., and Menkes, H. A. (1976). Local regulation of collateral ventilation by oxygen and carbon dioxide. *J. Appl. Physiol.,* **40**:819-823.

Traystman, R. J., Terry, P. B., and Menkes, H. A. (1978). Carbon dioxide–

a major determinant of collateral ventilation. *J. Appl. Physiol.*, **45**: 69-74.

Uylings, H. B. M. (1977). Optimization of diameters and bifurcation angles in lung and vascular tree structures. *Bull. Math. Biol.*, **39**:509-520.

Weibel, E. R. (1963). *Morphometry of the Human Lung.* Berlin: Springer-Verlag, p. 139.

Willson, H. G. (1922). The terminals of the human bronchiole. *Am. J. Anat.*, **30**:267-295.

Wilson, T. A. (1967). Design of the bronchial tree. *Nature*, **213**:668-669.

Woldehiwot, Z., and Horsfield, J. (1978). Diameter, length and branching angles of the upper airways in the dog lung. *Respir. Physiol.*, **33**:213-218.

3

Gas Transport in the Conducting Airways

JAMES S. ULTMAN

The Pennsylvania State University
University Park, Pennsylvania

I. Scope

The first step in the oxygenation of blood by the lungs is the transport of fresh air through the conducting airways, from the mouth and nose to the alveolar membranes. This transport occurs by a combination of bulk flow and mixing. Whereas mixing is defined as the relative motion of one gas species, such as oxygen, with respect to another gas species, such as nitrogen, bulk flow refers to the movement of all gas species at the mean velocity of the airstream. Therefore, in the absence of mixing, bulk flow can only transport inspired air over its tidal volume. For a typical tidal volume of 0.5 liter, fresh air could reach only about 10% of all alveoli in the lung by bulk flow alone.

Clearly, the presence of longitudinal mixing is critical for normal ventilation. Even more dramatic is the fact that alveolar ventilation can be de-

---

This work was supported in part by National Institutes of Health Grant HL-20347.

tected at tidal volumes which are only one-third of the normal Fowler dead space, and the use of such low tidal volumes in high-frequency mechanical ventilation can sustain normal blood gas compositions. The purpose of this chapter is to describe what is known about the underlying mixing mechanisms during normal breathing, with discussions focusing on those processes that occur within the conducting airways. Transport in the respiratory zone is described as a separate subject in Chapter 6. This chapter will also be limited to steady or quasi-steady interpretations of mixing and aerodynamics. Chapter 4 contains material dealing with the effect of respiratory frequency on gas transport.

Mixing can occur by diffusion processes associated with the molecular nature of the gas species or by dispersion processes which depend on local velocity patterns, and the relative importance of these contributing factors is strongly dependent on airway geometry. Therefore, this chapter begins in Section II with a brief overview of airway anatomy and aerodynamic characteristics and their implications in the identification of airway mixing mechanisms. Theoretical transport models, useful in the design and interpretation of mixing experiments, are described in Section III. In Section IV, mixing experiments in physical models and human subjects are classified according to the nature of their design, and the use of mass transfer theory for data interpretation is stressed. The chapter concludes with a short discussion of possible applications in Section V.

II. Background

A. Anatomical Features

The conducting airways are those segments of the pulmonary tree that do not contain alveoli and therefore are not directly involved in gas exchange. These airways may be subdivided into the *upper airways,* which extend from the lips and nares to the glottis, and the *tracheobronchial tree,* which encompasses 11 or more generations of branching from the carina to the terminal bronchioles. Most of what is known concerning airway anatomy has resulted from extensive measurements made on a select number of port-mortem lung casts and excised lung preparations, but the recent development of acoustic reflectance techniques offers the possibility of noninvasively evaluating the serial distribution of airway cross sections in individual subjects (e.g., Fredberg et al., 1980).

Inspired air normally enters the lungs through the nose, except under those conditions where nasal obstruction occurs or where high ventilatory demand necessitates a lower-resistance path through the mouth. In patients requiring mechanical ventilation or general anesthesia, the upper airways are

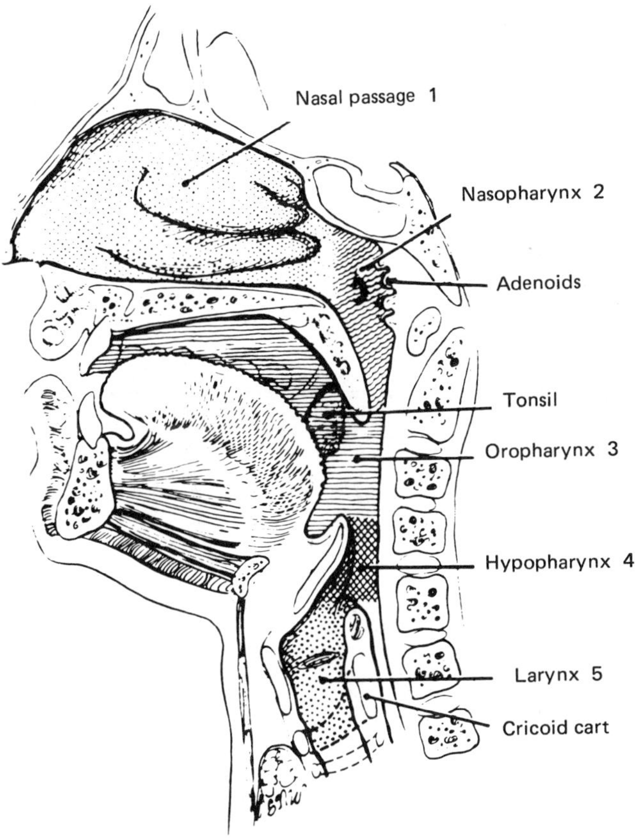

Figure 1 Upper airways. (From Proctor, 1966. Reprinted with the permission of the American Society for Microbiology.)

completely bypassed by intubation or tracheotomy. In addition to ambiguities in air access, gas transport in the upper airways is complicated by the complex array of converging and diverging conduits. Swift and Proctor (1977) have summarized the most important geometric characteristics of the upper airways (Fig. 1) during nasal breathing: the ostium internum, a 0.32-cm^2 constriction just beyond the nasal entrance, leads to a sharp vertical-to-horizontal bend; the nasal turbinates, which possess a flow cross-section of narrow width, contain the airflow within the main nasal passage and also communicate with quiescent gas in the paranasal sinuses; and a further bend and slight constriction in the nasopharynx conducts gas, by way of the

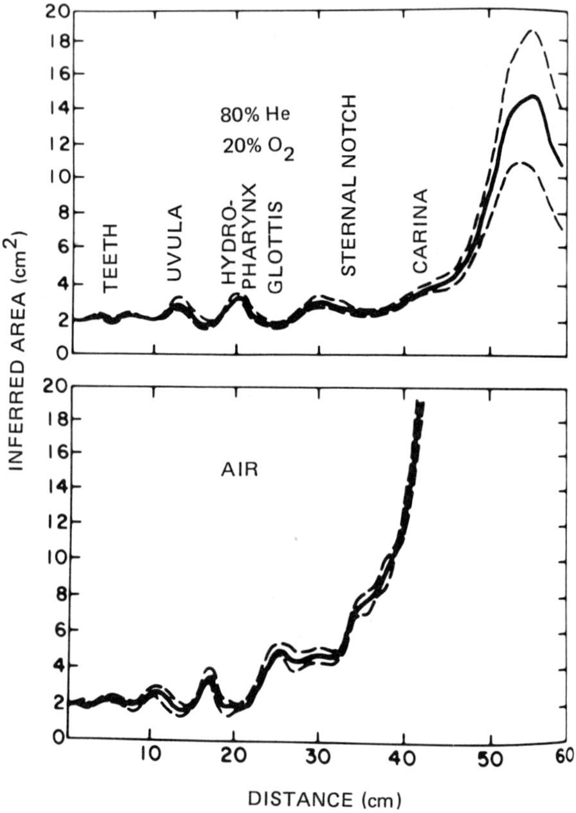

Figure 2 Airway summed cross-section (mean ± SD) inferred by acoustic reflectance. Features of the area inference have been identified with anatomical landmarks by using radiographs. (From Fredberg et al., 1980. Reprinted with the permission of the American Physiological Society.)

oropharynx, to the glottic constriction lying within the larynx. In gas mixing studies with human subjects, it has become accepted practice to use a nose clip to eliminate nasal flow and a mouthpiece which provides access to the lungs while simultaneously standardizing the position of the lips, the teeth, and to some extent, the cheeks. Under these conditions, nasal structures proximal to the oropharynx are bypassed so that the glottis is the primary flow constriction (Fig. 2), causing acceleration of respired air and generation of local turbulence in the upper airways.

The glottis is a triangular aperture whose area changes considerably during the respiratory cycle. Beginning late in expiration, the glottic aperture continually widens, reaching a maximum cross section at midinspiration; and during the last 25% of the inspiration phase, the glottis progressively narrows, reaching a minimum value at midexpiration. The amplitude of this oscillation in glottic cross section is inversely related to breathing frequency, the ratio of maximum (inspiration) to minimum (expiration) areas being reported as 1.32 (England et al., 1982) or 1.80 (Brancatisano et al., 1983) during quiet respiration and close to 1 during panting. On the other hand, the time-averaged glottic area is directly related to breathing frequency, having representative values of 0.66 cm^2 during quiet breathing, 0.75 cm^2 at an elevated frequency of about 100 breaths per minute, and 0.82 cm^2 during panting (Baier et al., 1977). Relative to the 2.5-cm^2 area of the adjacent trachea, this means that the glottis normally creates a 70% reduction in the cross section available for inspiratory flow and an 80% reduction during expiration.

The total volume of the upper airways depends on the type of air access. For mouth breathing in adult humans, volume estimates of the upper airways plus trachea range from 50 to 100 ml, with a suggested mean value of 80 ml (Horsfield and Cumming, 1968a), and the path length from lips to glottis is approximately 17 cm (Olson et al., 1973). Assuming a tracheal volume of 30 ml, it is reasonable to model the upper airways as a cylinder with a 2.9-cm^2 cross section and 17-cm length (Table 1, generation 000). Such a representation is also consistent with acoustic reflectance measurements (Fig. 2).

Once inspired air passes through the larynx, it reaches the trachea and then the bronchial tree. Weibel's model A (Weibel, 1963), a widely used geometric idealization of the tracheobronchial tree, consists of 23 generations of dichotomous branching originating at the trachea, but only the first 16 generations are conducting airways. Since the cylindrical branch segments of each generation are identical, all 2^{16} possible gas transport paths from the carina to the terminal bronchioles are geometrically equivalent. It follows that if airflow is uniformly distributed among the terminal bronchioles, gas velocities and species fractions will be unique functions of the generation number, or equivalently, the longitudinal distance measured from the carina.

Weibel's original model is based on a cadaveric lung hyperinflated to three-fourths of its total capacity of 4.8 liters; thus the branch dimensions are larger than expected for quiet breathing. Normally, the trachea and major bronchi are supported by inelastic cartilage rings which minimize radial distension, and although some lengthening of these airways occurs with lung inflation (Macklin, 1925), the relative volume increase of the smaller unsupported airways is far greater. Expansion of the unsupported airways is isotropic in that changes in their branch lengths and diameters are proportional to the cube root of changes in the total lung volume (Hughes et al., 1972).

Table 1 Flow Characteristics (υ = 0.167 cm^2/sec) in the Conducting Airway Branches

Symmetric conducting airway model					Quiet breathing ($\dot{V}$ = 0.4 liter/sec)		Moderate exercise ($\dot{V}$ = 1.6 liters/sec)	
Generation	Branch diameter, d (mm)	Branch length, ℓ (mm)	Summed cross-section, A (cm^2)	Cumulative volume, $\bar{V}$ (cm^3)	Reynolds number, Re	Entrance length fraction, ℓ/ℓ_e	Reynolds number, Re	Entrance length fraction, ℓ/ℓ_e
000 (mouth/pharynx)	19.0	170	2.8	48.0	1602	0.19	6409	0.05
00 (glottis)	9.0	—	0.7	—	3080	—	12320	—
0 (trachea)	18.0	120	2.5	78.5	1697	0.14	6789	0.03
1 (primary bronchi)	12.2	47.6	2.3	89.8	1254	0.11	5016	0.03
2 (secondary bronchi)	8.3	19.0	2.1	93.7	933	0.08	3733	0.02
3 (bronchioles)	4.8	6.5	1.5	94.7	786	0.06	3143	0.02
4	3.9	10.9	1.8	96.8	509	0.21	2038	0.05
5	3.0	9.2	2.3	98.9	316	0.34	1262	0.08
6	2.4	7.7	2.9	101	197	0.56	790	0.14

7	↓	2.0	6.5	3.7	104	127	0.90	506	0.23
8		1.6	5.5	5.1	106	75.0	1.6	300	0.40
9		1.3	4.6	7.0	110	45.3	2.7	181	0.67
10		1.1	3.9	9.8	113	27.1	4.6	109	1.14
11		0.93	3.3	14.3	118	15.6	7.9	62.4	1.98
12		0.81	2.8	21.1	124	9.2	13.5	36.9	3.38
13		0.70	2.3	32.5	132	5.2	23.0	20.7	5.75
14		0.63	2.0	50.7	142	3.0	37.2	12.0	9.29
15		0.56	1.7	82.6	156	1.6	62.0	6.5	15.5
16	↓	0.51	1.4	132	174	0.9	103	3.7	25.6
17 (respiratory bronchiole)		0.46	1.2	219	201	0.5	178	2.0	44.5

Thus, in order to scale down Weibel's model to a 3.0-liter lung, corresponding to normal midinspiratory conditions, the linear dimensions of all airway branches distal to the second generation should be reduced by a factor of 14%. In the resulting model (Table 1), individual branch diameters decrease with increasing generation number, but the corresponding values of the summed branch cross section increase (except over the first four generations, where the cross section decreases somewhat). This progressive and dramatic expansion of summed cross section, which is also apparent in acoustic reflectance measurements (Fig. 2), leads to a parallel decrease in longitudinal gas velocity from a value of 158 cm/sec in the trachea during a quiet respiratory flow of 0.4 liter/sec to a value of 3 cm/sec in the terminal bronchioles. Within the respiratory zone distal to the conducting airways, Weibel's model also predicts a continually increasing summed cross section. However, the more recent work of Hansen and Ampaya (1975) indicated that the cross section eventually tapers off due to the nonuniform termination of respiratory ducts.

It is important to recognize that the bronchial tree is actually an asymmetric structure and, as a result, the sequence of branch lengths and branch diameters is different among alternative transport paths. Horsfield and Cumming (1968a) reported that there are between 8 and 25 branchings from the carina to the respiratory lobules which they pruned off their lung cast. Since each lobule contained an additional three generations of conducting bronchioles (Horsfield et al., 1971), there were, on the average, 18 generations of conducting airways compared to Weibel's 16 generations. The corresponding path lengths measured by Horsfield and Cumming ranged from 7 to 23 cm with a mean value of 14 cm, similar to the 13-cm path length of the symmetric model. Because of this variation in path length and the concomitant variation in volume among the alternative transport paths, there results a finite distribution of gas transit times from the mouth to the terminal bronchioles, even when the flow is uniformly distributed among the terminal bronchioles (Fig. 3). The presence of this residence time distribution constitutes a form of longitudinal mixing induced solely by geometric asymmetries. Although Horsfield and Cumming's data were derived from a cadaveric lung inflated to a total volume 200 ml larger than that used by Weibel, the asymmetric model had a 106-ml volume from carina to terminal bronchioles, compared to the 144-ml volume of corresponding airways in the symmetric model.

The nature of gas transport in the tracheobronchial tree bears a subtle but important relationship to the detailed geometry of the individual branch points. Three geometric features that were noted by Horsfield et al. (1971) are: branches are not straight but instead tend to curve outward from the bifurcation point of their origin; daughter branches are separated from one another by a sharp dividing surface which projects upstream from the bifur-

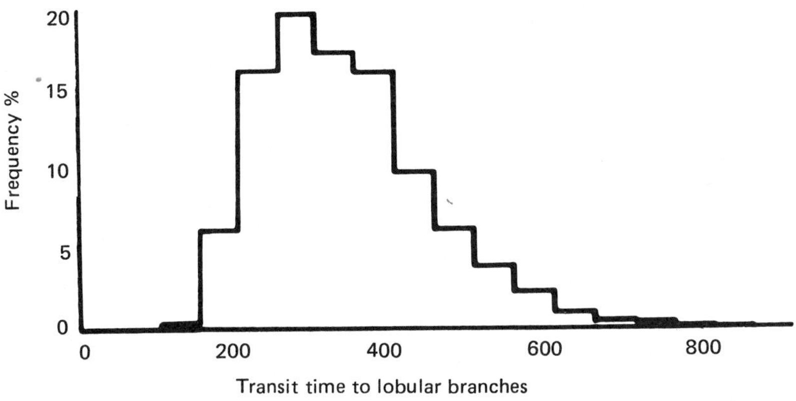

Figure 3 Frequency distribution of transit times to the respiratory lobule of an asymmetric lung. (From Horsfield and Cumming, 1968a. Reprinted with the permission of the American Physiological Society.)

cation of the airway walls; and beginning at midposition in a mother branch, there is a gradual transition in cross section which is accommodated by a continual change of shape until the bifurcation point is passed (Fig. 4). These investigators also found that the branching angle between the axis of a mother and its daughter branch ranged from 8 to 73° with an average value of 38°, and the radius of curvature of a branch relative to its diameter (R/d) ranged from 0.5 to 15 with an average value of 6.8. As will be discussed more fully in the next section, the existence of branch curvature creates centrifugal forces, resulting in radial circulation of the airflow, and the sharpness of the dividing surface causes a marked skewing of the peak gas velocity toward the inner wall of a daughter branch. The gradual transition of cross-sectional area probably serves to minimize the boundary layer separation characteristic of such abruptly diverging flows.

What has been described thus far is the anatomy of the human airways, but some of the most elucidating gas mixing experiments require a degree of invasion that is possible only by using animal models. The dog is by far the most popular animal used for this purpose, yet its airways are considerably less symmetric than those of humans (Ross, 1957). Moreover, when using open-chested procedures or excised lungs, the pleural pressure gradient is changed in such a way that the normal distribution of respired flow may be altered (Glaister et al., 1973). Therefore, caution must be used when comparing data from animal or cadaveric preparations to those obtained on intact humans.

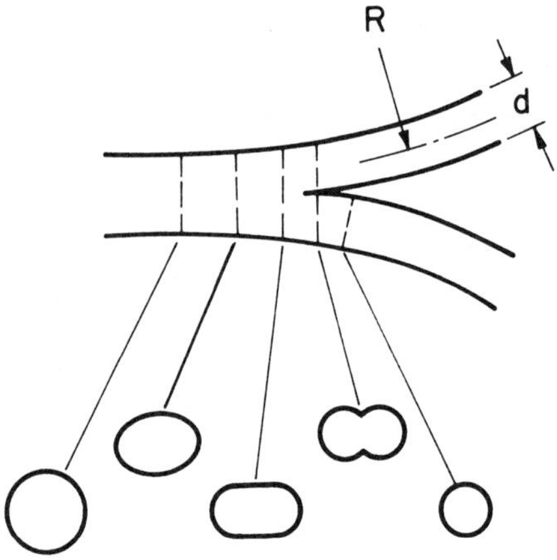

Figure 4 Typical geometry at a branch point. The transition in cross section from the mother to daughter branches is illustrated, and the daughter branch diameter d and radius of curvature R are labeled. (From Horsfield et al., 1971. Adapted with the permission of the American Physiological Society.)

B. Aerodynamics

Longitudinal mixing is the process by which one gas species is transported in the direction of flow relative to another gas species. Although mixing by molecular diffusion is present throughout the pulmonary airways, the magnitude of this process is comparatively small, except in the more distal airways, where the summed cross section is very large (Gomez, 1965). Through most of the conducting airways it is the radial distribution of axial velocity, or what is commonly called the *axial velocity profile,* that has the principal influence on mixing. That is, if the axial velocity profile were uniform, all molecules would be translated at the same speed and there would be no possibility for fresh inspired air to mix with residual air. What actually occurs, however, is that friction retards the translation of molecules near the airway walls so that the centrally located fresh air molecules move at greater than average speed and can thereby penetrate into the residual air. Understanding this type of mixing, called *longitudinal dispersion,* requires a comprehension of the aerodynamics within conducting airways.

Laminar and Turbulent Flow Regimes

A primary consideration in analyzing longitudinal dispersion is whether the flow is laminar (i.e., streamlined) or turbulent (i.e., possessing random velocity fluctuations). Flow will be turbulent when the inertial force, which is the source of turbulent energy, overcomes the viscous friction force, which acts to dissipate the turbulent eddies. The Reynolds number,

$$\mathrm{Re} = \frac{ud}{\upsilon} \tag{1}$$

expresses the ratio of the inertial to the viscous force. In a cylindrical airway, the flow will be laminar when Re is less than 2100, and turbulence will be generated when Re is greater than 4000. At values of Re intermediate between 2100 and 4000, the flow is in transition between laminar and turbulent regimes. In the tracheobronchial tree, both longitudinal velocity u and branch diameter d decrease toward the higher-order generations so that the maximum value of Re occurs in the trachea. During quiet respiration, Re is below 2100 in all generations (Table 1) and turbulence cannot be generated within the airway branches themselves. With moderate exercise, however, the respiratory flow is larger and turbulence does occur within the trachea and major bronchi.

In regions of the upper airways where the airstream is accelerated by a drastic change in the geometry, local turbulence can be generated even when the Reynolds numbers in the adjacent branches are below 2100. For example, Swift and Proctor (1977) reported that during a quiet inspiration of 0.42 liter/sec through a nasal airway cast, the narrowing of the ostium internum caused a jetting of fluid with accompanying turbulence that was propagated throughout the nasal turbinates to the oropharynx. Under these conditions, the tracheal Reynolds number was approximately 1800, while through the ostium internum Re was 2500. In an airway cast extending from the epiglottis to the primary bronchi, Dekker (1961) observed turbulence downstream of the laryngeal constriction for all inspiratory flows greater than a critical value of 0.1 liter/sec, which corresponds to a tracheal Reynolds number of roughly 430 and a glottic Re of 750. This is consistent with the observations of Weaver and Ultman (1980) that the onset of turbulent mixing in a constricted tube occurred at orifice Reynolds numbers in the range 500-1000. Even in tracheobronchial casts where the upper airways were absent, both Dekker (1961) and West and Hugh-Jones (1959) observed tracheal turbulence during inspiratory airflow at subcritical Reynolds numbers of 1800 and 800, respectively. It is conceivable that this was due to a destabilization of laminar flow by protrusion of the cartilage rings.

Once generated in the upper airways, local turbulence is transported downstream and continually decays by the dissipative action of viscous forces. Simone and Ultman (1982a,b) studied turbulence propagation downstream of a larynx cast mounted in a 1.6-cm-diameter straight tube. At a tube Reynolds number of 1100, laryngeal turbulence required 110 cm of downstream tubing for complete decay. Although this distance is eight times the total path length of the conducting airways, the rate of turbulence decay is proportional to tube diameter and to Reynolds number, so that within the tracheobronchial tree, where both variables decrease with increasing distal penetration, the decay length should be less. Owen (1969) has derived a specific formula to predict turbulence decay, but the simpler entrance length equation (Olson et al., 1970) serves as an adequate approximation:

$$\frac{\ell}{\ell_e} = \frac{34.8\,\ell}{d\ \mathrm{Re}} \tag{2}$$

When the length ℓ of an individual tube exceeds the entrance length ℓ_e, it is safe to assume that local turbulence will be dissipated, whereas an entrance length fraction ℓ/ℓ_e less than 1 implies that some turbulence will persist. Entrance length fractions can be computed with Eq. (2) for each airway branch (Table 1), and at that position in the bronchial tree where the cumulative value of ℓ/ℓ_e reaches unity it is probable that laryngeal turbulence has been dissipated. It appears that upper airway turbulence would be eliminated by the sixth generation during quiet inspiration, while the elevated airflow occurring with moderate exercise could carry turbulence as far as the eighth generation. In a conducting airway cast spanning the mouth to the fourth generation, Olson et al. (1972) did detect turbulence throughout the model at all inspiratory flows where the tracheal Reynolds numbers was above 300.

Although studied less extensively, it is clear that turbulence can exist in the trachea and the major bronchi during expiration. In a single-generation lung cast, Dekker (1961) observed the onset of tracheal turbulence at a critical flow of 0.122 liter/sec, corresponding to a tracheal Reynolds number of about 1000. Using a three-generation tracheobronchial cast, West and Hugh-Jones (1959) reported a critical airflow which was about six times larger than Dekker's value. Apparently, differences in the development of the flow from the most distal airway to the trachea have an important influence on turbulence generation.

Velocity Patterns

Given a sufficiently low flow rate or long entrance length of straight tube, the velocity profile is independent of axial position and is considered to be fully developed. Under laminar flow conditions, the fully developed velocity profile would have a parabolic shape with a peak (centerline) velocity u_p twice as large as the cross-sectional mean velocity u. For fully developed turbulent conditions, the velocity profile is considerably blunter, the ratio u_p/u having a value of roughly 1.25. Since longitudinal dispersion depends on the difference in speed between gas molecules at different radial positions, laminar dispersion is generally more extensive than is turbulent dispersion.

The state of development of a laminar velocity profile within a conducting airway branch can be judged from its entrance length fraction in Table 1. Where the entrance length fraction is greater than 1, in the distal airways, there is sufficient opportunity for the velocity profile to become fully developed. In the proximal airways, however, velocity disturbances caused by geometric transitions tend to persist, and as a result, velocity profiles are not necessarily parabolic. As an example of such a disturbance, consider flow through the larynx. When streamlines of air converge in order to negotiate the glottal constriction, the axial velocity is so greatly accelerated that a jet of gas, detached from the surrounding airway walls, is formed immediately downstream of the constriction. The space between the jet and the airway wall is filled with gas which continually circulates in the axial direction. Olson et al. (1973), employing inspiratory airflows of 600 ml/sec in upper airway casts designed to simulate mouth breathing, found that the peak velocity u_p at the center of the laryngeal jet reached four times the mean value u, and within the surrounding circulation region the reversed velocity was comparable in magnitude to u.

It is at the boundary between the laryngeal jet and the circulation region that shear rate (i.e., the slope of the velocity profile) is so large that turbulent velocity fluctuations are generated. Simone and Ultman (1982b) demonstrated that because of this turbulence, the pointed velocity profile ($u_p/u = 3.5$) associated with the jet of a larynx cast underwent a rapid transition to a blunter profile ($u_p/u = 1.4$) within 10 cm downstream of the glottis (Fig. 5). Further downstream, u_p/u gradually increased toward a fully developed laminar value of 2.0 as the turbulence was observed to decay.

Measurements of laminar flow through single-bifurcation models also reveal that velocity profiles are not parabolic. In fact, velocity profiles during inspiration and expiration are quite different (Schroter and Sudlow, 1969). During inspiration, the centerline velocity of the parent branch encounters a "no slip" (i.e., zero velocity) condition at the flow divider, and this creates a distinct velocity peak near the inner wall of the daughter branches in the plane of the bifurcation (Fig. 6). Perpendicular to the plane of the bifurcation, the velocity profile is blunter and quite symmetric, with some peaking of velocity near anterior as well as posterior tube walls. During expiration, velocity profiles are symmetric in both planes and are considerably blunter than during inspiration. For multiple airway branchings, velocity profiles are more complicated since the exiting profile from a daughter branch becomes the entering profile to its progeny. Then, in addition to the geometric details of a given branch, the relative orientation of branches (i.e., coplanar or rotated) becomes an important factor.

Chang and El Masry (1982) made extensive measurements of axial velocity in a three-generation planar model patterned after the asymmetric airway system of Horsfield et al. (1971). Inspiratory as well as expiratory

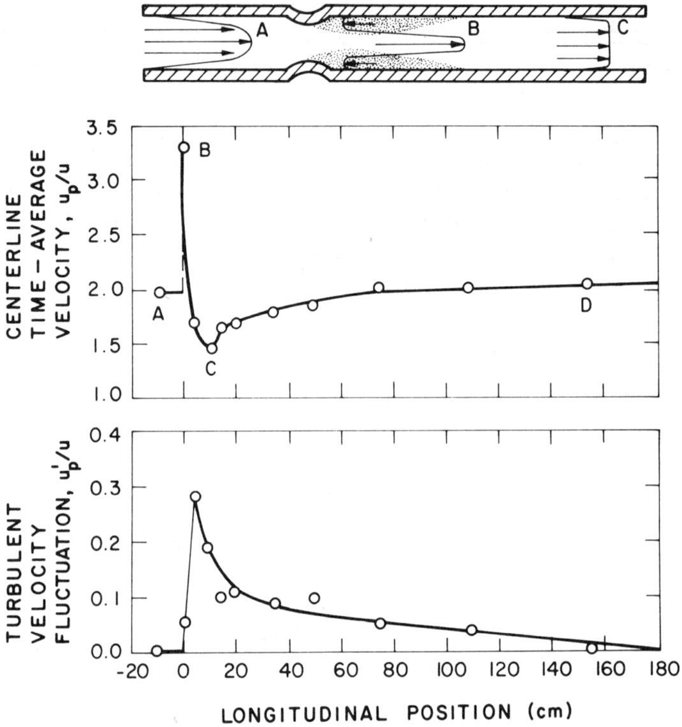

Figure 5 Aerodynamics of inspiratory airflow through a larynx cast at a subcritical tube Reynolds number of 1110. The uppermost panel is a sketch of the velocity profiles associated with a glottal jet which is surrounded by a longitudinally circulating separation (stippled) region. In the two lower panels, the centerline time-averaged velocity, u_p, and root-mean-square turbulent fluctuations, u_p', of these velocity profiles are shown. Note that a longitudinal position of zero corresponds to the point of maximum constriction, and both u_p and u_p' are normalized by the time-averaged cross-sectional velocity, u. As air approaches the glottis in fully developed laminar flow (A), the normalized centerline velocity is 2, and there are no velocity fluctuations. Both the turbulent fluctuations and centerline velocity increase markedly as air is accelerated within the glottal jet (B). Downstream of the jet, the centerline velocity falls below 2 because of turbulent flattening of the velocity profile (C), and then recovers to a value of 2 (D) as the turbulent fluctuations decay to zero and fully developed flow is reestablished. (Adapted from Simone and Ultman, 1982a.)

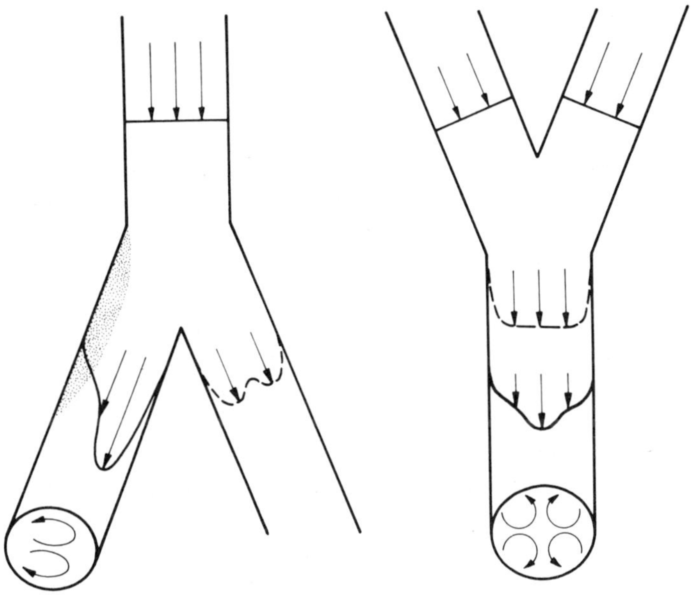

Figure 6 Flow downstream of a single bifurcation with a flat entrance profile at a parent tube Reynolds number of 700. Velocity profiles are shown in the plane of the bifurcation (solid line) and perpendicular to it (dashed line). A longitudinally circulating separation (stippled) region and radial circulation pattern are also shown. (Adapted from Schroter and Sudlow, 1969.)

flows were employed at tracheal Reynolds numbers characteristic of quiet breathing, $Re_t = 2100$, and moderate exercise, $Re_t = 8000$. At both airflows, tracheal velocity profiles were flat during inspiration, with u_p/u having a value of about 1.1, and this is suggestive of turbulent flow conditions. Tracheal velocity profiles were somewhat more pointed during expiration than during inspiration. Velocity profiles in the primary and secondary bronchi resembled those previously observed for single bifurcations, with the higher Reynolds number velocity profiles generally being smoother than those observed at the lower airflow. In select experiments, the trachea was preceded by a narrow constriction simulating the effect of the larynx. Although the constriction had no obvious influence on velocity profiles in the bronchi, the tracheal value of u_p/u during inspiration was 60% larger than that measured in the open-ended trachea. This was undoubtedly caused by jetting of air through the constricted tracheal inlet.

In addition to characterizing axial velocity profiles, it is important to consider the gas circulation patterns that result from additional radial and circumferential velocity components. Circulating flows in the longitudinal direction can act as "dead zones" in which a gas species is temporarily trapped, thereby adding to the nonuniformity of axial transport rates and enhancing dispersion. Within the upper airways, the large-scale standing eddies that have been observed in the nasal passages and oropharynx (Proetz, 1951) are examples of longitudinal circulation. In the trachea, the gas that surrounds the laryngeal jet constitutes a longitudinal circulation region whose role in enhancing dispersion has been established (Weaver and Ultman, 1980). Also, when air flowing through a bronchial bifurcation possesses too much linear momentum to negotiate the sudden bend at the outer wall, a separated flow region similar in nature to the laryngeal gas circulation region can be formed (Fig. 6).

Circulation patterns may also occur in a lateral or radial plane. Such secondary flows tend to limit longitudinal dispersion because they continually interchange gas molecules at different radial positions, thereby diminishing the effect of the axial velocity profile. It is well known that when fluid flows through a curved tube, the presence of centrifugal force generates a matched pair of secondary flow circulations. Indeed, Schroter and Sudlow (1969) observed such paired circulations during inspiratory flow in single-bifurcation models (Fig. 6). During expiration, the circulation pairs of the two daughter branches combined at the bifurcation point to form a quadruple vortex pattern. Schroter and Sudlow characterized the strength of these circulations at parent tube Reynolds numbers of 290 and 700 by indicating that secondary flows caused air molecules to complete at least one helical cycle within three diameters of downstream travel. In a multiple-branched model, Isabey and Chang (1982) concluded that secondary flow effects were diminished because of branch interactions. At a tracheal Reynolds number of 1000, they found that three branch diameters were not sufficient for an air molecule to complete one helical cycle in any airway. Moreover, in the major bronchi, secondary flow velocities were only 10 or 20% of the mean axial velocity, and there was a tendency of secondary flows to become even smaller toward the higher-order generations.

A discussion of velocity patterns in the conducting airways would not be complete without reference to the subtle but possibly important effect of cardiac pulsations. Although the exact nature of their origin is not understood, small oscillations of respiratory flow occurring at the same frequency as the heartbeat are routinely observed. Employing a specially designed bronchoscopic flowmeter, West and Hugh-Jones (1961) were able to estimate the value of such cardiogenic flows within lobar and sublobar bronchi. Although not detected in all 60 patients they examined, cardiogenic flow amplitude were generally found to be from 0.5 to 1.5 liters/min relative to a typical peak lobar flow of 5.0 liters/min. This corresponded to volumetric displacements of 1-5 ml, with the larger values occurring in the left lung. These investigators had the impression that cardiogenic pulsations forced gas out of some lung lobes and into others, and they concluded that direct displacement of the lungs by volume variations of the heart is responsible for the measured flow oscillations.

C. Mixing Mechanisms

The total rate of longitudinal transport of a gas species results from the movement of gas by bulk flow and by mixing. This can be expressed mathematically by a one-dimensional form of Fick's law which has been averaged over the flow cross section:

$$\dot{V}_T = F\dot{V} - A(\kappa + D)\frac{\partial F}{\partial x} \tag{3}$$

$$\text{Total transport} = \text{bulk transport} + \text{longitudinal mixing}$$

where F is the cross-sectionally averaged species fraction and x is distance measured in the flow direction. Bulk transport is simply the translation of gas molecules at the mean flow velocity. Thus its magnitude is proportional to the volumetric flow $\dot{V}$, but independent of the nature of the gas species. For gases to mix, a gradient or difference in species gas fraction must exist in the flow direction. Longitudinal mixing is proportional to the magnitude of this gradient, $\partial F/\partial x$, and to the sum of the diffusion coefficient D and the longitudinal dispersion or mixing coefficient κ.

Since diffusion results from the random thermal agitation of gas molecules, D is inversely related to the molecular weights of the interdiffusing species. For example, at body temperature and pressure (BTP) conditions the diffusivity of helium (MW = 4) in pure nitrogen (MW = 28) is 0.729 cm^2/sec while the diffusivity of sulfur hexafluoride (MW = 146) in nitrogen is only 0.103 cm^2/sec (Worth et al., 1978). Thus it is possible to infer the importance of diffusion by experimentation with inert gases of different molecular weights. Strictly speaking, Eq. (3) only applies to binary gas mixtures and one must exercise care in designing multicomponent gas transport experiments. Since the natural respired species (N_2, O_2, CO_2, H_2O) have similar molecular weights, they can be treated collectively as one pure species, and the diffusion of a single foreign gas of a markedly different molecular weight can usually be characterized by an effective binary coefficient (Worth and Piiper, 1978). However, if two foreign gases are introduced simultane-

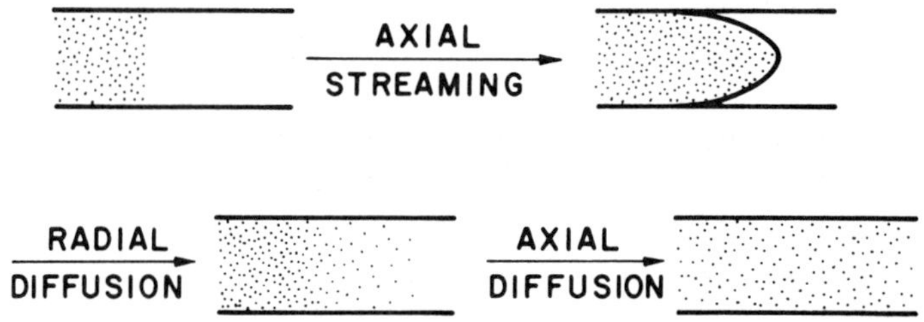

Figure 7 Development of dispersion in laminar flow through a tube. An initially planar front is first distorted by the velocity profile, resulting in axial streaming. This generates radial gas fraction differences leading to radial diffusion. Axial diffusion, which always occurs in parallel with this dispersion process, causes a continuous blurring of the front. (Adapted from Wilson and Lin, 1970.)

ously, there can be ternary as well as binary molecular interactions, and this might invalidate the use of Fick's law (e.g., Chang et al., 1975).

As explained in the preceding section, longitudinal dispersion is a mixing process that relies on nonuniformities in the axial velocity profile to propel gas molecules that are near to the tube centerline ahead of those near the tube wall. Suppose, for example, that a planar dividing front separates pure oxygen on the upstream side of the front from pure nitrogen on the downstream side (Fig. 7). To eliminate the effect of bulk flow, imagine that you are moving with the dividing front at the mean gas velocity. In that case, the front will become distorted such that oxygen near the centerline of the tube will move downstream of you, while near the tube wall oxygen appears to move upstream. In terms of the cross-sectionally averaged oxygen fraction, this implies that the initial discontinuity represented by the planar front is transformed by the velocity profile into a finite longitudinal distribution of oxygen. To complete the description of longitudinal dispersion, it is necessary to recognize that the distortion of the dividing front leads to radial differences in the species fraction, and these differences act as a driving force for radial transport. Radial transport, which can occur by molecular diffusion, turbulent eddy diffusion, or by the action of secondary flow circulation, interchanges molecules on slow streamlines with those on fast streamlines. In effect, this limits the extent to which dispersion can occur.

The design of experiments to elucidate the nature and importance of dispersion requires that the dispersion coefficient be known as a function of relevant geometric and gas transport parameters. In this respect, the most comprehensive theory is available for dispersion in a tube. By dimensional analysis it can be shown that the dispersion coefficient of a gas flowing at a velocity u through a straight tube of diameter d and length ℓ has the general form

$$\frac{\kappa}{D} = f(Re, Sc, \frac{\ell}{d}) \tag{4}$$

The variable f denotes a functional dependence on the geometric aspect ratio ℓ/d, the Reynolds number, and the Schmidt number,

$$Sc \equiv \frac{\upsilon}{D} \tag{5}$$

which is the ratio of the kinematic gas viscosity υ to the diffusivity. In a fully developed laminar flow, the shape of the velocity profile does not depend on υ, so that Re and Sc must appear as the Péclet number product. That is,

$$\frac{\kappa}{D} = f_d(Pe, \frac{\ell}{d}) \tag{6}$$

where the Péclet number,

$$Pe \equiv ReSc = \frac{ud}{D} \tag{7}$$

represents the ratio of the axial velocity to the characteristic radial diffusion velocity (D/d).

Gill and Sankarasubramanian (1970) formulated a general expression for the function f_d. Their result can be described in terms of the dimensionless product Pe(d/ℓ), representing the ratio of radial diffusion time (d^2/D) to mean transit time of inert gas in the tube (ℓ/u). Under those conditions where

$$Pe\left(\frac{d}{\ell}\right) > 200 \tag{8}$$

the inert gas passes through the tube in such a short time that radial diffusion does not have an opportunity to occur. Dispersion then occurs by a mechanism called *axial streaming,* in which gas particles are confined to fixed streamlines and an initially planar dividing front is progressively distorted by the action of the velocity profile. The resulting axial streaming coefficient,

$$\frac{\kappa}{D} = k_{as} Pe\left(\frac{\ell}{d}\right) \tag{9}$$

increases linearly with axial velocity and tube length. At smaller values of the Pe(d/ℓ) product, radial diffusion becomes important and κ increases less dramatically with tube length until, in the limit that

$$\mathrm{Pe}\left(\frac{\mathrm{d}}{\ell}\right) < 10 \tag{10}$$

a constant and maximum value of the dispersion coefficient is reached:

$$\frac{\kappa}{\mathrm{D}} = \mathrm{k_{td}Pe^2} \tag{11}$$

This asymptotic limit, known as Taylor dispersion (Taylor, 1953), corresponds to a situation where the evolution of radial gas fraction gradients by axial streaming is in balance with their relaxation by radial diffusion. For a parabolic velocity profile, k_{as} and k_{td} have values of 0.167 and 1/192, respectively. For velocity profiles having a more pointed shape, the values are larger, while for blunter profiles, the values are smaller (Subramanian and Gill, 1976).

It is useful as a first approximation to apply these formulas to the cylindrical branches of the symmetric airway model given in Table 1. According to calculations using the laminar classification criteria given by Eqs. (8) and (10), dispersion should occur by axial streaming from the lips to the third generation during quiet breathing and to the fifth generation during moderate exercise; Taylor dispersion should occur distal to the eighth generation during quiet breathing and distal to the eleventh generation during exercise; and in the intermediate generations, dispersion is in transition between these two mechanisms (Table 2). Corresponding values of the κ/D ratio computed from Eqs. (9) and (11) are very large in the proximal airways, but distal to the tenth generation during quiet breathing and the thirteenth generation during exercise, κ/D falls below unity. This indicates that axial molecular diffusion dominates over dispersion in the smallest airways. Wilson and Lin (1970) developed a similar classification of mixing mechanisms but did not compute values for the dispersion coefficient.

The dispersion coefficient values in Table 2 should be regarded as crude estimates since airway velocity profiles are not fully developed as was assumed in choosing values for the axial streaming, k_{as}, and Taylor dispersion, k_{td}, constants. Moreover, because it occurs in the absence of diffusion, axial streaming is a process that is reversible with respect to changes in flow direction. In the most extreme case, when flow is reversed in a long straight tube, the velocity profile will retain its shape but point in the opposite direction, so that no net axial streaming would occur over a complete cycle of oscillation; in the pulmonary airways, the axial streaming induced by the

Table 2 Longitudinal Mixing Characteristics of Natural Respired Gases (D = 0.25 cm^2/sec) During Steady Fully Developed Flow

Generation	Quiet breathing					Moderate exercise				
	Laminar classification, Pe(d/ℓ)		Laminar coefficient, κ/D		Turbulent coefficient, κ/D	Laminar classification, Pe(d/ℓ)		Laminar coefficient, κ/D		Turbulent coefficient, κ/D
000	120	Axial streaming	1610		392	481	Axial streaming	6435		1365
00	—		—		—	—		—		—
0	170		1262		413	680		5046		1438
1	212		538		315	847		2153		1095
2	278		242		241	1111		972		839
3	386		119		207	1546		475		719
4	110	Transition	—		140	439		588		487
5	69		—		91	278		434		316
6	41		—			165	Transition	—		207
7	26		—			103		—		139
8	15		—			58		—		87
9	8.6	Taylor dispersion	4.77			35		—		
10	5.1		1.71			20		—		
11	2.9		0.57	Diffusion		12		—		
12	1.7		0.20			6.9	Taylor dispersion	3.16		
13	1.0		0.06			4.0		0.99		
14	0.6		0.02			2.5		0.33	Diffusion	
15	0.4		0.006			1.5		0.10		
16	0.2		0.002			0.9		0.03		
17	0.1		0.001			0.5		0.01		

pointed velocity profiles during inspiration is only partially reversed by the flattened profiles during expiration, and thus some net axial streaming occurs (Haselton and Scherer, 1980). Since Eq. (9) applies to dispersion in a steady flow and does not provide at all for flow reversal effects, the tabulated axial streaming coefficients probably represent an upper bound of those values averaged over a complete respiratory cycle.

The occurrence of secondary flows can reduce Taylor dispersion coefficient values below those predicted in Table 2. To demonstrate this, consider the similarity of the secondary flows in curved tubes to those occurring downstream of an airway bifurcation during inspiratory flow. Nunge et al. (1972) formulated the Taylor dispersion coefficient for fully developed flow in a curved tube in which the relative curvature is large. The simplified form of the dispersion coefficient for intermediate values of Reynolds numbers is appropriate for present purposes.

$$\frac{\kappa}{D} = \frac{Pe^2}{192} - [3.06Sc^2 - 0.048]\left[\frac{10^{-9}Re^6 Sc^2 d^2}{R^2}\right] \tag{12}$$

The first term on the right-hand side of Eq. (12) is the Taylor dispersion coefficient for a straight tube and the group of bracketed terms comprises a secondary flow correction which decreases the value of κ/D as Reynolds number increases. Using a typical respiratory gas Schmidt number of 0.7 and a relative curvature of 6.8, mixing coefficients have been recomputed in those generations where Taylor dispersion is presumed to dominate. The resulting values of κ/D are from 1 to 30% less than the straight-tube values listed in Table 2, the biggest reductions occurring in the largest airways, wherein the Reynolds number is the largest.

The presence of turbulence also has the tendency to reduce dispersion since the improved radial transport of momentum causes a blunting of the velocity profile as well as increased radial mass transport. Taylor (1954) formulated the fully developed turbulent dispersion coefficient in terms of a friction factor which has here been replaced by a conventional engineering correlation (Bennet and Myers, 1974), so that

$$\frac{\kappa}{D} = 0.766Pe^{0.9}Sc^{0.1} \tag{13}$$

Employing this equation, κ/D has been computed in those airways where turbulence is suspected to occur (Table 2). Notice that the turbulent dispersion and unidirectional axial streaming coefficients depend on Péclet number in a similar manner and have similar values distal to the primary bronchi. From the lips to the carina, however, axial streaming is predicted to be much larger. Using a more comprehensive velocity profile than Taylor, Flint and

Eisenklam (1970) computed κ over a wide range of Reynolds numbers, including the turbulent transition region. In their graphs, κ/D is roughly proportional to Pe^{-1} at Re between 2000 and 6000 while the $Pe^{0.9}$ dependence in Eq. (13) is closely followed for Re greater than 6000.

One of the least understood factors that contributes to airway mixing is the inhomogeneity in both branch geometry and tissue mechanics, which imposes a nonuniform distribution of transit times along alternative transport paths. Based on their asymmetric airway model, Horsfield and Cumming (1968a,b) inferred the transit-time distribution (Fig. 3) and indicated how it could affect the outcome of a single-breath washout test. Yu (1975), on the other hand, used a more general statistical theory to formulate the dispersion coefficient for a dichotomously branching network in which the branch lengths of each generation were randomly distributed with a coefficient of variation ϵ^2.

$$\frac{\kappa}{D} = \frac{1}{2}\epsilon^2 \mathrm{Pe}\left(\frac{\ell}{d}\right) \tag{14}$$

Based on Weibel's data, Yu suggested using a value of 0.422 for ϵ^2. In that case, Eq. (14) predicts values which are virtually identical to those of the unidirectional axial streaming equation (9).

As outlined above, there is such a wide variety of mechanisms by which longitudinal mixing can occur that an unambiguous interpretation of gas mixing experiments is difficult to achieve. As a guide in designing such experiments, Ultman and Thomas (1979) noted that Eqs. (9), (11), (13), and (14) suggest that the dispersion coefficient can often be expressed in a "power law" form:

$$\kappa = \alpha[D]^m[\dot{V}]^{n+1} \tag{15}$$

where α is a function of geometric parameters, while m and n are constant exponents corresponding to a particular mixing mechanism (Table 3). By

Table 3 Longitudinal Mixing Parameters

Mechanisms	α	m	n
Axial molecular diffusion	1.0	1	-1
Unidirection axial streaming	$0.167\ell/A$	0	0
Laminar Taylor dispersion	$d^2/192A^2$	-1	1
Turbulent Taylor dispersion	$0.766\upsilon^{0.1}(d/A)^{0.9}$	0	-0.1
Mixing by asymmetry	$0.211\ell/A$	0	0

performing experiments in which molecular diffusion constant D and/or respiratory flow $\dot{V}$ are changed, the values of the exponents can be determined, and in so doing the mixing mechanism can be identified. This approach is not without ambiguity, however. For example, the (m,n) pairs for axial streaming and mixing by asymmetry are equal.

III. Theoretical Basis of Mixing Experiments

A. Residence Time Distribution

Mixing in the conducting airways can alternatively be deduced by direct or indirect measurements. With indirect methods, a physiologic end point such as gas uptake or A-a difference is measured in different carrier gases or in different respiratory maneuvers. Although indirect measurements certainly depend on airway mixing, the dependence may be quite weak and difficult to define. On the other hand, there is a class of measurements, including the single-breath washin or washout test and the inert gas bolus response, where mixing is directly inferred by observing the time-varying inert gas fraction as carrier gas flows into and out of the system of interest.

The most straightforward protocol for such a measurement is to inject an aliquot of an inert gas, all at the same instant of time. In the engineering literature, this is known as an impulse response. Since all inert gas molecules were injected at the same time, the gas fraction monitored at the flow outlet is equivalent to the residence time distribution (RTD) of inert gas molecules within the system. If all molecules had the same residence time, the gas fraction curve would be an impulse function, and it could be concluded that no mixing (i.e., relative motion) of molecules occurred. However, the inert gas molecules normally exit over a finite time interval and, when referred to a flow volume variable (Fig. 8A), the RTD is a bell-shaped curve whose essential features can be characterized by its mean value $\bar{V}$, or normalized first moment, and its variance $\sigma_V{}^2$, or normalized second moment. While $\bar{V}$ is a measure of the volume through which the inert gas passed by bulk flow, $\sigma_V{}^2$ specifies the broadness of the RTD and is a direct measure of mixing. In fact, a simple relationship between the variance and the dispersion coefficient exists and will be discussed in Section III.D. Another useful protocol for determining the RTD is to continuously infuse an inert species into the flow inlet, beginning at some predetermined time. This procedure is referred to by engineers as a step response. Within the context of pulmonary function analysis, the impulse response is called the bolus-response method, and the step response is usually identified as the single-breath washin or washout test.

In the engineering literature, RTD theory is quite developed (Himmel-

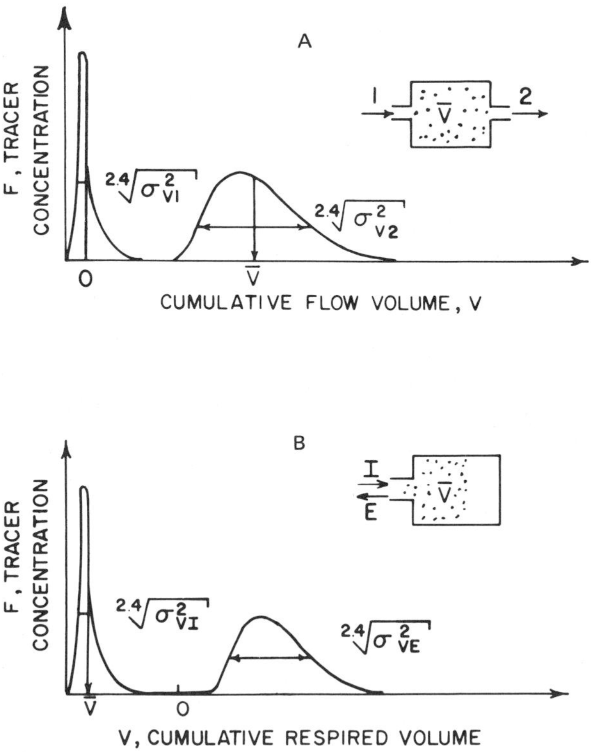

Figure 8 Bolus-response experiment. Where the gas fraction distributions are approximated as gaussian curves, their width at one-half peak height is equal to 2.4 times their standard deviation, $\sqrt{\sigma_V{}^2}$. For a unidirectional flow system (A), the mean flow volume, $\bar{V}$, is identical to the system volume, and mixing can be characterized by the net increase in variance $\sigma_{V2}{}^2 - \sigma_{V1}{}^2$. For a reversing flow system (B), the cumulative volume of air between the bolus peak and the end of inspiration is equivalent to the bolus penetration volume, $\bar{V}$, and mixing is characterized by the cyclic increase in variance, $\sigma_{VE}{}^2 - \sigma_{VI}{}^2$. (Adapted from Ultman, 1981.)

blau and Bishoff, 1968) since it is the accepted method of determining mixing dynamics within chemical process vessels. Three general results of RTD theory are especially useful to adapt to the analysis of pulmonary mixing experiments.

Property 1. The mean value $\bar{V}$ of the impulse response is a bulk flow parameter that is equivalent to the volume of the system being tested, while the variance $\sigma_V{}^2$ represents the extent of mixing.

Property 2. Consider a system such as the bronchial tree comprised of a series of subsystems, the generations. If there is no mixing between the subsystems, the values of $\bar{V}$ and $\sigma_V{}^2$ for the entire system are equal to the sum of the corresponding subsystem values.

Property 3. The integral with respect to time of the impulse response is identical to the step response.

Strictly speaking, the foregoing results apply only to unidirectional steady flow conditions. In the pulmonary system, flow is bidirectional, and the blind-ended alveolar sacs can affect gas mixing. For example, in breathing maneuvers at normal tidal volumes, an impulse or step input penetrates so close to the terminal airways that inert gas is accumulated in the respiratory zone, resulting in significant "back-diffusion" effects. During shallow breathing, however, the penetration of a bolus or step input may be sufficiently small that the terminal airways do not exert a strong influence on the measured RTD. In that case, Properties 1 to 3 may be applied as an approximation.

B. The Bohr Model

The simplest theoretical representation of pulmonary gas transport is the Bohr Model (1891), which consists of a dead space and an alveolar compartment, representing the conducting airways and the respiratory zone, respectively. Rather than providing a detailed account of airway mixing, the Bohr Model provides a limiting condition in which the alveolar compartment is completely mixed while no mixing occurs in the dead space. For an inspiratory tidal volume V_I which is greater than the dead-space volume V_D, the Bohr Model predicts that the dead space is entirely filled with fresh gas and the alveolar region is ventilated with a volume $(V_I - V_D)$ of fresh gas. In that case, the expired volume of a particular inert gas species, $\bar{F}_E V_E$, equals the sum of the species volume originating from the dead space, $V_D F_I$, and that from the alveolar compartment, $(V_E - V_D)F_A$. Thus the dead space may be computed as

$$V_D = \frac{V_E(\bar{F}_E - F_A)}{F_I - F_A} \tag{16}$$

This equation can be evaluated using the expired gas fraction curve from either a single-breath washin or washout test, the most critical step being the selection of a unique value for the alveolar gas fraction, F_A.

When inspired volumes are less than V_D, the Bohr Model predicts that the alveoli are not ventilated with fresh gas. But in reality, some inspired gas is transported into the alveolar region even at very small tidal volumes.

Presumably this occurs because of longitudinal mixing within the dead space and intercompartmental mixing between the dead space and alveolar regions. The volume of air that ventilates the alveoli, V_{TA}, can be determined by a single-breath washin of inert gas. At the end of inspiration, the volume of inert gas in the alveolar compartment, $(V_A + V_{TA})F_A$, is equal to the inert gas that entered during the course of inspiration, $V_{TA}F_I$, and therefore,

$$V_{TA} = \frac{V_A F_A}{F_I - F_A} \tag{17}$$

where F_A is the alveolar fraction of inert gas measured during the expiration immediately following washin. The Bohr Model is implicit in Eq. (17) in the sense that the alveolar compartment volume V_A is a basic parameter of the model that must be determined during a normal tidal volume maneuver.

Contemporary researchers recognize that because it does not account for airway mixing, the Bohr Model cannot simulate many interesting and potentially important characteristics of expired gas fraction distributions. To circumvent this difficulty, some investigators have extended the Bohr Model to include a larger number of well-mixed compartments. For example, Saidel et al., (1971) developed a five-compartment model consisting of one common upper airway compartment which branches into two parallel paths, each comprised of a conducting airway in series with an alveolar compartment. On the other hand, Sikand et al. (1976) employed a pure series model in which the alveolar and dead space compartments were further divided into two subcompartments. There was a fundamental difference in the way in which intercompartmental transport was accounted for in these models: Saidel et al. stipulated that gas was transported between compartments by bulk flow alone, whereas Sikand et al. utilized an intercompartmental mass conductance expression derived from Fick's law. In the former case the compartment sizes and regional flow ratio could be adjusted to simulate experimental data, but the latter method was superior in the sense that derived values of the mass conductance could be directly correlated with fundamental mixing parameters such as the diffusion coefficient.

C. Distributed Parameter Models

Even these extended Bohr Models do not realistically account for airway geometry, and therefore Fick's law cannot be applied in a rigorous manner. Rauwerda (1946) was the first to combine a spacially varying anatomic model with Fick's law, his objective being to estimate the time necessary for diffusion to homogenize longitudinal gas fraction gradients. In modeling the respiratory zone, Rauwerda assumed that the longitudinal distribution of summed cross section was linear and he ignored the contribution of individual airway dimensions and branching characteristics. In the continual development of this style of analysis, the major improvements have included more realistic representation of the summed cross-section distribution (LaForce and Lewis, 1970), the incorporation of bulk transport by the tidal airflow (Cumming et al., 1971), and attempts to account for dispersion in the conducting airways (Pack et al., 1977) and diffusion between unequally ventilated parallel units (Paiva and Engel, 1979).

The basis of all these analyses is a differential conservation of mass equation written for the transported species of interest. Baker et al. (1974) describe in detail how Fick's law [Eq. (3)] is applied to two longitudinal airway positions, x and (x + Δx), in order to determine the net rate of longitudinal transport into the intervening airway region, Δx. This net transport is equated to the rate of accumulation of material in the Δx region, and then the mathematical limit Δx → 0 is taken in order to transform the equation into a differential form. In the conducting airways, where corrections for the presence of the alveolar septa are not necessary, the resulting conservation of species equation is given by

$$\underbrace{\frac{\partial F}{\partial t}}_{\text{Accumulation}} + \underbrace{\frac{\dot{V}}{A}\frac{\partial F}{\partial x}}_{\text{Bulk transport}} = \underbrace{\frac{1}{A}\frac{\partial}{\partial x}\left[A(\kappa + D)\frac{\partial F}{\partial x}\right]}_{\text{Longitudinal mixing}} \qquad (18)$$

This equation is considered to be a "distributed parameter" representation since, unlike the Bohr Model, gas fraction is continuously distributed with respect to the longitudinal penetration distance x. Once the airway cross section A(x) and dispersion coefficient $\kappa(x)$ functions have been specified, the respiratory flow pattern $\dot{V}(t)$ has been selected, and the boundary and initial conditions have been prescribed, Eq. (18) can be integrated for the species fraction F(x,t) as a function of longitudinal position and time. Although an analytical solution is possible for some A, κ, and $\dot{V}$ functions (Scherer et al., 1972), it is generally necessary to use computerized numerical algorithms to solve for F.

By employing such numerical techniques, Scherer et al. (1972), Paiva (1973), and Baker et al. (1974) all simulated the Fowler (1948) single-breath nitrogen washout test, chosing Weibel's anatomical model to specify A(x) and neglecting the effect of dispersion relative to longitudinal diffusion. The first two of these studies presented internal gas fraction distributions (Fig. 9) which show how the inspired oxygen/residual nitrogen front penetrates the airways, reaching a position and shape after about 0.8 sec (inspired volume of 200 ml) which is virtually unchanged until inspiration ends at 2.0 sec (inspired volume of 500 ml). Engel et al. (1973b) predicted that

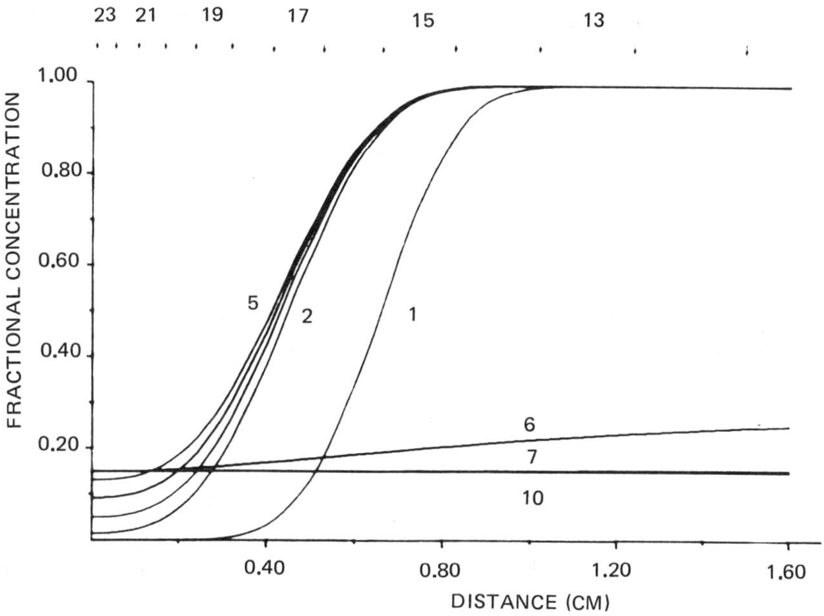

Figure 9 Simulated nitrogen distribution within a modified Weibel model during a single cycle of oxygen breathing. Respiratory flow is constant at 0.25 liter/sec and tidal volume is 0.5 liter. Distance is measured from the terminal alveolar sacs, with generation number indicated on upper axis. Each distribution is labeled with the appropriate number of 0.4-sec time intervals. Notice the stability of the O_2/N_2 front from 0.8 sec (curve 2) until the end of inspiration at 2.0 sec (curve 5). (From Paiva, 1973. Reprinted with the permission of the American Physiological Society.)

this *quasi-stationary gas front* should exist because the distal transport of nitrogen by bulk flow reaches a balance with proximal transport by molecular diffusion. Mathematically, this condition corresponds to a quasi-steady state that can be formulated by directly integrating Fick's law (Fukuchi et al., 1976), or alternatively, by equating the time derivative in Eq. (18) to zero (Paiva et al., 1976). Employing the latter method, the conservation of species equation becomes

$$\left[\dot{V}_I - (\kappa + D)\frac{dA}{dx}\right]\frac{dF}{dx} = A(\kappa + D)\frac{d^2F}{dx^2} \tag{19}$$

The second derivative, d^2F/dx^2, will have a value of zero when the slope of the gas fraction distribution, dF/dx, assumes its maximum value. Judging from the numerical simulation (Fig. 9), this occurs near the middle of the stationary front. Therefore, the position of the front may be characterized by that x position where the left-hand side of Eq. (19) is equal to zero. This implies that the quasi-stationary front is positioned such that

$$\dot{V}_I = (\kappa + D)\,\frac{dA}{dx} \tag{20}$$

This equation indicates that A must be an increasing function of x (as it is in the lungs) if a stationary position is to exist.

Distributed parameter simulations also indicated that washout of the quasi-stationary front occurs with little mixing so that its midpoint position, expressed as cumulative airway volume, is a useful approximation of the dead space. Equation (20) demonstrates that when inspiratory flow is increased, the front must shift to a more distal position where dA/dx has an appropriately larger value, and therefore V_D must increase. Conversely, when a gas having a larger mixing coefficient $(\kappa + D)$ is used, the front shifts proximally to effect a compensating reduction in dA/dx, and V_D is thereby reduced. Similarly, because an increase in lung volume is accommodated more by an increase in branch cross section than by an increase in branch length, the derivative dA/dx will increase after lung expansion and the front must recede toward the mouth to reestablish the original dA/dx value.

In both Paiva's (1973) solution of the complete conservation equation, and the direct integration of Fick's law by Fukuchi et al. (1976), the quasi-stationary front occupied airways between the fifteenth and twentieth Weibel generations. Since dispersion is negligible within these small airways, it would appear that the shape of internal as well as expired gas fraction distributions is strongly determined by diffusion in the respiratory zone and in the last few generations of the conducting airways. This conclusion is supported by the fact that Paiva's simulation of expired nitrogen fraction at the proximal end of the trachea resulted in a reasonable value of 115 ml for the Fowler dead space, on the basis of diffusion alone. More recent distributed parameter simulations have incorporated a laminar Taylor dispersion coefficient in order to estimate the maximum impact of dispersion effects. In simulations of oxygen and carbon dioxide transport as well as the single-breath nitrogen washout (Pack et al., 1977), internal gas fraction distributions that were computed for simultaneous axial diffusion and Taylor dispersion were virtually the same as those obtained when dispersion was omitted. Moreover, although the dead space-to-alveolar transitions in expired gas fractions were somewhat steeper and total expired nitrogen was slightly smaller in the absence of dispersion, the rate of oxygen uptake, carbon dioxide excretion, and nitrogen dead space volume were unaffected. In a simulation of multiple breath SF_6 washout, Lacquet et al. (1975) also found that dispersion effects were small, the dead-space volume being decreased by only 1 ml in 200 when Taylor dispersion was added to axial diffusion. Engel et al. (1979) examined the effect of a dispersion coefficient having the form of Eq. (9) in the simultaneous single-breath washin of He and SF_6. Computing the ratio of the internal inert gas distributions, they observed only a minor change in the relative separation of He and SF_6 when dispersion was superimposed on diffusion.

Paiva and Engel (1979) modified the previous distributed parameter model of Paiva (1973) by incorporating two parallel airway units, each having its own cross-sectional area function A(x), distal to a single proximal airway segment. With such a model, the effect of unequal flow distribution as well as geometric differences between the distal parallel units could be evaluated. Simulating the simultaneous washin of He and SF_6, it was always apparent that the position of the quasi-stationary front is more proximal for the species of higher molecular diffusion coefficient, and this resulted in a smaller dead space and better alveolar ventilation for that species. When the distal units were of equal volume but respiratory flow was unequally distributed to them, the asymmetry in gas fraction distribution depended on the point of origin of the parallel units. When the origin was located proximal to the end inspiratory position of the inert/residual gas front, gas fractions were distributed between the distal units in proportion to their flow. On the other hand, when the origin of parallel units was located distal to the end inspiratory front, the gas fraction differences between them tended to be equalized. This Paiva and Engel regarded as an "interdependence" of gas transport caused by molecular diffusion of the inert gases between the distal airway units.

D. Network Models

Because of the extensive computational effort required, it is impractical to use a distributed parameter model routinely to interpret the large number of data sets produced in pulmonary function experiments and in standard clinical tests. On the other hand, network models are able to utilize the results of RTD theory in such a way that geometric features as well as mixing characteristics can be incorporated into an analysis requiring a minimum of computation.

The network model treats the tracheobronchial tree as a symmetric bifurcating system containing a series of distinct airway generations, each having its own volume $\bar{V}_j$ and impulse-response variance σ_{Vj}^2. If mixing between adjacent generations is neglected, Property 2 of RTD theory can be employed to predict the impulse response of the entire network under unidirectional flow conditions (Ultman and Blatman, 1977a,b).

$$\sigma_{VN}^2 = \sum_{j=0}^{J} \sigma_{Vj}^2 \tag{21}$$

where J is the total number of generations and j = 0 designates the trachea. During respiration, an inert gas bolus injected at the lips penetrates to volume $\bar{V}$ during inspiration and is then washed out by the reversed expiratory flow. If mixing during the instant of flow reversal is ignored, Eq (21) can be applied separately to inspiration (subscript I) and to expiration (subscript E) and the result summed in order to obtain the impulse response for the network over a complete respiratory cycle (Ultman et al., 1978):

$$\sigma_{VN}^2 = \sum_{j=0}^{J(\bar{V})} [(\sigma_{Vj}^2)_I + (\sigma_{Vj})_E] \tag{22}$$

The summation limit $J(\bar{V})$ corresponds to the number of generations that the bolus traverses when it penetrates to a volume $\bar{V}$. In a bolus-response experiment, $\bar{V}$ is predetermined by selection of the inspired volume at which the bolus is injected.

In order to incorporate branch geometry and mixing properties, it is necessary to consider the impulse response that is predicted by the distributed parameter equation (18) for steady flow through an individual tube branch. Levenspiel and Smith (1957) solved this problem analytically and presented the equation for the gas fraction distribution inside the tube. According to this result, the inert gas molecules comprising the bolus are, at any instant of time, distributed about their center of mass in a gaussian manner. Since two standard deviations of a gaussian curve must contain all but 5% of the distributed species, it follows that an air volume equal to $2\sqrt{\sigma_V^2}$ contains 95% of the inert gas molecules. Provided that bulk flow dominates mixing at the branch junctions, the variance of Levenspiel and Smith's distribution equation may be expressed as

$$\sigma_{Vj}^2 = 2(\kappa_j + D)\frac{A_j^2 \bar{V}_j}{\dot{V}} \tag{23}$$

Therefore, the air volume in which inert gas is dispersed is directly related to branch cross section A_j, branch volume $\bar{V}_j$, and mixing coefficient (κ_j + D), but it is inversely related to volumetric flow rate $\dot{V}$ of the air. In reality, gas fraction distributions (Fig. 8) are not perfectly gaussian but are usually skewed toward the larger flow volumes. With excessive skewness, the use of Eq. (23) is questionable.

Network theory can be employed to analyze data both from physical models and living systems. Inert gas mixing in physical models of normal respiration has traditionally been studied with a steady unidirectional flow of carrier gas. In that case, Eq. (23) is combined with (21) in order to predict the network variance.

$$\sigma_{VN}^2 = 2\sum_{j=0}^{J} (\kappa_j + D)\frac{A_j^2\bar{V}_j}{\dot{V}} \tag{24}$$

This equation demonstrates that the contribution to mixing by each generation, besides being proportional to its mixing coefficient (κ_j + D), is weighted by the geometric factor $A_j^2\bar{V}_j$. Since this factor becomes increasingly important toward the distal generations, the predicted extent of mixing increases dramatically with increasing airway penetration (Fig. 10), even though the value of the mixing coefficient tends to decrease. Thus it is clear that, because of the expanding cross section of the lung, diffusion in the small airways can be more important than dispersion in the larger airways, even though the dispersion coefficients may be hundreds of times greater than the diffusion coefficient.

Rather than reporting data as σ_V^2 values, it is often useful to define a mean network dispersion coefficient κ_N by visualizing the tracheobronchial tree as a single tube of total volume $\bar{V}_N$ and hypothetically uniform cross section equal to that of the trachea, A_t. In that case, Eq. (23) can be rewritten by replacing the branch properties (subscript j) with the corresponding network properties such that

$$\kappa_N = \frac{\sigma_{VN}^2\dot{V}}{2\bar{V}_N A_t^2} \tag{25}$$

where the contribution of longitudinal diffusion has been neglected. A formulation for κ_N in terms of individual branch properties can be obtained by substituting σ_{VN}^2 from Eq. (24) into (25).

$$\kappa_N = \sum_{j=0}^{J} \kappa_j \left(\frac{A_j}{A_t}\right)^2 \frac{\bar{V}_j}{\bar{V}_N} \tag{26}$$

This equation indicates that κ_N is a weighted sum of the branch κ_j values, and if the form of κ_j is specified by a particular mixing mechanism, then κ_N can be computed from Eq. (26). For example, in a proximal segment of the bronchial tree in which axial streaming predominates, κ_j can be formulated by Eq. (9) so that (26) becomes

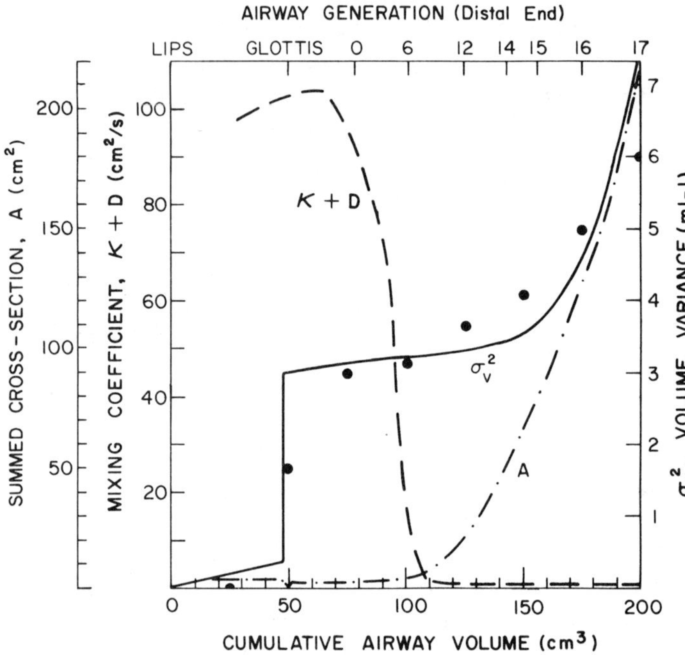

Figure 10 Comparison of summed cross section and branch mixing coefficient to the predicted single-breath volume variance for nitrogen in air at a flow of 0.4 liter/sec. The $\sigma_V{}^2$ values were obtained by doubling the unidirectional prediction of Eq. (24) and then adding a variance of 2.6 ml^{-1} to account for jet dispersion at the glottis (Fig. 12, region B). Branch geometry was specified from Table 1, and mixing coefficients were taken from Table 2 for turbulent dispersion in the first seven generations and laminar Taylor dispersion plus axial diffusion in the more distal airways. The solid points are representative values selected from available human subject data (Fig. 13).

$$\frac{\kappa_N}{D} = Pe_t\left(\frac{\ell_t}{d_t}\right) \sum_{j=0}^{J} (\kappa_{as})_j \left(\frac{\bar{V}_j}{\bar{\bar{V}}_t}\right)^2 \frac{\bar{V}_t}{\bar{\bar{V}}_N} \tag{27}$$

Thus, when axial streaming is important, the network dispersion coefficient should be proportional to the Péclet number in the tracheal branch, Pe_t. Scherer and Haselton (1979) presented an alternative method of treating axial dispersion in symmetric tube networks, and they have also suggested a means by which geometric asymmetries might be incorporated into a network model (Scherer and Haselton, 1980).

For the analysis of data from human subjects, Eqs. (22) and (23) are combined in order to formulate the relationship between the network variance and the branch mixing coefficients:

$$\sigma_{VN}^2 = 2\sum_{j=0}^{J} A_j^2 \bar{V}_j \left[\left(\frac{\kappa_j + D}{\dot{V}}\right)_I + \left(\frac{\kappa_j + D}{\dot{V}}\right)_E\right] \tag{28}$$

where it has been recognized that the dispersion coefficient as well as the respired flow may have different values during inspiration and expiration. A useful experimental protocol for taking advantage of this equation is to measure the variance values, σ_V^2 and $(\sigma_V^2 + \sigma_{Vj}^2)$, corresponding to two different bolus penetrations, $\bar{V}$ and $\bar{V} + \bar{V}_j$. The incremental variance, σ_{Vj}^2, is associated with mixing in the intermediate airway region, $\bar{V}_j$, and by applying Eq. (28) to each measurement, σ_{Vj}^2 can be formulated. When inspiratory and expiratory flows are equal, this leads to an equation by which the branch dispersion coefficient averaged over the respiratory cycle can be computed directly.

$$\frac{(\kappa_j)_I + (\kappa_j)_E}{2} = \frac{\dot{V}}{A_j^2 \bar{V}_j} \sigma_{Vj}^2 - D \tag{29}$$

Notice that the longitudinal distribution of the summed cross section A_j is required to perform this computation.

From the form of Eq. (28), it might first appear that the network variance decreases as either inspiratory or expiratory flow increases. In fact, the dispersion coefficients themselves depend on flow rate, so that this is not necessarily the case. To demonstrate this, Eq. (28) can be combined with (15) to obtain a more basic form of the network variance,

$$\sigma_{VN}^2 = 2\sum_{j=0}^{J} A_j^2 \bar{V}_j [(\alpha_j D^m \dot{V}^n)_I + (\alpha_j D^m \dot{V}^n)_E] \tag{30}$$

where the significance of α_j, m, and n are given in Table 3. The variation in σ_{VN}^2 in response to changes in airflow or inert gas diffusivity will depend on the mixing mechanisms dictating the (m,n) parameter values. Only in the case of axial diffusion does σ_{VN}^2 decrease significantly with flow rate. For laminar Taylor dispersion n is positive, and the variance actually increases with flow rate.

IV. Mixing Experiments

A. Physical Models

A straight tube of uniform cross section is the simplest physical system in which longitudinal mixing can be studied. For example, Van Liew and Mazzone (1977) passed a gas mixture of 3% He:3% Ne:3%SF_6:21% O_2:70% Ar through a 102-cm-long 1.27-cm-diameter tube initially filled with N_2, and they then monitored the gas fraction of each species as it emerged at the tube exit. In such a step-response experiment, the planar interface that separates nitrogen from the inert gas mixture at the tube entrance is transformed by mixing into a continuous transition in gas fraction as the gases flow toward the sampling point. Data indicated that the normalized slope (NS) at the midpoint of the gas fraction transition was inversely related to the gas flow-rate and directly related to the binary diffusion coefficient of the inert gas in nitrogen. Using Property 3 of residence-time distribution theory, it can be shown that NS is proportional to the peak value of the gaussian impulse-response distribution such that

$$\mathrm{NS} = \left[\frac{\ell\dot{V}}{4\pi A(\kappa + D)}\right]^{1/2} \times 100\% \tag{31}$$

Because the Pe(d/ℓ) product was less than 10 under almost all experimental conditions, Taylor dispersion should have been the dominant mixing mechanism and Eq. (31) can be combined with (11).

$$\mathrm{NS} = \left(\frac{D\ell}{16k_{td}\dot{V}}\right)^{1/2} \times 100\% \tag{32}$$

Employing a k_{td} value corresponding to fully developed laminar flow, the values for NS have been computed from Eq. (32). These predicted values follow the same trends with respect to $\dot{V}$ and D (Table 4) as do the experimental measurements, but the data are underpredicted by about 30% for the lowest diffusivity species, SF_6, and overpredicted by 50% for the highest diffusivity component, helium.

It is instructive to consider why these deviations from the theory occur. First, the aerodynamic entrance length computed with Eq. (2) was between 19 and 50 cm, so that the velocity profile in the first 17-45% of the tube was flatter than in a fully developed parabola. This leads to smaller values of κ than expected, which may explain why the NS values for SF_6 are larger than predicted. On the other hand, when the inert gas mixture is introduced at the tube entrance, some initial mixing is unavoidable, and this may explain why the NS values for helium are smaller than expected; the fact that the mass spectrometer used to monitor the gas fractions had a

Table 4 Comparison of the Normalized Slope of Straight-Tube Step-Response Data (Van Liew and Mazzone, 1977) to Taylor Dispersion Calculations [Eq. (32)]

		Inert gas		
	Airflow (liters/sec)	SF_6	O_2	He
Pe(d/ℓ)	0.083	10	3.8	1.4
	0.150	18	6.9	2.5
	0.217	26	10	3.6
NS (theory)	0.083	119	192	320
	0.150	88	143	240
	0.217	74	119	199
NS (data)	0.083	145	165	170
	0.150	120	135	150
	0.217	105	117	123

finite rise time created a similar effect. Finally, because five inert gases were used simultaneously, multicomponent interaction effects could cause the effective values of the diffusion coefficients to group closer together than would be expected from binary diffusion theory.

Whereas the experiments cited above were limited to conditions within the Taylor dispersion limit, Ultman and Blatman (1977a,b) performed experiments that covered a sufficiently broad range, $1500 > Pe(d/\ell) > 0.5$, that mixing by axial streaming as well as laminar Taylor dispersion could be detected. In this bolus-response study, a "calming section" long enough to ensure fully developed laminar flow was located upstream of the bolus injection site, and the inert gases, O_2 and SF_6, were always used in separate experiments to avoid multicomponent diffusion effects. Gas fraction distributions were sampled both immediately downstream of the injection site and at the tube exit, and the variance of each gas fraction distribution was computed by numerical integration according to the definition

$$\sigma_V^2 = \dot{V}^2 \left[\frac{I_2}{I_0} - \left(\frac{I_1}{I_0} \right)^2 \right] \tag{33}$$

where

$$I_i = \int_0^\infty Ft^i dt \qquad (i = 0, 1, 2) \tag{34}$$

By characterizing mixing in the intervening tube segment as the increase in variance between the two sampling points, the effect of the gas analyzer rise time and the intrinsic variance of the injected bolus were subtracted out

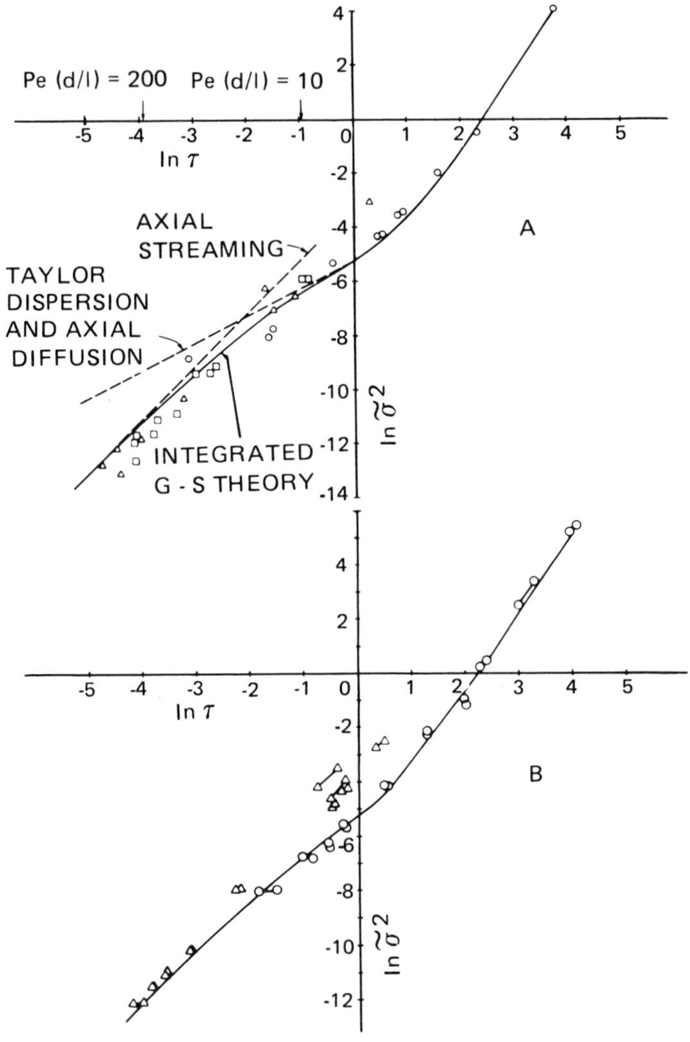

Figure 11 Bolus response for airflow through a 1.6-cm-diameter straight tube (A), and a two-generation symmetric tube network (B). Experimental data for boluses of He (open circle), SF_6 (open triangle), and O_2 (open square), at airflows in the range 1-400 ml/sec are compared to the dispersion theory (solid line) of Gill and Sankarasubramanian (1970). The asymptotic limits of axial streaming and Taylor dispersion are also shown (dashed line). The nondimensional variables are related to those in the text by equations $\tilde{\sigma}^2 = 2\tilde{\sigma}_V^2/d_t^2 A_t Pe_t^2$ and $\tau = 4/\sum_j Pe_j(d_j/\ell_j)$. (Adapted from Ultman and Blatman, 1977b.)

(Ultman and Weaver, 1979). The resulting data were in good agreement with the variances predicted by the dispersion theory of Gill and Sankarasubramanian (1970), and the data reached the appropriate asymptotic limits of axial streaming at small values of τ [$= 4/\mathrm{Pe}(d/\ell)$] and Taylor dispersion at large values of this dimensionless residence time parameter (Fig. 11A).

Scherer et al. (1975) were the first to study longitudinal mixing in a physical model of the tracheobronchial tree. They determined the bolus response of benzene in nitrogen flowing through a five-generation tube network. Although steady laminar flow conditions were used in each experiment, data were separately obtained during inspiratory flow after bolus injection into the tracheal branch and during expiratory flow after injection into a fifth-generation branch. Rather than using the exact definition of $\sigma_V{}^2$ [Eq. (33)], the benzene distribution was presumed to be gaussian, and the variance was determined from the width of the curve at nine-tenths of its peak height. The network dispersion coefficients were calculated from the measured variance by using Eq. (25), and they were separately correlated for inspiration,

$$\frac{\kappa_N}{D} = 1.08\mathrm{Pe}_t \tag{35}$$

and for expiration,

$$\frac{\kappa_N}{D} = 0.37\mathrm{Pe}_t \tag{36}$$

over a range of airflows from 0.04 to 0.70 liter/sec.

The fact that these equations are linearly related to tracheal Péclet number suggests a strong influence of axial streaming. In fact, the tracheal values of $\mathrm{Pe}(d/\ell)$ which varied from 60 to 1200, were usually within the limit for axial streaming. Since the tube network employed by Scherer et al. had constant branch volumes and a branch aspect ratio (ℓ_j/d_j) of six, Eq. (27) can be simplified to predict the network dispersion coefficient due to axial streaming. That is,

$$\frac{\kappa_N}{D} = 3k_{as}\mathrm{Pe}_t \tag{37}$$

where it has been assumed that k_{as} has the same value in all generations. Comparing Eq. (37) to Eqs. (35) and (36) suggests that k_{as} has a value of 0.360 during inspiration and 0.123 during expiration. Since k_{as} is equal to 0.167 for fully developed laminar flow in a single tube, these results can be explained by a velocity profile which is, on the average, more pointed than a parabola during inspiratory flow and considerably flattened during expiration. There is a distinct problem in applying Eqs. (35) and (36) to normal respiration since, as pointed out in Section II.C, axial streaming is a reversible process and the net dispersion over a complete respiratory cycle would probably be overestimated.

Although axial streaming may be important in the first three to six generations of the tracheobronchial tree, branch values of Pe(d/ℓ) are as low as 0.2 in the distal conducting airways. Thus Ultman and Blatman (1977a, b) performed bolus-response studies in two- and four-generation uniform tube networks, with steady flow conditions and inert gases, He, O_2, and SF_6, chosen so that the tracheal values of Pe(d/ℓ) spanned a broad range of values, from 0.2 to 1100. As in their straight-tube experiments, the variance of the gas fraction distribution was computed at both upstream and downstream sampling sites using definition (33). The resulting variance increases (Fig. 11B) were in general agreement with those predicted by network dispersion theory [Eq. (24)] using κ values from Gill and Sankarasubramanian's (1970) straight-tube theory. This supports the view that a finite transition, from axial streaming in the proximal airways to Taylor dispersion in the distal airways, can occur in tube networks with open tracheal branches. Scherer and Haselton (1979) attempted to explain both the data of Scherer et al. (1975) and Ultman and Blatman (1977a) on the basis of axial streaming alone. However, they did not consider variance data at the lowest values of Pe(d/ℓ), and it was those data that were most strongly influenced by Taylor dispersion.

Ultman and Blatman (1977b) also observed that the bolus response measured at a branch angle of 70° was the same during inspiratory and expiratory flows, indicating that differences in the velocity profile may have been less than those implied by data obtained in 35° bifurcations by Scherer et al. (1975). Perhaps the greater centrifugal force associated with the more severe branch angle tended to equalize the inspiratory and expiratory velocity profiles. In addition, Ultman and Blatman found that a reduction in the branch aspect ratio (ℓ_j/d_j) leads to an increase in mixing, presumably because the most pointed velocity profiles occur closest to the branch flow divider and therefore have a larger relative effect as the branch length is decreased.

The mixing properties of the upper airways have received little attention in physical model studies, yet the jetting of fluid through the larynx is bound to have a significant effect. Weaver and Ultman (1980) studied the mixing of O_2 and He in the air flowing through three different circular orifices with β values (the ratio of orifice to tube diameter) of 0.2, 0.33, and 0.5. Each orifice was mounted in a long tube, and bolus responses were measured at orifice Reynolds numbers Re_0 from 10 to 5000 and at several sampling sites both upstream and downstream of the point of minimum constriction. Because of the highly pointed velocity profile associated with the jet, the variance of the gas fraction distributions underwent a sudden increase immediately downstream of the constriction. This enhancement had its maximum value at an intermediate value of Re_0 between 500 and 1000, depending on the orifice diameter.

Weaver and Ultman reasoned that mixing enhancement depends directly upon the residence time of gas inside the glottic jet, or in other words, the reattachment length of the jet. When a jet is laminar its length is proportional to Re_0, whereas the length of a turbulent jet is inversely related to Re_0. Thus enhancement should be maximized at the orifice Reynolds number associated with the laminar-to-turbulent transition. This critical Re_0 has a typical value of 400 when β is 0.5 (Iribarne et al., 1972). Below this critical Re_0, Weaver and Ultman were able to predict their data with a Taylor dispersion analysis that idealized the jet as a cylindrical plug of fast-moving fluid surrounded by a quiescent dead zone. In terms of the dispersion parameter of Eq. (11), the analysis predicted that

$$k_{td} = \frac{\beta^2 - 1 - 2 \ln \beta}{16} \tag{38}$$

For example, the glottic constriction, which obstructs half the diameter of the trachea ($\beta = 0.5$), would have a k_{td} of 0.082, which is 7.6 times larger than the corresponding value of 1/192 for an unobstructed tube.

Simone and Ultman (1982a,b) performed similar experiments with a cast of a cadaveric larynx positioned in an inspiratory configuration with a β value of 0.4. At physiological airflows of 200-700 ml/sec, corresponding to supercritical Re_0 values from 2500 to 9600, the larynx induced significant mixing enhancement by Taylor dispersion, up to 2 cm downstream of the glottis (Fig. 12B). However, for an additional downstream distance of 20-50 cm, the variance of the gas fraction distribution was essentially constant (Fig. 12C). This leveling out of dispersion was attributed to a blunting of downstream velocity profiles by the propagation of jet-induced turbulence. Thus the larynx produces two opposing effects during inspiration: an enhancement of mixing by the confined jet in the vicinity of the glottis, and a retardation of mixing by turbulence as the gas moves downstream. Simone and Ultman found that for the mixing of oxygen in air flowing at 0.5 liter/sec, the net effect of the larynx was to reduce the extent of mixing relative to that of an empty tube once the gas was 30 cm or more downstream of the glottis (Fig. 12D).

Horsfield et al. (1977) mounted a pinched-tube model of the glottis at the proximal end of a tracheobronchial cast of the first few generations of a pig lung. Performing a step-response experiment in which a mixture of 60% air:20% SF_6:20% He flowed into an initially air-filled system, they con-

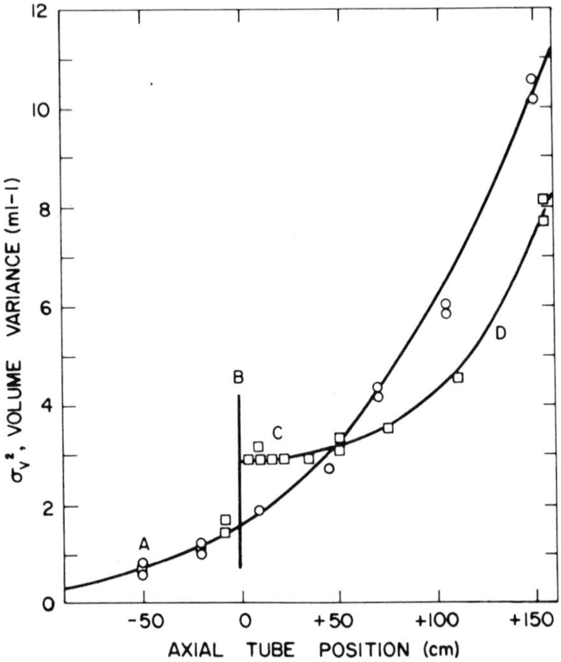

Figure 12 Bolus response of oxygen in air flowing through on open tube (open circle) compared to a tube containing a larynx cast (open square). The steady inspiratory airflow of 0.46 liter/sec corresponded to a tube Reynolds number of 2310 and an orifice Reynolds number of 5250. The point of maximum constriction was located at tube position zero, and the glottic jet was estimated to be 2.8 cm long. The evolution of the mixing process in the constricted tube (A,B,C,D) can be compared to the underlying aerodynamics in Figure 5. (Adapted from Simone and Ultman, 1982a.)

cluded that Taylor dispersion was a dominant mixing mechanism during inspiratory-directed flow. That this is contrary to the implication of axial streaming in the open-ended model of Scherer et al. (1975) may be due to the influence of the glottis. In particular, at the small gas flow of 0.13 liter/sec (corresponding Reynolds number is unknown) where the effects observed by Horsfield et al. were most obvious, the contribution of laryngeal turbulence was probably minimal so that enhanced Taylor dispersion in the glottal jet could have dominated the observed mixing for several generations downstream.

B. Dead Space

As Krogh and Lindhard (1917) described, pioneering investigators believed that dead-space volume is equivalent to the anatomically measured volume of the conducting airways. With the development of high-speed gas analysis apparatus, it became possible to study the details of expired gas fraction curves, and this led to the modern view that both airway mixing and geometry are determinants of V_D. That is, increased mixing, whether caused by elevation of the diffusion coefficient, a larger available diffusion cross section, or a shorter diffusion path, will lead to a decrease in dead space just as certainly as will a decrease in the conducting airway volume.

Fowler's (1948) description of the single-breath nitrogen washout curve divides the expired gas into three parts: phase I, representing the first 20-100 ml of expired air, is comprised of pure inspired oxygen and water vapor originating from the upper respiratory tract; phase II, which designates the next 100-300 ml of expired gas, is characterized by a rapid but finite rise in N_2 fraction and results from the mixing of inspired gas with residual alveolar gas; and phase III, encompassing the remainder of expired air during a normal expiration, exhibits a linear alveolar plateau in N_2 fraction. Because the boundary between phase II and phase III is not distinct and because the alveolar plateau exhibits a slight positive slope, the separation between dead space and alveolar gas is somewhat arbitrary, and the selection of an alveolar gas fraction to use in the Bohr equation [Eq. (16)] is somewhat ambiguous. To overcome this problem, Fowler developed a simple graphical technique which provides reproducible values of V_D, and for a series of normal male subjects he determined a mean dead space volume of 156 ml.

Fowler and others who followed him studied the effects of lung volume, respiratory maneuver, and inert gas type on dead space in humans. The fact that V_D increased by only 40-60% when lung volume was increased by 100% (Fowler, 1948; Shepard et al., 1957) was due, in part, to a true nonlinearity in the airway anatomy. That is, the conducting airways from which the dead space gas originates are less compliant and undergo smaller volume changes than does the lung as a whole. Increases in dead space are also attenuated because the cross-sectional area derivative, dA/dx, increases with lung expansion, causing the position of the quasi-stationary front to recede mouthward.

An increase in the total period of a breath, whether due to prolonged inspiration, prolonged expiration, lowered breathing frequency, or end-inspiratory breath holding pauses, caused a decline in measured dead space (Roos et al., 1954). This can be explained by the increase in the time available for mixing, a conclusion that is further supported by distributed parameter model simulation studies (Paiva, 1973; Baker et al., 1974), in which mixing was represented by axial diffusion alone.

The effect of inspiratory flow, per se, was found to be negligible when VD was measured at the lips (Fowler, 1948; Roos et al., 1954; Shepard et al., 1957). However, by measuring dead space at sites located within the eleventh to fifteenth generations (i.e., 4- to 16-mm-diameter airways) of open-chested dogs, Engel et al. (1973b) were able to establish a correlation between nitrogen dead space and the inspiratory flow rate. This positive correlation, Engel et al. were the first to point out, can be predicted by a quasi-stationary-front model [Eq. (5)]. That is, when the inspiratory flow of oxygen is increased, the stationary front must move to a more distal position in order to cause a compensatory increase in dA/dx. This results in a delayed appearance of phase II and thus an increase in the dead space observed during expiration.

The single-breath washout experiments of Bartels et al. (1954) on human subjects did not reveal a difference between the dead space of alternative inert gases, such as He and N_2. On the other hand, a more recent single-breath study on dogs (Meyer et al., 1983) indicated that He dead space was 16% less than that of SF_6. Mulitple-breath washouts in humans confirm that VD is directly related to the molecular weight of the inert carrier gas: Lacquet et al. (1975) reported a dead space for H_2 which is about 12% less than for SF_6; Wagner et al. (1972) found that He dead space was 9% less than that of SF_6; Sikand et al. (1976) presented dead-space values of He and Ar which were 17% and 7%, respectively, less than SF_6 dead space. These results imply that dead space is inversely related to the inert gas diffusion coefficient and is not strongly influenced by dispersion. The fact that VD is only moderately sensitive to the magnitude of the diffusion coefficient can be explained by the stationary front theory [Eq. (20)]. When D is increased, the front must assume a more proximal location in order for dA/dx to undergo a compensatory decrease. However, dA/dx is very sensitive to longitudinal position, so that a large increase in D can be accommodated by a small mouthward shift of the front.

Okubo and Piiper (1974) performed multiple-breath washouts of 10% He:10% SF_6:80% air mixtures in excised dog lungs. At a fixed breathing frequency of 15 breaths per minute and tidal volumes varying from 2 to 40% of total lung volume, the washout rate of He was as much as 65% faster than that of SF_6 at the lowest tidal volumes, while the rates were similar at the largest tidal volumes. Using an extended Bohr model, these results were explained on the basis of diffusion as the sole means of longitudinal mixing. However, when they repeated this experiment on human subjects, Kawashiro et al. (1976) found that computed mass conductances were frequency dependent and could not be explained by diffusion alone. The results reported by

Lacquet et al. (1975) for the multiple-breath washout of a 3% He:3% SF_6: 94% air mixture from human subjects were consistent with those of Okubo and Piiper (1974). Over a wide range of tidal volumes from 200 to 1800 ml as well as breathing periods from 1.2 to 4.0 sec, Lacquet et al. found that SF_6 dead space was always greater than He dead space. The significance of this difference became greatest under conditions when the residence time available for mixing was the least (i.e., at the lowest breathing period) and when the penetration volume was the smallest (i.e., at the smallest tidal volumes). This work was unique in that the data were predicted, without the use of any adjustable parameters, by a distributed parameter model. In the final form of the simulation (Paiva et al., 1976), mixing occurred by axial diffusion in a Weibel anatomic model containing a lower airway modification suggested by the measurements of Hansen and Ampaya (1975). These results demonstrated that the detailed geometry of the small airways is crucial in the determination of dead space volume, but dispersion in the conducting airways has little effect.

Some of the most interesting measurements of dead space regard its behavior during breath holding. The value of V_D decreases exponentially with end-inspiratory breath-holding time, the rate of decrease being greater at larger lung volumes (Shepard et al., 1957). During 5 sec of breath holding, V_D may drop by as much as 70%, and this should certainly be a consideration in all experiments where, whether intentionally or unintentionally, an end-inspiratory pause is present. To understand the effect of breath holding, consider first that a quasi-stationary O_2/N_2 front is established during inspiration. Then, when inspiration ends, there is no longer a distal transport of N_2 by bulk flow to counteract the proximal transport induced by mixing, and the front must migrate mouthward. The rate of this migration is directly proportional to the local value of the summed airway cross section and is inversely proportional to airway length. As the front moves mouthward the cross section for mixing is reduced, the rate of migration progressively decreases, and this explains why V_D decreases exponentially with breath-holding time. Moreover, because an increase in airway volume is accomplished more by an increase in branch cross section than in branch length, this explains why the rate of V_D decrease is faster at larger lung volumes.

Because of the absence of flow during breath holding, it would seem that mixing should occur by diffusion alone. It is therefore surprising that Bartels et al. (1954), who measured dead space volumes at breath-holding times from 2 to 60 sec, found no systematic differences between a high-diffusivity inert gas, He, and a much lower diffusivity gas, N_2. The authors attributed this to the fact that mixing was due to the "churning action" of the heart. Engel et al. (1973a) supported this hypothesis by demonstrating that V_D was normally about 15% greater in dogs postmortem than in the same dogs during life. Moreover, the rate of VD decrease during breath holding in live dogs was faster than postmortem, but when the heart of the dead dogs was manually oscillated the rate of VD decrease approached the value measured in vivo. Using catheter sampling probes within airways from 2 to 6 mm in diameter, Engel et al. also observed the proximal migration of the O_2/N_2 front, which, as one would expect, occurred more quickly during life than postmortem. The study of Wagner et al. (1972) further supported the notion of cardiogenic mixing by demonstrating that differences between the pattern of decline in He and SF_6 dead space with breath-holding time were reversed, when a comparison was made between normal human subjects and isolated dog lungs. A recent study by Horsfield et al. (1982) indicated that the nitrogen dead space in dogs is, on the average, 22% greater postmortem than during life. But these investigators were unable to demonstrate a correlation of VD with either cardiac stroke volume or heart rate. It appears that cardiogenic mixing is an "all or nothing" process, which Horsfield et al. concluded is more effective in the conducting airways than in the respiratory zone.

Sikand et al. (1976) used a 10% He:10% Ar:30% SF_6:50% O_2 mixture to obtain multigas breath-holding data from human subjects. They analyzed these data with an extended Bohr Model to determine the magnitude of cardiogenic mixing, and to partition its influence between a distal and a proximal airway compartment. Whereas the dead-space values at small breath-holding times were inversely related to the inert gas diffusion coefficients, after 20 sec the dead space of the three inert gases decreased to essentially the same value. By matching the model simulation to the SF_6 and He data, the cardiogenic mass conductance was found to be from 2.4 to 4.2 times larger than diffusional conductance in the 2000-ml proximal compartment, and from 5.8 to 6.2 times larger than its diffusional counterpart in the 2500-ml distal compartment.

Fukuchi et al. (1976) deduced a coefficient of cardiogenic mixing by monitoring the nitrogen fraction within canine airways during single-breath O_2 inspiration, both in life and postmortem. They determined the inspiratory flow postmortem, $\dot{V}_I'$, necessary to produce the same end-inspiratory nitrogen fraction that occurred at a flow rate $\dot{V}_I$ during life. Since the value of dA/dx is constant at a fixed sampling point, quasi-stationary-front equation (20) can be applied to compute the ratio of cardiogenic mixing to pure diffusion coefficient:

$$\frac{\dot{V}_I}{\dot{V}_I'} = \frac{\kappa + D}{D} \tag{39}$$

where it has been assumed that the postmortem dispersion coefficient is insignificant. Fukuchi et al. reported an average value of 5.6 for this ratio in central airways from 2.5 to 8.5 mm in diameter. Although theirs is a more direct method of inferring cardiogenic enhancement than that of Sikand et al., the numerical values of the κ/D ratios are similar.

Theoretical analyses have resulted in two plausible explanations of cardiogenic mixing. Using a symmetric network model of the dog lung, Slutsky (1981) demonstrated that oscillatory airflows generated by cardiac pulsation could cause sufficient longitudinal dispersion to elevate mixing coefficients as much as 50 times above the molecular diffusion coefficient. In the larger airways where the Reynolds number is above a critical value, assumed to be 30, dispersion by combined axial and secondary flow was stipulated by an equation essentially equivalent to Eq (35); but in the smaller airways where Reynolds number is below this critical value, laminar Taylor dispersion was prescribed by a formulation similar to Eq. (11). In sharp contrast to this model, Paiva and Engel (1982) used a distributed parameter analysis to show that cardiogenic flow oscillations could produce significant mixing by the interaction of longitudinal diffusion processes between parallel asymmetric lung units. Slutsky's symmetric dispersion model and Paiva and Engel's parallel-unit diffusion analysis were both capable of predicting cardiogenic mixing coefficients similar to the measured values, but in both cases this required the use of adjustable parameters.

C. Alveolar Ventilation and Gas Uptake

From the measurement as well as the simulation of dead space, it appears that the critical process in establishing V_D is the evolution of the quasi-stationary front, primarily by molecular diffusion within the distal airways. To measure mixing in the upper and central airways, it is necessary to limit the penetration of the front by using small tidal volumes on the order of or less than the normal dead-space value of 160 ml. In that case, the phase II region of gas washin or washout data is only mildly affected by diffusion processes within the respiratory zone. However, as Worth et al. (1977) pointed out, the direct measurement of V_D at such small tidal volumes presents technical difficulties which are best avoided by measuring alveolar ventilation instead.

Based on the visual observation of axial streaming in smoke-filled tubes, Henderson et al. (1915) first suggested that dispersion in conducting airways could lead to significant alveolar ventilation when tidal volumes are less than the normally measured dead space. Forty years later, the development of high-resolution gas analysis techniques made it possible to monitor the low level of inert gas which accumulates in the alveolar region during small inspiratory volumes. Briscoe et al. (1954) studied the washin of an 80% He: 20% O_2 mixture in normal human subjects. Alveolar He fraction was recorded from the phase III plateau of the expired gas distribution, and the alveolar ventilation equation (17) was used to determine V_{TA}; this computation required a separate evaluation of alveolar volume in which a measured amount of He was thoroughly washed into the alveolar region and then washed out in order to determine its dilution. In a subject whose normal dead space was 170 ml, the alveolar ventilation ranged from 10 to 47 ml when tidal volume was varied from 60 to 150 ml. Although these results demonstrated that alveolar ventilation can be substained when inspired volume is less than V_D, it is not clear by what mechanism this occurred. In particular, the observations of Henderson et al. regarding axial streaming of smoke may not apply to a highly diffusible gas such as He, for which radial transport would tend to reduce longitudinal dispersion. Moreover, Briscoe et al. utilized an end-inspiratory pause of several seconds which may have introduced additional longitudinal mixing by cardiogenic effects.

Following virtually the same experimental design, Power (1969) used a 15% H_2:5% SF_6:80% air mixture to determine simultaneously the alveolar ventilation of H_2 and SF_6. Contrary to what would be expected from axial streaming or Taylor dispersion, at tidal volumes smaller than V_D, a greater proportion of H_2 reached the alveolar region. Worth et al. (1977) used a 40% SF_6:10% He:20% O_2:30% N_2 mixture to measure the difference between He and SF_6 ventilation,

$$\Delta V_{TA} = V_{TA}(\text{He}) - V_{TA}(\text{SF}_6) \tag{40}$$

as a function of inspiratory flow, expiratory flow, and total lung volume. Their results are consistent with those of Power in that ΔV_{TA} was positive under all conditions, indicating that the more diffusible gas always exhibited the greatest alveolar ventilation.

One cannot conclude on the basis of these results alone that mixing in the conducting airways is dominated by diffusion. In reality, alveolar ventilation is a manifestation of a compound series of mixing phenomena which occur in the conducting airway region, in the alveolar region, and at the boundary between them. This can be illustrated by normal tidal volume washin simultations (Paiva and Engel, 1979) in which increasing the severity of a distal flow inhomogeneity increased the alveolar gas fraction, even though mixing in the conducting airways was unchanged. Therefore, alveolar ventilation is only indirectly related to dispersion processes in the upper and central airways. Similarly, the dynamics of gas exchange may not be strongly related to mixing in the conducting airways. For example, Kvale et al. (1975) reported an inverse relationship between the diffusion coefficient of CO in alternative carrier gases, N_2, He, and SF_6, and its rate of uptake in the pulmonary circulation. While these authors attributed this result solely to Taylor dispersion effects, Nixon and Pack (1980) used a distributed parameter simulation to demonstrate that an alternative explanation could be based on the coupling of pure axial diffusion with the stratification of blood flow in the respiratory zone.

In similar experiments, Wood et al. (1976) found that the arterial-to-alveolar (a-A) oxygen difference in humans was reduced by the use of SF_6 as a carrier gas rather than N_2, and Worth et al. (1976) obtained the same result in anesthetized dogs. Johnson and Van Liew (1974) used He and N_2 as alternative carrier gases and reported that arterial PO_2 with the latter gas declined faster during breath holding and recovered more quickly after resuming ventilation than with the former gas. It is tempting to interpret these results strictly in terms of longitudinal airway dispersion, as did Johnson and Van Liew. That is, the smaller A-a gradients and the more responsive arterial PO_2 observed in the presence of higher-molecular-weight carrier gases can be explained by an inverse dependence of airway mixing on diffusion coefficient, and this is indicative of Taylor dispersion. However, several other investigators feel that the real effect of a higher-molecular-weight carrier gas is to improve ventilation perfusion matching either by more uniform flow distribution (Worth et al., 1976), by increased cardiogenic mixing (Wood et al., 1976), or by diminished molecular diffusion between parallel lung units (Paiva and Engel, 1979).

D. Inert Gas Bolus Response

By measuring the "growth" of an inert gas bolus as it traverses a known airway region, this technique provides a direct characterization of mixing in the conducting airways. Most of the ambiguities associated with the interpretation of indirect measurements, such as alveolar ventilation and gas uptake, are thereby eliminated.

The noninvasive bolus-response method consists of introducing from 1 to 20 ml of inert gas into inspired air at a predetermined time and simultaneously monitoring the time-integrated flow and the inert gas fraction during the remainder of that single breath. The region of the lung being interrogated by the bolus is called the penetration volume $\bar{V}$. It corresponds to the volume of air that passes the lips, between the time at which the maximum inspired gas fraction is recorded and the time that inspiration ends (Fig. 8B). Because the subject is trained to maintain the same tidal volume in each single-breath measurement, it is possible to impose a desired penetration volume by appropriately timing the injected bolus, relative to the initiation of the breath.

Cumming et al. (1969) were the first to publish bolus-response data. They computed the integral of the expired gas fraction curves to evaluate the effect of lung asymmetry on alveolar ventilation, but they overlooked the potential of more subtle distribution characteristics such as the volume variance.

Ultman et al. (1978), being aware of the direct relationship between σ_V^2 and airway mixing, performed an experiment to determine the relationship between the volume variance and the penetration of both He and SF_6 boluses. In this work, the inert gases were introduced in separate experiments to avoid multicomponent diffusion effects, and the amount of pure inert gas used in each experiment was only 20 ml, so that there was an insignificant modification of the overall gas density and viscosity. The resulting gas fraction distributions were assumed to be gaussian curves, and volume variance was computed from their widths at half the peak height. Even though the shape of the inspired gas fraction distributions was quite reproducible and its volume variance was quite small, its effect was minimized by computing σ_V^2 as the difference $(\sigma_{VE}^2 - \sigma_{VI}^2)$ between the variances of the inspired and expired distributions.

As the penetration volume increased and the bolus was transported farther into the lungs, the resulting response curves broadened, and thus their variances progressively increased (Fig. 13A-C). A complete set of variances for He and for SF_6 is shown in Figure 13D. These data are strikingly similar to values that were predicted on the basis of turbulent dispersion in the first five airway generations (Fig. 10), and it is therefore possible that this mechanism underlies the human subject measurements. However, distal to the trachea the predicted values of turbulent dispersion, axial streaming, and asymmetric mixing coefficients are all similar, and any one of these could conceivably explain the data. Moreover, all three of these mechanisms are independent of the inert gas diffusion coefficient, and this is consistent with the experimental result that σ_V^2 for He and SF_6 are virtually identical at penetrations of less than 150 ml.

The data for He in Figure 13D terminate at a penetration of 240 ml, since beyond that volume, mixing is so great that the gas fraction distribution is essentially flat, and the variance could not be computed. The fact that SF_6 variance can be determined at still higher penetrations implies that beyond 240 ml, mixing of SF_6 is less than that of He. This could be due to axial diffusion effects. To clarify this point, Ultman et al. (1978) used their data with Eq. (29) to estimate the mean mixing coefficients over penetration intervals of 40 ml (Table 5). As expected, the coefficient values are the same for He and SF_6 until, at a penetration of 240 ml, the He calculation terminates close to its molecular diffusion value of 0.7 cm^2/sec while the SF_6 coefficient continues to decrease toward its lower diffusivity value of 0.1 cm^2/sec. The order of magnitude and downward trend of the mixing coefficients in Table 5 are comparable to those estimated for quiet breathing from straight-tube theory (Table 2).

Ben Jebria et al. (1981a,b) performed argon bolus-response experiments over a range of penetrations from 93 to 163 ml and at a nominal respiratory

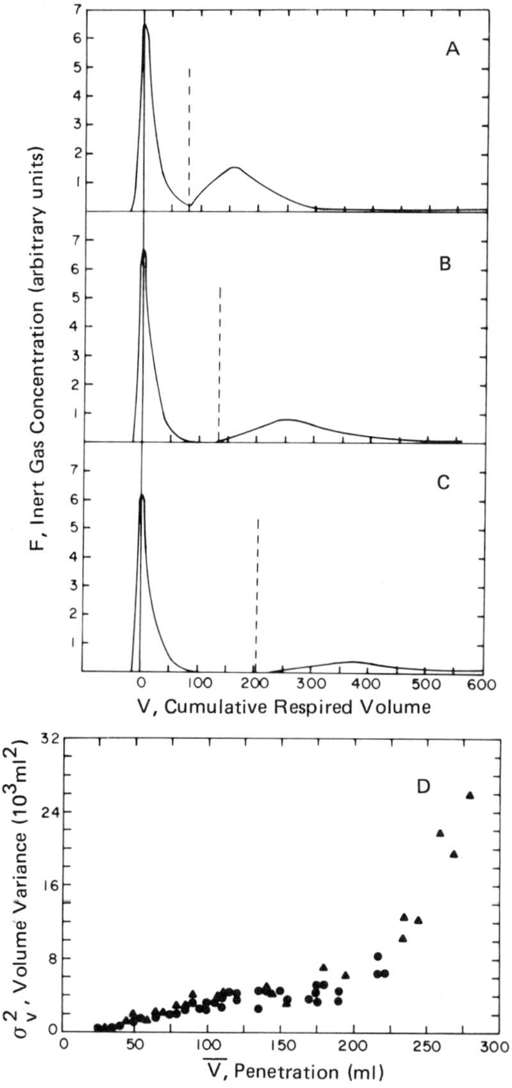

Figure 13 Bolus-response data for healthy male subject DWW at a constant respiratory flow of 0.4 liter/sec. The progressive spreading of the expired SF_6 distribution is shown at penetrations of 80 ml (A), 135 ml (B), and 205 ml (C). The dashed lines demark the end of inspiration. The composite relationship between volume variance and bolus penetration is given (D) for both He (closed circle) and SF_6 (closed triangle) inert gases. (From Ultman et al., 1978. Reprinted with the permission of the American Physiological Society.)

Table 5 Mean Mixing Coefficients Measured with the Bolus-Response Method in Five Healthy Subjects During Respiration at 0.4 liter/sec (Ultman et al., 1978)[a]

Airway penetration region (cm^3)	Inclusive generations	Summed cross section, A (cm^2)	Mean mixing coefficient, κ (cm^2/sec) He	Mean mixing coefficient, κ (cm^2/sec) SF_6
0-39	(Upper airways)	3.1	312	390
40-79	(Upper airways)	3.1	290	390
80-119	0-1	2.4	430	560
120-159	1-10	7.9	44	51
160-199	11-13	32	3.2	3.7
200-239	14-15	91	0.60	0.75
240-279	16-17	240	–	0.60

[a]Airway dimensions have been estimated from Weibel's unmodified airway model (Weibel, 1963).

flow of 0.4 liter/sec. Rather than applying network theory, however, their goal was to simulate data by repetitive solution of distributed parameter equation (18). They used the inspired bolus distribution as an input function, and the mixing coefficient was treated as an adjustable constant to force the simulation to match the expired gas fraction distribution. A modified Weibel model was incorporated to specify the serial distribution of cross section A(x) for both subjects tested. As it turned out, the noninvasive data were not adequately simulated because, the authors suspected, local mixing effects in the upper airways were not specifically accounted for. To prove this, they repeated the experiment on a normal volunteer in which upper airway mixing was eliminated by intubation. The resulting data could be simulated, and the longitudinally averaged mixing coefficients assumed values from 9 to 2.5 cm^2/sec for inclusive generations ranging from 0-9 to 0-15, respectively. Ben Jebria et al. pointed out that these results were numerically consistent with the empirical correlations, Eqs. (35) and (36), that were developed by Scherer et al. (1975) for an open-ended-tube network model. However, these values are much smaller than those presented in Table 5 for mouth breathing, implying that the upper airways do make a significant contribution to mixing.

Engel and Macklem (1977) reported the results of invasive experiments in which the dispersion of oxygen boli, between the trachea and a peripheral airway, was measured in dogs during lung inflation. The mixing coefficients that they computed from these data were an order of magnitude or more greater than those found by Ben Jebria et al. in intubated human subjects. In all likelihood this was due to differences in the structure of the dog's bronchial tree or in the method of intubation. Although in many lungs there was no clear relationship between the value of κ and the rate of inspiratory flow, in some of Engel's experiments a linear relationship was evident. This trend, which was also found in Scherer's model studies, corresponds to a flow parameter n of zero in Eq. (15), implying the existence of axial streaming, asymmetric mixing, or at sufficiently high tracheal Reynolds number, the possible action of turbulent dispersion.

To better evaluate mixing in the upper airways of humans, Ben Jebria et al. (1982) designed a noninvasive experiments to isolate this process from dispersion in the bronchial tree. The gas fraction distribution of ^{133}Xe was measured both at the lips and at the level of the proximal opening of the trachea, using two external radiation counters. By introducing a tracer gas bolus proximal to the lips during a single inspiration of normal tidal volume, the ^{133}Xe distribution could be separately monitored during inspiration and during expiration at both sampling sites. Then, applying the distributed parameter simulation, each of the appropriate input-output pairs of ^{133}Xe gas fraction curves could be analyzed for separate values of the inspiratory and the expiratory mixing coefficients. Over the range of respiratory flows tested, 0.18-0.38 liter/sec, the mixing coefficient values were linearly correlated with tracheal Péclet number, both during inspiration and expiration. Since turbulent dispersion coefficients have a Pe dependence that is very close to being linear, it is quite possible that these results were due to local turbulence of the type that has been observed in upper airway models. As to why the inspiratory κ values (mean of 570 cm^2/sec) were so much larger than expiratory values (mean of 70 cm^2/sec), this may have been due to the intensification of turbulence during expiration when the glottic aperture is reduced. The average of inspiratory and expiratory κ values found by Ben Jebria et al. was 320 cm^2/sec, and this is similar to the value of 390 cm^2/sec reported by Ultman et al. (1978) at a penetration volumes up to 80 ml (Table 5).

In an attempt to distinguish between inspiratory and expiratory mixing mechanisms in the upper and central airways combined, Ultman and Thomas (1979) measured the bolus response of SF_6 at a fixed 160-ml penetration, while separately varying the inspiratory and the expiratory flows. With the expiratory flow fixed at 0.4 liter/sec, the volume variance exhibited a slight negative inspiratory flow dependence of $\dot{V}_I^{-0.21}$ and $\dot{V}_I^{-0.16}$ in two of the three subjects tested (Fig. 14). This result is consistent with the action of turbulent dispersion, for which network theory [Eq. (30)] prescribes a flow exponent of -0.1 (Table 3); the data from all three subjects might also be explained by axial streaming or mixing by asymmetry for which the flow

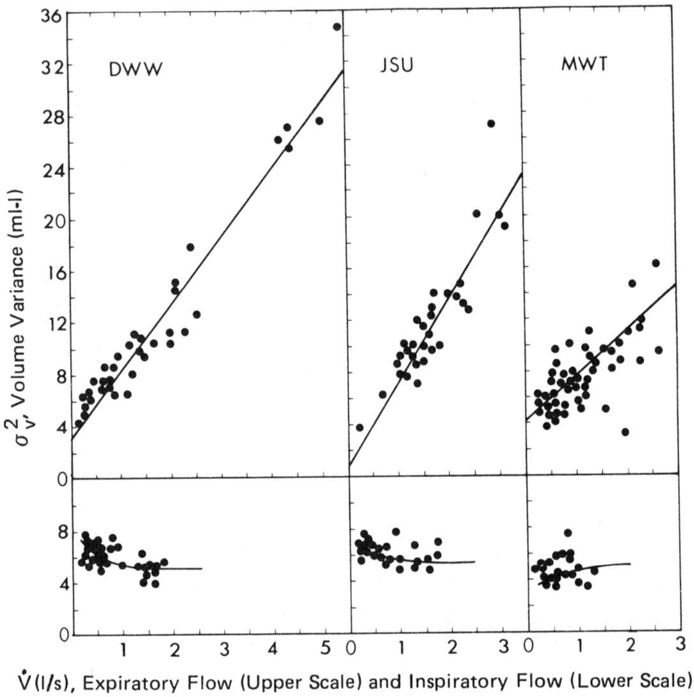

Figure 14 Bolus response of SF_6 of a fixed penetration of 160 ml. When the expiratory flow was varied (upper panel), the inspiratory flow was maintained at 0.4 liter/sec, and when the inspiratory flow was varied (lower panel), the expiratory flow was 0.4 liter/sec. (From Ultman and Thomas, 1979. Reprinted with the permission of the American Physiological Society.)

exponent is zero. At a fixed inspiratory flow, the volume variance was found to vary linearly with expiratory flow. This corresponds to a flow exponent n of unity, which can be attributed to laminar Taylor dispersion.

The basis of this directional sensitivity of mixing mechanisms—turbulent dispersion during inspiration and laminar Taylor dispersion during expiration—is possibly related to differences in the way in which the inert gas distribution develops. For example, during inspiration, local turbulence generated within the upper airways is propagated to higher-order generations so that the bolus will continually be subjected to turbulent dispersion as it is transported distally; but during expiration, the bolus is transported proximally from a penetration of 160 ml (corresponding to about the fifteenth generation) to the glottis before the effects of upper airway turbulence are felt. Another possible difference between inspiratory and expiratory mixing relates to the effect of the glottic jet. That is, during inspiration, any Taylor dispersion occurring in the jet is masked by turbulence that the bolus encounters as it moves through the next 15 generations, but during expiration, the jet is sufficiently close to the lips that Taylor dispersion effects can be recognized.

V. Applications

Based on theoretical simulations as well as mixing experiments, it can be concluded that gas transport during normal respiration in healthy lungs occurs primarily by bulk transport in the conducting airways, by diffusion in the respiratory zone, and by simultaneous bulk transport and diffusion in an intermediate region which Gomez (1965) has referred to as the "critical zone." Although experiments in both physical models and human subjects have uncovered dispersion effects in the conducting airways, the relatively small summed cross section of these generations limits the overall contribution of dispersion to normal lung function. There are, however, three special circumstances where dispersion in the conducting airways may be of importance: (1) the existence of pathological limitations or elected mechanical ventilation procedures, which impose low tidal volume breaths on the order of the conducting airway volume or less; (2) the existence of lung diseases, which modify the distribution of summed cross section and of flow; and (3) the presence of environmental pollutants or the use of inhalation therapy, which introduce aerosol particles of very low diffusivity into the respiratory tract.

A. Low-Tidal-Volume Ventilation

During long-term breathing at low tidal volumes, elevated breathing frequencies as well as abnormally large minute volumes are required to sustain tolerable gas exchange rates. At these high frequencies, gas flow in the core of the airway branches may undergo such rapid changes in momentum that the velocity profiles will be flattened, causing a reduction in dispersion below the steady-state value. In straight rubes it is well known that frequency effects become important when the Womersley unsteadiness parameter,

$$\mathrm{Wo} \equiv d\sqrt{\frac{2\pi f}{\upsilon}} \tag{41}$$

is greater than 1. Calculations indicate that this would be the case in the majority of conducting airway branches at typical high-frequency ventilation conditions, where f is on the order of 10 cycles per second. In branching networks, however, the shape of the velocity profile may depend on other frequency parameters besides Wo (Pedley, 1977; Isabey and Chang, 1981), and it is not clear to what extent flattening of the profile will occur. Moreover, the elevation of minute volumes above their normal values can result in turbulent flow, in which case network dispersion may be independent of Wo (Azhar and Tarbell, 1983).

To the extent that frequency effects are not important, aerodynamics can be considered to be quasi-steady, and the dispersion equations presented in this chapter can be applied. For example, Fredberg (1980) used a distributed parameter simulation to demonstrate that augmentation of mixing by a dispersion coefficient of the form

$$\frac{\kappa}{D} \propto Pe \tag{42}$$

could be responsible for normal gas exchange during low tidal volume/high frequency conditions. Under quasi-steady conditions, a formulation of this type could be attributed to mixing by axial streaming [Eq. (9)] or by anatomic asymmetries [Eq. (14)].

Whether or not quasi-steady conditions exist, axial dispersion in the conducting airways does play a central role in low-tidal-volume ventilation, and this is discussed more fully in Chapter 4.

B. Pulmonary Disease

Pulmonary disease can cause changes in airway geometry which modify the distribution of airflow and local mechanisms of mixing. Gomez (1965) presented a classification of obstacles to transport that might exist in the critical zone, where it is anticipated that gas fraction gradients will be steepest. These obstacles are (Fig. 15): a reduction of conducting airway cross section (K2), either by narrowing of the diameter such as during asthmatic bronchospasm, or by partial plugging with secretions as often occurs in bronchitis; dilation of the respiratory airways (K3), as can be produced by centrilobular emphysema; and either isotropic expansion (K4) or elongated expansion (K5) of the respiratory airways, as happens in panacinar emphysema.

Using the single-breath nitrogen washout test, Comroe and Fowler (1951) observed that the positive slope of the phase III alveolar plateau rises from a normal value of 1% (N_2 per liter of expired gas) to a value of from 3 to 7% in patients suffering from a variety of lung diseases. For many years it was thought that the phase III slope was the result of regional inhomogeneity in flow distribution, with delayed emptying of the poorly ventilated nitrogen-enriched regions. It now appears that a finite alveolar slope can exist even if regional emptying is synchronous, provided that diffusion occurs in parallel lung units having different flow-to-volume ratios (Paiva and Engel, 1981). In either case, it is plausible that the existence of partial air-

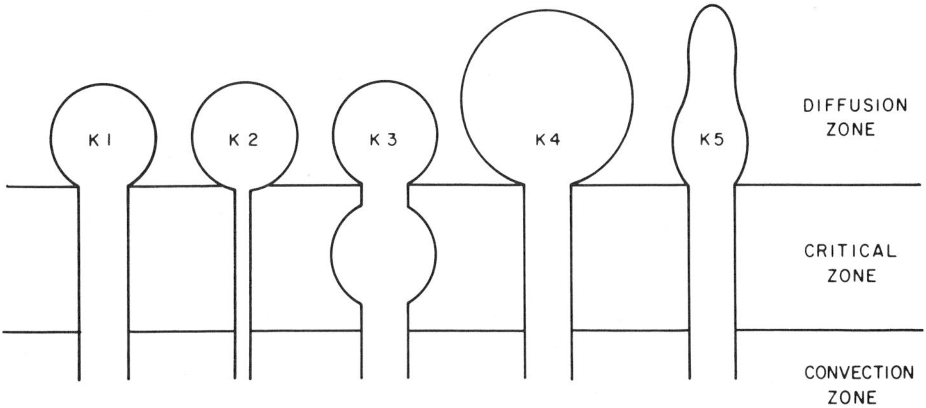

Figure 15 Geometric idealizations of "obstacles" in the abnormal lung (K2, K3,K4,K5) compared to the normal lung (K1). (Adapted from Gomez, 1965.)

way obstruction (K2) at select sites within the critical zone could lead to increased parallel ventilation inhomogeneity and thus to an elevated phase III slope. In multiple-breath washout measurements as well, there is evidence of an unevenness in ventilation that is produced by several lung diseases (Fowler et al., 1952; Briscoe and Cournand, 1959).

To understand better the effect of disease on the mechanisms of gas transport, Georg et al. (1965) monitored the expired SF_6/He gas fraction ratio in response to a single 0.5-liter inspiration of air containing a mixture of 10% SF_6 and 30% He. In normal subjects, the expired SF_6/He ratio (normalized to the inspired ratio) was equal to 1.2 at an expired volume of 0.5 liter, but steadily dropped to a value of 0.95 after 2.0 liters of air was expired. For emphysematous subjects, the decline in SF_6/He was steeper, with the initial value of the ratio being 1.3 and its final value being 0.8. Georg et al. argued that if there was a nonuniform regional distribution of airflow and if diffusion played no role, the inert gas species should not separate, and the expired SF_6/He ratio should be constant. On the other hand, the presence of a longitudinal diffusion limitation would result in greater stratification of the lower diffusivity gas and hence a continual decrease in SF_6/He ratio from the mouth to the respiratory zone. It was concluded that the progressive decline in SF_6/He observed during expiration was a manifestation of this internal stratification. These investigators further postulated that the more marked decline in emphysematous subjects was the result of an increased diffusion path length, perhaps as a result of condition (K5).

Hogg et al. (1972) used a similar dual inert gas method to characterize transport in isolated dog lungs in which 0.29-cm steel beads were insufflated to produce partial airway obstruction. Prior to obstruction they found that the SF_6/He ratio either decreased continually, as Georg et al. had observed in humans, or remained constant during an expiration from vital capacity (VC) to 26% of VC. After obstruction, however, SF_6/He increased as expiration progressed from about 80% VC to residual volume. Additional data from both single-breath and multiple-breath nitrogen washouts suggested that insufflation of beads created unevenness in ventilation. Hogg et al. reasoned that the beads were unequally distributed among parallel pathways, such that velocities in the unobstructed branches were elevated by the redistribution of flow away from the occluded airways, and this led to enhanced Taylor dispersion. Since Taylor dispersion is inversely related to inert gas diffusivity, SF_6 would undergo more mixing and less longitudinal stratification than He, and this could explain the increasing SF_6/He ratios that were observed.

Kelly et al. (1982) employed the dual inert gas washin to evaluate the effect of pharmacological bronchoconstriction in dogs and in pigs. Using continuous gas analysis, they were able to monitor SF_6 and He throughout expiration, but they focused attention on the phase III portion of the data, that is, after the dead space was washed out. The individual SF_6 and He gas fraction data both exhibited negative phase III slopes in pigs as well as in dogs. In dogs, the SF_6/He ratio declined continuously during phase III, a trend that became more pronounced in the presence of the bronchoconstrictive agent. In pigs, on the other hand, the SF_6/He ratio was normally quite constant, but after bronchoconstriction, the ratio continuously increased. Whereas the results for dogs parallel those reported by Georg et al. for humans, the trends in pigs are similar to the insufflation data of Hogg et al.

Kelly et al. pointed out that the negative phase III slopes normally found with dogs were consistent with a distributed parameter analysis (Paiva and Engel, 1981) of diffusional interaction between parallel lung units which originate in the critical zone and receive unequal (but not necessarily asynchronous) flow. Because SF_6 is less diffusive than He, its gas fraction gradient equalizes more slowly during expiration, and this is the source of the decreasing SF_6/He ratio. The normally present nonuniformity in flow distribution was attributed to geometric asymmetries that occur naturally in the dog lung and presumably, in the human lung as well. It was further hypothesized that the use of a bronchoconstrictive agent caused a partial obstruction which impeded diffusion in some but not all of the possible parallel pathways. Such a parallel asymmetry in diffusion cross section could produce the exaggerated decline in the SF_6/He ratio that was observed during bronchoconstriction.

In the normal pig lung, a diffusion model could not explain why the measured phase III slopes of SF_6 and He were equal. Kelly et al. speculated that the pig lung is geometrically symmetric, and the existence of finite phase III slopes is due to a mechanically induced asynchrony of flow to parallel lung units. They also postulated that the bronchoconstrictive agent had a greater effect in the more proximal airways where the quasi-stationary front of He resided. In that way, a parallel asymmetry in diffusion cross section induced by bronchoconstriction would have a greater effect on He than on SF_6, and the SF_6/He ratio would increase.

As indicated by the discussion above, the presence of a partial airway obstruction is generally viewed as an impedance to mixing, to flow, or to both mixing and flow. It is not widely recognized that a local constriction in branch cross section can actually enhance mixing by the formation of a downstream jet. Suppose, for example, that the diameter of a diseased airway is two-thirds obstructed. Then Eq. (38) predicts that Taylor dispersion in the downstream jet will have a mixing coefficient that is almost 16 times greater than in the unobstructed tube, and this could conceivably compensate for restricted bulk flow through the narrowed airway branch. Thus, in a central airway such as a twelfth-generation branch, where axial diffusion rates are normally five times the dispersion rates, it is possible for Taylor dispersion to become the dominant mixing process after bronchoconstriction or partial obstruction occurs. With respect to the dual inert gas washin, such a shift in mechanism from diffusion to Taylor dispersion could be a factor in the appearance of increasing SF_6/He ratios in bronchoconstricted pigs lungs.

C. Aerosol Transport

There is a need to understand the infiltration and ultimate disposition of particulate matter in the lungs, whether it occurs because of atmospheric pollution, occupational factors, or an elected regime of respiratory therapy. The diverse geometry, physical properties, and chemical properties of solid and liquid aerosols preclude experimental evaluation of each specific type, so predictive methods to assess both the total rate of deposition and its internal distribution are required. Progress toward this goal could be accelerated by a better understanding of aerosol transport mechanisms in the complex geometry of the human airways.

As Altshuler (1969) pointed out, the deviation of particle flow from the velocity field of the carrier gas is caused by three mechanisms: diffusion, sedimentation, and inertial force. Diffusion results from a balance between inherent thermal energy and the frictional restraining force of air on the particle surface. The rate of sedimentation is driven by gravitational force and opposed by air friction. The inertia of a particle depends directly on its mass, and when inertia greatly exceeds air friction, the particle possesses so much momentum that it cannot negotiate the curvature of gas streamlines. Whereas diffusion is inversely proportional to particle diameter, both sedimentation and inertial effects are proportional to the squared diameter. Thus for large particles greater than 1 μm in diameter, diffusion is unimportant relative to inertial and sedimentation effects, whereas for small particles of less than 0.2 μm, diffusion dominates. (These particle sizes have been estimated by Altshuler by using representative respiration conditions and airway dimensions.)

There is an intermediate diameter, 0.5 μm, at which aerosol particles follow the gas flow throughout most of the lung, with little opportunity for deposition on airway walls. Yet there is considerable interest in ½-μm particles because of their apparent persistence in the residual gas. Altshuler (1959) estimated that of all such particles that deposit during the course of one breath, half actually originated from the inspired aerosol of previous breaths. Given the exceedingly small diffusion coefficient of these particles, 6.3×10^{-7} cm^2/sec (Davies, 1972), the smallest Péclet number expected in the human airways is somewhere in excess of 2000, and thus longitudinal dispersion more than likely occurs throughout the lungs. Moreover, because of their low diffusivity, inhaled aerosols do not establish a quasi-stationary position of the inspired/residual aerosol front. That is, unlike gases that establish a quasi-stationary front at a penetration of about 150 ml with little sensitivity to the inspired tidal volume, an aerosol front penetrates to a tidal volume which is essentially equal to the inspired volume (Fig. 16).

Heyder and Davies (1971) performed both step-response (i.e., "single inhalation") and bolus-response experiments with ½-μm liquid aerosols. They varied penetration volumes from 300 to 1200 ml and reported their data in terms of the expired volume at which the aerosol droplet concentration reached 1% of its peak inspired level. Since the expired aerosol distribution in the bolus-response experiments closely resembled a gaussian curve, these data could be reinterpreted in terms of volume variance. By assuming that Property 3 is satisfied, the volume variance could also be computed from the single-inhalation data. The resulting $\sigma_V{}^2$ values (Fig. 17) are similar for the two experimental methods at the lower penetrations but deviate significantly at the higher penetrations. These differences could very well be associated with the small (up to 11%) but progressive retention of aerosol, which is not accounted for in the conventional RTD theory.

The explanation that Davies (1972) proposed for his data began with the concept that "mechanical mixing" of aerosols is induced by the coupling of axial streaming with radial mixing by turbulence or laminar secondary flows. Such mixing is largely confined to the anatomic dead space, where the branch Reynolds numbers are sufficiently large that inertial forces out-

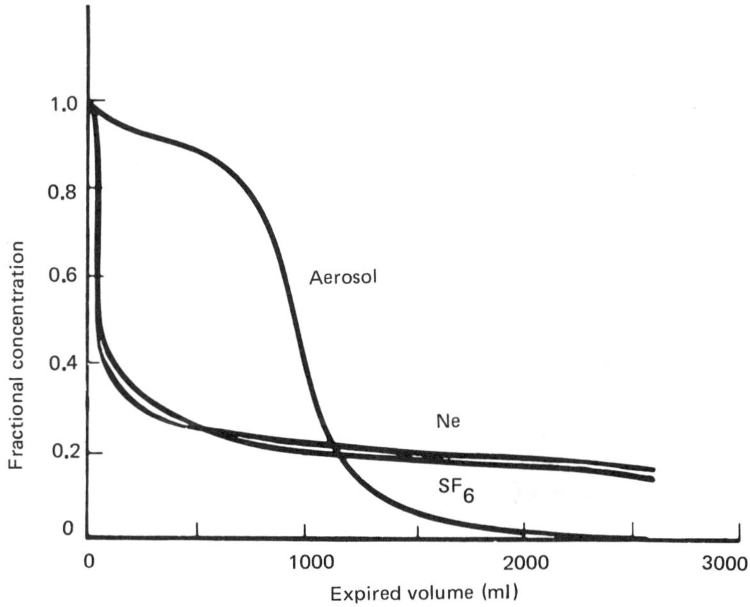

Figure 16 Comparison of the single-breath washin of inert gases to a ½-μm aerosol at an inspired tidal volume of 1 liter. The position of phase II in the aerosol data is centered at an expired volume which is equal to the inspired tidal volume of 1 liter. This indicates that a quasi-stationary front was not established during inhalation. The inert gas data, on the other hand, appear to establish a quasi-stationary front at a penetration of about 0.15 liter. (From Cumming et al., 1967.)

weigh viscous forces. On the other hand, flow in the respiratory zone is viscous in nature, resulting in a streamlined velocity field which follows the contours of the airway walls with a minimum of radial movement. When an aerosol is inhaled, the inspired aerosol/residual air front is distorted by axial streaming, and radial interchange of the aerosol with residual gas occurs, as long as the front remains in the dead space. Once inspiration proceeds to the point where the front is washed out of the dead space, however, there can be no further dispersion, because of the absence of radial mixing in the respiratory zone. This two-zone model is supported by the experimental finding that aerosol recovery in the tidal air of single inhalations is 80%, regardless of tidal volume. Presumably this is the case because dispersion of aerosol occurs within the dead space during a fixed initial inspired volume, regardless of the total inspired tidal volume.

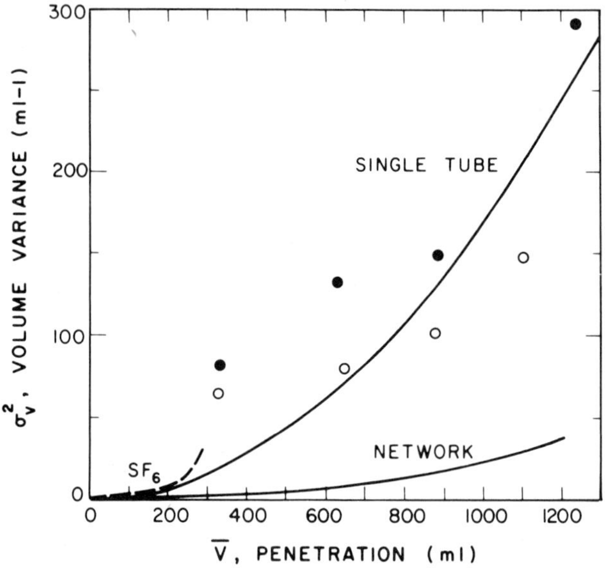

Figure 17 Dispersion of ½-μm aerosols computed from bolus-response (open circle) and single-inhalation (closed circle) experiments. These data are compared to the predictions (solid line) of network dispersion theory and a single-tube dispersion analysis. The data from the bolus response of SF_6 (dashed line) are also shown.

Haselton and Scherer (1980) have advanced an alternative explanation of aerosol transport, which is based on irreversibilities in axial streaming and which disregards radial mixing. As discussed in Section II.C, by virtue of the reversibility of oscillating laminar flow in a straight tube, there can be no net transport by axial streaming. In the bronchial tree, however, the branching structure imparts a directional asymmetry to the flow field, manifested by a difference in shape between the velocity profiles during inspiration and expiration. Because the velocity profile is generally more pointed during inspiration than during expiration, aerosol particles near the centerline of airway branches undergo a net displacement toward the distal airways over each respiratory cycle. Conversely, particles near the airway walls migrate closer to the mouth with each breath. The net result of this opposing motion of the particles is a "countercurrent exchange" of material between the upper and lower airways, and this can occur even in the absence of a net flow. Haselton and Scherer presented photographic records of flow marker studies in tube network models which graphically illustrated this mechanism. However, these models were open-ended, so that possible effects of velocity profile flattening by upper airway turbulence could not be observed.

In support of Haselton and Scherer's proposed mechanism, it is useful to consider the potential contribution of axial streaming to the dispersion data of Figure 17. As a first approximation, these investigators suggested that velocity profiles be considered parabolic during inspiration and completely flat during expiration. In that case, the axial streaming that occurs during inspiration is not at all reversed during expiration. Altshuler (1959) postulated an equation for the particulate distribution originating from such unidirectional axial streaming, but this relationship had a different form than that of the corresponding theoretical formulation of Taylor (1953). On the contrary, Eq. (9) is entirely rigorous for axial streaming in straight tubes, and when substituted into the tube network theory [Eq. (24)] results in a prediction of the volume variance for unidirectional axial streaming in a parabolic velocity field.

$$\sigma_{VN}^2 = 0.167 \sum_{j=0}^{J(\bar{V})} (\bar{V}_j)^2 \tag{43}$$

After substitution of the generation volumes, $\bar{V}_j$, from Weibel's anatomical model, it is obvious that Eq. (43) drastically underestimates the aerosol dispersion data (Fig. 17; lower curve).

One explanation for this is that the network theory treats each airway branch as if it acts independently of all others. At the opposite extreme, one can assert that the branches are interactive to the extent that the branch points may be disregarded and the airways considered as a single tube of expanding cross section. Then the volume variance is obtained by combining the mixing coefficient equation (9) directly with the single-tube relationship [Eq. (23)]. That is,

$$\sigma_V^2 = 0.167\bar{V}^2 \tag{44}$$

where $\bar{V}$ represents the cumulative airway volume at which σ_V^2 is measured. The agreement of this prediction with the aerosol dispersion data is quite reasonable (Fig. 17; upper curve).

Although axial streaming appears to be a possible explanation of both aerosol bolus-response and step-response mixing data, some basic considerations appear to limit its range of influence. In the respiratory zone, the increase in the entrance length fraction to above unity (Table 1) implies that irreversibilities in velocity profiles should be much smaller than presumed in Eq. (44). Moreover, in the large airways the presence of the turbulence will act to flatten velocity profiles, particularly during inspiration, thereby diminishing axial streaming. Clearly, further work is required in which the measurement of aerosol dispersion is accompanied by the observation of velocity patterns in realistic models of the tracheobronchial tree.

VI. Summary

The Bohr Model (1891) idealizes gas transport by subdividing the pulmonary airways into a dead space (i.e., conducting airways) wherein air is translated by bulk convection alone, and an alveolar compartment in which incoming fresh air is perfectly mixed with residual gas. Gomez (1965), who considered the relative magnitude of bulk flow and longitudinal molecular diffusion, was also of the opinion that mixing in the conducting airways was negligible. He further argued that although deep within the respiratory zone bulk convection could be disregarded in favor of molecular diffusion, there is an intermediate critical zone in which transport by bulk flow and by diffusion are of the same order of magnitude. Wilson and Lin (1970), who evaluated the effect of longitudinal dispersion processes in addition to molecular diffusion, agreed with Gomez's conclusions regarding the dominance of molecular diffusion in the most distal airways. Within the conducting airways, however, Wilson and Lin indicated that dispersion by axial streaming or Taylor dispersion would result in more mixing than is predicted by molecular diffusion. The uncertainty still remained as to whether such dispersion effects were large enough to affect overall lung function.

In the decade that followed these initial observations, considerable evidence from both mathematical simulations and inert gas mixing studies indicated that axial diffusion in the terminal conducting bronchioles and respiratory zone can normally explain the behavior of physiological end points such as dead space and gas exchange, and conversely, dispersion processes in the larger conducting airways have little effect. Yet another experiments, particularly those using the inert gas bolus-response method, have shown that mixing coefficients, κ, in the conducting airways of both physical models (Scherer et al., 1975) and human subjects (Ultman et al., 1978) may be hundreds of times greater than those expected from pure diffusion. To resolve this apparent contradiction, one must recognize that the summed airway cross section A available for mixing drastically increases, while the characteristic distance ℓ over which mixing occurs decreases, with airway penetration. Thus the product $(\kappa A/\ell)$, representing the characteristic mixing rate, is far greater in the respiratory zone than in the conducting airways, even though the magnitudes of the κ values themselves are in the reverse order.

A significant step in improving our understanding of lung function was the realization that during a quiet inspiration of three times the Fowler dead space volume, a quasi-stationary fresh/residual air front is quickly established within the critical zone, where the convective inflow of gas species is balanced by diffusive outflow (Engel et al., 1973b). The shape of this front serves as a controlling factor in the determination of gas exchange and Fowler dead space during normal respiration. There are, however, special conditions where this situation is modified.

During mechanical ventilation at tidal volumes less than the Fowler dead space, the front never reaches the critical zone, so that mixing within the conducting airways must play a role in establishing adequate gas exchange. Pathologies in airway geometry can also alter mixing patterns. For example, in centrilobular emphysema, the enlargement of airways in the critical zone might result in the a mouthward shift of the quasi-stationary front toward the conducting airways; and in acute bronchial asthma the constriction of airways within the critical zone could result in jetting of fluid with a concomitant enhancement of axial dispersion. Also, in considering the transport of both atmospheric and pharmaceutical aerosols, one is faced with a situation where molecular diffusion is essentially nonexistent so that dispersion effects, particularly axial streaming and turbulent dispersion, should play an important role in the conducting airways as well as in the respiratory zone.

There is strong evidence that the upper airways are an important factor in gas dispersion. In inert gas bolus-response measurements in both open-ended physical models (Scherer et al., 1975) and in an intubated human subject (Ben Jebria et al., 1981b), the derived dispersion coefficients were always linearly correlated with respiratory flow. In the presence of the upper airways, however, mixing coefficients in the lungs of normal subjects was correlated with the squared respiratory flow (Ultman and Thomas, 1979). Whereas the linear flow dependence in open-ended tube networks may be indicative of axial streaming, the greater sensitivity to flow during expiration through the upper airways might be due to enhanced mixing by Taylor dispersion within a laryngeal jet (Weaver and Ultman, 1980).

Nomenclature

A	Summed airway cross section (cm^2)
d	Tube or airway diameter (cm)
D	Binary molecular diffusion coefficient (cm^2/sec)
f	Oscillation or breathing frequency (cycles/sec)
F	Species gas fraction
$\bar{F}_E$	Mean expired species gas fraction
I_0, I_1, I_2	Zeroth, first, and second moments of inert gas bolus-response distributions (s, s^2, s^3)
J	Total number of generations
k_{as}, k_{td}	Axial streaming coefficient and Taylor dispersion coefficient parameters, respectively
ℓ	Length of a tube or an airway branch (cm)
ℓ_e	Entrance length for development of parabolic laminar velocity profile (cm)
m	Diffusion exponent in power law dispersion formulation

M	Volume of inert gas in bolus (liters)
n	Flow exponent in power law dispersion formulation
Pe	Péclet number
R	Radius of curvature of an airway branch (cm)
Re	Reynolds number
Sc	Schmidt number
t	Time (sec)
u	Sectionally averaged axial velocity (cm/sec)
u_p	Peak axial velocity (cm/sec)
V	Tidal or cumulative flow volume (liters)
V_D	Fowler dead space (liters)
V_{TA}	Tidal volume that reaches alveolar compartment (liters)
$\bar{V}$	Penetration or airway volume (liters)
$\dot{V}$	Volumetric rate of airflow (liters/sec)
$\dot{V}'$	Volumetric rate of airflow, postmortem (liters/sec)
$\dot{V}_T$	Total rate of transport of a particular species (liters/sec)
Wo	Womersley unsteadiness parameter
x	Longitudinal distance (cm)

Greek Symbols

α	Parameter in power law dispersion formulation
β	Orifice aspect ratio, the ratio of the constriction diameter to the tube diameter
Δ	Incremental increase
ϵ^2	Coefficient of variation of branch length distribution
κ	Dispersion coefficient (cm^2/sec)
υ	Kinematic viscosity, ratio of shear viscosity to density (cm^2/sec)
$\sigma_V{}^2$	Volumetric variance, the squared standard deviation of the inert gas bolus-response distribution (ml-liter)

Subscripts

A	Alveolar value
E	Expiration
I	Inspiration
j	Airway generation order or airway region
N	Value for the entire network
0	Evaluated at point of maximum constriction
t	Evaluated for trachea

References

Altshuler, B. (1959). Calculation of regional deposition of aerosol in the respiratory tract. *Bull. Math. Biophys.*, **21**:257-270.

Altshuler, B. (1969). Behavior of airborne particles in the respiratory tract. In *Circulatory and Respiratory Mass Transport.* Edited by G. F. Wolstenholme and J. Knight. Boston, Little, Brown, pp. 215-235.

Azhar, N., and Tarbell, J. M. (1983). Axial dispersion during oscillatory flow in a lung model. *Proc. Annu. Conf. Eng. Med. Biol.*, **25**:36.

Baier, H., Wanner, A., Zarzecki, S., and Sackner, M. A. (1977). Relationship among glottis opening, respiratory flow and upper airway resistance in humans. *J. Appl. Physiol. Respir. Environ. Exercise Physiol.*, **43**: 603-611.

Baker, L. G., Ultman, J. S., and Rhoades, R. A. (1974). Simultaneous gas flow and diffusion in a symmetric airway system: a mathematical model. *Respir. Physiol.*, **21**:119-138.

Bartels, J., Severinghaus, J. W., Forster, R. E., Briscoe, W. A., and Bates, D. V. (1954). The respiratory dead space measured by single-breath analysis of oxygen, carbon dioxide, nitrogen or helium. *J. Clin. Invest.*, **33**:41-48.

Ben Jebria, A., Mallet, A., Steimer, J. L., Boisvieux, J. F., and Hatzfeld, C. (1981a). Quantitative analysis of gas transport in the central airways. *Prog. Respir. Res.*, **16**:96-102.

Ben Jebria, A., Mallet, A., Steimer, J. L., Hatzfeld, C., and Boisvieux, J. F. (1981b). Finite element simulation of gas transport in proximal respiratory airways: comparison with experimental data. *Comp. Biomed. Res.*, **14**:493-505.

Ben Jebria, A., Bedig, G., Mensch, B., and Hatzfeld, C. (1982). Dispersion d'un embole radioactif dans l'oropharynx et le larynx: recherche de la fonction de transfert. *J. Biophys. Med. Nucl.*, **6**:51-57.

Bennet, C. O., and J. E. Myers (1974). *Momentum, Mass and Heat Transfer*, New York, McGraw-Hill, p. 164.

Bohr, C. (1891). Uber die Lungenatmung. *Skand. Arch. Physiol.*, **2**:236-268.

Brancatisano, T., Collett, P. W., and Engel, L. A. (1983). Respiratory movements of the vocal cords. *J. Appl. Physiol. Respir. Environ. Exercise Physiol.*, **54**:1269-1276.

Briscoe, W. A., and Cournand, A. (1959). Uneven ventilation studied by an open-circuit method. *J. Appl. Physiol.*, **14**:284-290.

Briscoe, W. A., Forster, R. E., and Comroe, J. H. (1954). Alveolar ventilation at very low tidal volumes. *J. Appl. Physiol.,* 7:27-30.

Chang, H. K., and El Masry, O. A. (1982). A model study of flow dynamics in human central airways. *Respir. Physiol.,* **49**:75-95.

Chang, H. K., Tai, R. C., and Farhi, L. E. (1975). Some implications of ternary diffusion in the lung. *Respir. Physiol.,* **23**:109-120.

Comroe, J. H., Jr., and Fowler, W. S. (1951). Detection of uneven ventilation during a single breath of O_2. Am. J. Med., **10**:408-413.

Cumming, G., Horsfield, K., Jones, J. G., and Muir, D. C. F. (1967). The influence of gaseous diffusion on the alveolar plateau at different lung volumes. *Respir. Physiol.,* **2**:386-398.

Cumming, G., Jones, J. G., and Horsfield, K. (1969). Inhaled argon boluses in man. *J. Appl. Physiol.,* **27**:447-451.

Cumming, G., Horsfield, K., and Preston, S. B. (1971). Diffusion equilibrium in the lungs examined by nodal analysis. *Respir. Physiol.,* **12**:329-345.

Davies, C. N. (1972). Breathing of half-micron aerosols: II. Interpretation of experimental results. *J. Appl. Physiol.,* **35**:601-611.

Dekker, E. (1961). Transition between laminar and turbulent flow in human trachea. *J. Appl. Physiol.,* **16**:1060-1064.

Engel, L. A., and Macklem, P. T. (1977). Gas mixing and distribution in the lung. In *International Review of Physiology: Respiratory Physiology II,* Vol. 14. Edited by J. G. Widdicombe. Baltimore, University Park Press, pp. 37-82.

Engel, L. A., Menkes, H., Wood, L. D. H., Utz, G., Joubert, J., and Macklem, P. T. (1973a). Gas mixing during breath holding studies by intrapulmonary gas sampling. *J. Appl. Physiol.,* **35**:9-17.

Engel, L. A., Wood, L. D. H., Utz, G., and Macklem, P. T. (1973b). Gas mixing during inspiration. *J. Appl. Physiol.,* **35**:18-24.

Engel, L. A., Paiva, M., Siegler, D. I. M., and Fukuchi, Y. (1979). Dual tracer single breath studies of gas transport in the lung. *Respir. Physiol.,* **36**:103-119.

England, S. J., Bartlett, D., and Daubenspeck, J. A. (1982). Influence of human vocal cord movements on airflow and resistance during eupnea. *J. Appl. Physiol. Respir. Environ. Exercise Physiol.,* **52**:773-779.

Flint, L. F., and Eisenklam, P. (1970). Dispersion of matter in transitional flow through straight tubes. *Proc. R. Soc. Lond.,* **315A**:519-533.

Fowler, W. S. (1948). Lung function studies: II. The respiratory dead space. *Am. J. Physiol.,* **154**:405-416.

Fowler, W. S., Cornish, E. R., Jr., and Kety, S. S. (1952). Lung function studies: VIII. Analysis of alveolar ventilation by pulmonary N_2 clearance curves. *J. Clin. Invest.,* **31**:40-50.

Fredberg, J. J. (1980). Augmented diffusion in the airways can support pulmonary gas exchange. *J. Appl. Physiol. Respir. Environ. Exercise Physiol.,* **49**:232-238.

Fredberg, J. J., Wohl, M. E., Glass, G. M., and Dorkin, H. L. (1980). Airway area by acoustic reflections measured at the mouth. *J. Appl. Physiol. Respir. Environ. Exercise Physiol.,* **48**:749-758.

Fukuchi, Y., Roussos, C. S., Macklem, P. T., and Engel, L. A. (1976). Convection, diffusion and cardiogenic mixing of inspired gas in the lung, an experimental approach. *Respir. Physiol.,* **26**:77-90.

Georg, J., Lassen, N. A., Mellemgaard, K., and Vinther, A. (1965). Diffusion in the gas phase of the lungs in normal and emphysamatous subjects. *Clin. Sci.,* **29**:525-532.

Gill, W. N., and Sankarasubramanian, R. (1970). Exact analysis of unsteady convective diffusion. *Proc. R. Soc. Lond.,* **316A**:341-350.

Glaister, D. H., Schroter, R. C., Sudlow, M. F., and Milic-Emili, J. (1973). Transpulmonary pressure gradient and ventilation distribution in excised lungs. *Respir. Physiol.,* **17**:365-385.

Gomez, D. M. (1965). A physico-mathematical study of lung function in normal subjects and in patients with obstructive diseases. *Med. Thorac.,* **22**:275-294.

Hansen, J. E., and Ampaya, E. P. (1975). Human air spaces, sizes, areas and volumes. *J. Appl. Physiol.,* **38**:990-995.

Haselton, F. R., and Scherer, P. W. (1980). Bronchial bifurcation and respiratory mass transport. *Science,* **208**:69-71.

Henderson, Y., Chillingworth, F. P., and Whitney, J. L. (1915). The respiratory dead space. *Am. J. Physiol.,* **38**:1-19.

Heyder, J., and Davies, C. N. (1971). The breathing of half-micron aerosols: III. Dispersion of particles in the respiratory tract. *Aerosol Sci.,* **2**:437-452.

Himmelblau, D. M., and Bishoff, K. B. (1968). *Process Analysis and Simulation: Deterministic Systems.* New York, Wiley, pp. 59-129.

Hogg, W., Brunton, J., Kryger, M., Brown, R., and Macklem, P. (1972). Gas diffusion across collateral channels. *J. Appl. Physiol.,* **33**:568-575.

Horsfield, K., and Cumming, G. (1968a). Morphology of the bronchial tree in man. *J. Appl. Physiol.,* **24**:373-383.

Horsfield, K., and Cumming, G. (1968b). Functional consequences of airway morphology. *J. Appl. Physiol.,* **24**:384-390.

Horsfield, K., Dart, G., Olson, D. E., Filley, G. F., and Cumming, G. (1971). Models of the human bronchial tree. *J. Appl. Physiol.,* **31**:207-217.

Horsfield, K., Davies, A., and Cumming, G. (1977). Role of conducting airways in partial separation of inhaled gas mixtures. *J. Appl. Physiol. Respir. Environ. Exercise Physiol.,* **43**:391-396.

Horsfield, K., Gabe, I., Mills, C., Buckman, M., and Cumming, G. (1982).

Effect of heart rate and stroke volume on gas mixing in dog lung. *J. Appl. Physiol. Respir. Environ. Exercise Physiol.*, **53**:1603-1607.

Hughes, J. M. B., Hoppin, F. G., and Mead, J. (1972). Effect of lung inflation on bronchial length and diameter in excised lungs. *J. Appl. Physiol.*, **32**:25-35.

Iribarne, A., Frantisak, F., Hummel, R. L., and Smith, J. W. (1972). An experimental study of instabilities and other properties of a laminar pipe jet. *Am. Inst. Chem. Eng. J.*, **18**:689-698.

Isabey, D., and Chang, H. K. (1981). Steady and unsteady pressure-flow relationships in central airways. *J. Appl. Physiol. Respir. Environ. Exercise Physiol.*, **51**:1338-1348.

Isabey, D., and Chang, H. K. (1982). A model study of flow dynamics in human central airways: Part II. Secondary flow velocities. *Respir. Physiol.*, **49**:97-113.

Johnson, L. R., and Van Liew, H. D. (1974). Use of arterial pO_2 to study convective and diffusive gas mixing in the lungs. *J. Appl. Physiol.*, **36**: 91-97.

Kawashiro, T., Sikand, R. S., Adaro, F., Takahashi, H., and Piiper, J. (1976). Study of intrapulmonary gas mixing in man by simultaneous wash-out of helium and sulfur hexafluoride. *Respir. Physiol.*, **28**:261-275.

Kelly, S., Paiva, M., and Engel, L. A. (1982). Bronchoconstriction and gas mixing in canine and pig lungs. *Bull. Eur. Physiopathol. Respir.*, **18**: 229-237.

Krogh, A., and Lindhard, J. (1917). The volume of the dead space in breathing and the mixing of gases in the lungs of man. *J. Physiol.*, **51**:59-90.

Kvale, P. A., Davis, J., and Schroter, R. C. (1975). Effect of gas density and ventilatory pattern on steady state CO uptake by the lung. *Respir. Physiol.*, **24**:385-398.

LaForce, R. C., and Lewis, B. M. (1970). Diffusional transport in the human lung. *J. Appl. Physiol.*, **28**:291-298.

Lacquet, L. M., Van der Linden, L. P., and Paiva, M. (1975). Transport of H_2 and SF_6 in the lung. *Respir. Physiol.*, **25**:157-173.

Levenspiel, O., and Smith, W. K. (1957). Notes on the diffusion-type model for the longitudinal mixing of fluids in flow. *Chem. Eng. Sci.*, **6**:227-233.

Macklin, C. C. (1925). X-Ray studies on bronchial movements. *Am. J. Anat.*, **35**:303-329.

Meyer, M., Hook, C., Rieke, H., and Piiper, J. (1983). Gas mixing in dog lungs studied by single-breath washout of He and SF_6. *J. Appl. Physiol. Respir. Environ. Exercise Physiol.*, **55**:1795-1802.

Nixon, W., and Pack, A. (1980). Effect of altered gas diffusivity on alveolar gas exchange—a theoretical study. *J. Appl. Physiol. Respir. Environ. Exercise Physiol.,* **48**:147-153.

Nunge, R. J., Lin, T.-S., and Gill, W. N. (1972). Laminar dispersion in curved tubes and channels. *J. Fluid Mech.,* **51**:363-383.

Okubo, T., and Piiper, J. (1974). Intrapulmonary gas mixing in excised dog lung lobes studied by simultaneous wash-out of two inert gases. *Respir. Physiol.,* **21**:223-239.

Olson, D. E., Dart, G. A., and Filley, G. F. (1970). Pressure drop and fluid flow regime of air inspired into the human lung. *J. Appl. Physiol.,* **28**:482-494.

Olson, D. E., Iliff, L. D., and Sudlow, M. F. (1972). Some aspects of the physics of flow in the central airways. *Bull. Eur. Physiopathol. Respir.,* **8**:391-408.

Olson, D. E., Sudlow, M. F., Horsfield, H., and Filley, G. F. (1973). Convective patterns of flow during inspiration. *Arch. Intern. Med.,* **131**:51-57.

Owen, P. R. (1969). Turbulent flow and particle deposition in the trachea. In *Circulatory and Respiratory Mass Transport.* Edited by G. F. Wolstenholme and J. Knight. Boston, Little, Brown, pp. 236-252.

Pack, A., Hooper, M. B., Nixon, W., and Taylor, J. C. (1977). A computational model of pulmonary gas transport incorporating effective diffusion. *Respir. Physiol.,* **29**:101-124.

Paiva, M. (1973). Gas transport in the human lung. *J. Appl. Physiol.,* **35**:401-410.

Paiva, M., and Engel, L. A. (1979). Pulmonary interdependence of gas transport. *J. Appl. Physiol. Respir. Environ. Exercise Physiol.,* **47**:296-305.

Paiva, M., and Engel, L. A. (1981). The anatomic basis for the sloping N_2 plateau. *Respir. Physiol.,* **44**:325-337.

Paiva, M., and Engel, L. A. (1982). Influence of bronchial asymmetry on cardiogenic gas mixing in the lung. *Respir. Physiol.,* **49**:325-338.

Paiva, M., Lacquet, L. M., and Van der Linden, L. P. (1976). Gas transport in a model derived from Hansen-Ampaya anatomical data of the human lung. *J. Appl. Physiol.,* **41**:115-119.

Pedley, T. J. (1977). Pulmonary fluid dynamics. *Annu. Rev. Fluid Mech.,* **9**:229-274.

Power, G. G. (1969). Gaseous diffusion between airways and alveoli in the human lung. *J. Appl. Physiol.,* **5**:701-709.

Proctor, D. (1966). Airborne disease and the upper respiratory tract. *Bacteriol. Rev.,* **30**:498-513.

Proetz (1951). Air currents in the upper respiratory tract and their clinical significance. *Ann. Otol.,* **60**:439-467.

Rauwerda, P. E. (1946). Unequal ventilation of different parts of the lungs and the determination of cardiac output. Ph.D. dissertation, University of Groningen, Groningen, The Netherlands.

Roos, A., Dahlstrom, H., and Murphy, J. P. (1954). Distribution of inspired air in the lungs. *J. Appl. Physiol.,* **7**:645-659.

Ross, B. B. (1957). Influence of bronchial tree structure on ventilation in the dog's lung as inferred from measurements of a plastic cast. *J. Appl. Physiol.,* **10**:1-14.

Saidel, G. M., Militano, T. C., and Chester, E. H. (1971). Pulmonary gas transport characterization by a dynamic model. *Respir. Physiol.,* **12**: 305-328.

Scherer, P. W., and Haselton, F. R. (1979). Convective mixing in tube networks. *Am. Inst. Chem. Eng. J.,* **25**:542-544.

Scherer, P. W., and Haselton, F. R. (1980). A network theory of bronchial gas mixing applied to single breath nitrogen washout. *Lung,* **158**:201-220.

Scherer, P. W., Shendalman, L. H., and Greene, N. M. (1972). Simultaneous diffusion and convection in single-breath lung washout. *Bull. Math. Biophys.,* **34**:393-412.

Scherer, P. W., Shendalman, L. H., Greene, N. M., and Bouhuys, A. (1975). Measurement of axial diffusivities in a model of the bronchial airways. *J. Appl. Physiol.,* **38**:719-723.

Schroter, R. C., and Sudlow, M. F. (1969). Flow patterns in models of the human bronchial airways. *Respir. Physiol.,* **7**:341-355.

Shepard, R. H., Campbell, E. J. M., Martin, H. B., and Enns, T. (1957). Factors affecting the pulmonary dead space as determined by single-breath analysis. *J. Appl. Physiol.,* **11**:241-244.

Sikand, R. S., Magnussen, H., Scheid, P., and Piiper, J. (1976). Convective and diffusive gas mixing in human lungs: experiments and model analysis. *J. Appl. Physiol.,* **40**:362-371.

Simone, A. F., and Ultman, J. S. (1982a). Longitudinal mixing of oxygen with air during steady flow through the larynx. *Bull. Eur. Physiopathol. Respir.,* **18**:389-393.

Simone, A. F., and Ultman, J. S. (1982b). Longitudinal mixing by the human larynx. *Respir. Physiol.,* **49**:187-203.

Slutsky, A. S. (1981). Gas mixing by cardiac oscillations: a theoretical quantitative analysis. *J. Appl. Physiol. Respir. Environ. Exercise Physiol.,* **51**:1287-1293.

Subramanian, R. S., and Gill, W. N. (1976). Unsteady convective diffusion in non-Newtonian flows. *Can. J. Chem. Eng.,* **54**:121-125.

Swift, D. L., and Proctor, D. F. (1977). Access of air to the respiratory tract. In *Lung Biology in Health and Disease: Respiratory Defense Mechanisms,* Vol. 5 (Part 1): *Respiratory Defense Mechanisms.* Edited

by D. F. Proctor and L. M. Reid. New York, Marcel Dekker, pp. 63-93.
Taylor, G. I. (1953). Dispersion of soluble matter in solvent flowing slowly through a tube. *Proc. R. Soc. Lond.*, **219A**:186-203.
Taylor, G. I. (1954). The dispersion of matter in turbulent flow through a pipe. *Proc. R. Soc., Lond.*, **223A**:446-466.
Ultman, J. S. (1981). Gas mixing in the pulmonary airways. *Ann. Biomed. Eng.*, **9**:513-527.
Ultman, J. S., and Blatman, H. S. (1977a). A compartmental model for the analysis of mixing in tube networks. *Am. Inst. Chem. Eng. J.*, **23**: 169-176.
Ultman, J. S., and Blatman, H. S. (1977b). Longitudinal mixing in pulmonary airways. Analysis of inert gas dispersion in symmetric tube network models. *Respir. Physiol.*, **30**:349-367.
Ultman, J. S., and Thomas, M. W. (1979). Longitudinal mixing in pulmonary airways: comparison of inspiration and expiration. *J. Appl. Physiol. Respir. Environ. Exercise Physiol.*, **46**:799-805.
Ultman, J. S., and Weaver, D. W. (1979). Concentration sampling methods in relation to the computation of a dispersion coefficient. *Chem. Eng. Sci.*, **34**:1172-1174.
Ultman, J. S., Doll, B. E., Spiegel, R., and Thomas, M. W. (1978). Longitudinal mixing in pulmonary airways—normal subjects respiring at a constant flow. *J. Appl. Physiol. Respir. Environ. Exercise Physiol.*, **44**: 297-303.
Van Liew, H. D., and Mazzone, R. W. (1977). Mixing in flowing gas. *Respir. Physiol.*, **30**:27-34.
Wagner, P. D., Gaines, R. A., Mazzone, R. W., and West, J. B. (1972). Mechanism of intrapulmonary gas mixing during breath holding in man. *Physiologist,* **15**:295.
Weaver, D. W., and Ultman, J. S. (1980). Axial dispersion through tube constrictions. *Am. Inst. Chem. Eng. J.*, **26**:9-15.
Weibel, E. R. (1963). *Morphology of the Lung.* New York, Academic Press, Chap. 11.
West, J. B., and Hugh-Jones, P. (1959). Patterns of gas flow in the upper-bronchial tree. *J. Appl. Physiol.*, **14**:753-759.
West, J. B., and Hugh-Jones, P. (1961). Pulsatile flow in the bronchi caused by the heart beat. *J. Appl. Physiol.*, **16**:697-702.
Wilson, T. A., and Lin, K. (1970). Convection and diffusion in the airways and the design of the bronchial tree. In *Airway Dynamics.* Edited by A. Bohuys. Springfield, Ill., Charles C Thomas, pp. 5-19.
Wood, L. D. H., Bryan, A. C., Bau, S. K., Weng, T. R., and Levison, H. (1976). Effect of increased gas density on pulmonary gas exchange in man. *J. Appl. Physiol.*, **41**:206-210.

Worth, H., and Piiper, J. (1978). Diffusion of helium, carbon monoxide and sulfur hexafluoride in gas mixtures similar to alveolar gas. *Respir. Physiol.,* **32**:155-166.

Worth, H., Takahashi, H., Willmer, H., and Piiper, J. (1976). Pulmonary gas exchange in dogs ventilated with mixtures of oxygen with various inert gases. *Respir. Physiol.,* **28**:1-15.

Worth, H., Adaro, F., and Piiper, J. (1977). Penetration of inhaled He and SF_6 into the alveolar space at low tidal volumes. *J. Appl. Physiol. Respir. Environ. Exercise Physiol.,* **43**:403-408.

Worth, H., Nüsse, W., and Piiper, J. (1978). Determination of binary diffusion coefficients of various gas species used in respiratory physiology. *Respir. Physiol.,* **32**:15-26.

Yu, C. P. (1975). On equation of gas transport in the lung. *Respir. Physiol.,* **23**:257-266.

4

Alveolar Ventilation at High Frequencies Using Tidal Volumes Smaller than the Anatomical Dead Space

ARTHUR S. SLUTSKY*

Harvard Medical School
Boston
and West Roxbury Veterans
Administration Medical Center
West Roxbury, Massachusetts

ROGER D. KAMM

Massachusetts Institute of Technology
Cambridge, Massachusetts

JEFFREY M. DRAZEN

Harvard Medical School
and Brigham and Women's Hospital
Boston, Massachusetts

I. Introduction

The process of gas transport in the lung has traditionally been viewed as occurring by two relatively distinct mechanisms: (1) convection in the airways (dead space), and (2) molecular diffusion in the alveolar zone. Based on this concept effective alveolar ventilation can be maintained only if the tidal volume (V_T) exceeds the anatomical dead space (V_D). This traditional view has long been established and has been supported by a large body of experimental data in studies on spontaneously breathing subjects and mechanically ventilated patients.

Sponsored in part by the Research Service of the U.S. Veterans Administration, National Heart, Lung and Blood Institute Grants 26566 and 32333, and National Science Foundation Grant CME-7913092.

**Present affiliation:* Mount Sinai Hospital and University of Toronto, Toronto, Ontario, Canada.

In recent years, evidence has been advanced indicating that effective gas exchange can occur with tidal volumes smaller than the dead space if the respiratory frequency is sufficiently high (Lunkenheimer et al., 1972; Bohn et al., 1980; Slutsky et al., 1980, 1981; Wright et al., 1981; Rossing et al., 1981). These data have stimulated researchers to investigate this interesting phenomenon, which has been labeled high-frequency ventilation (HFV). The purpose of this chapter is to summarize some of the basic theoretical and experimental studies related to the mechanisms of gas exchange by HFV. We will not concern ourselves with the issue of an exact definition of HFV, but rather will limit the scope of this review to include studies relevant to explaining how effective alveolar ventilation ($\dot{V}_A$) is possible with $V_T < V_D$.

II. Historical Review

The concept that it is possible to achieve adequate $\dot{V}_A$ using $V_T < V_D$ is not a new one. In 1915, Yandell Henderson and colleagues (Henderson et al., 1915) came to the conclusion that "there may easily be a gaseous exchange sufficient to support life even when the tidal volume is considerably less than the dead space." This conclusion was based on flow visualization experiments of tracer smoke blown into one end of a glass tube and the observation was used to explain why panting dogs remain eucapnic even though they breathe with tidal volumes less than their dead space.

Henderson and colleagues observed that when they blew smoke into one end of a glass tube, the smoke penetrated the tube as a very thin spike and that the tip of this spike began to leave the tube before the tube was filled with smoke (Fig. 1). Thus they suggested that in the lung, a similar parabolic tongue could extend directly into the alveolar region and produce adequate gas exchange. Although this hypothesis is graphic and quite attractive, it is overly simplistic due to the effects of turbulence and secondary swirling flows found in the upper airways as well as the mixing due to diffusion. Thus the idea of a continuous parabolic tongue that extends from the airway opening to the alveolar zone is unrealistic. However, the general concept that axial convection plays an important role is a feasible one (see Sec. III).

The first evidence that it was possible to support human life while breathing very low tidal volumes was provided by Comroe et al. (1950). They presented data in a patient with emphysema who was alive (albeit with a PCO_2 of 150) while breathing 100% O_2 for 2-4 hr with a tidal volume of 120 ml. This observation stimulated Briscoe et al. (1954) to investigate this phenomenon further by calculating the volume of helium entering the alveo-

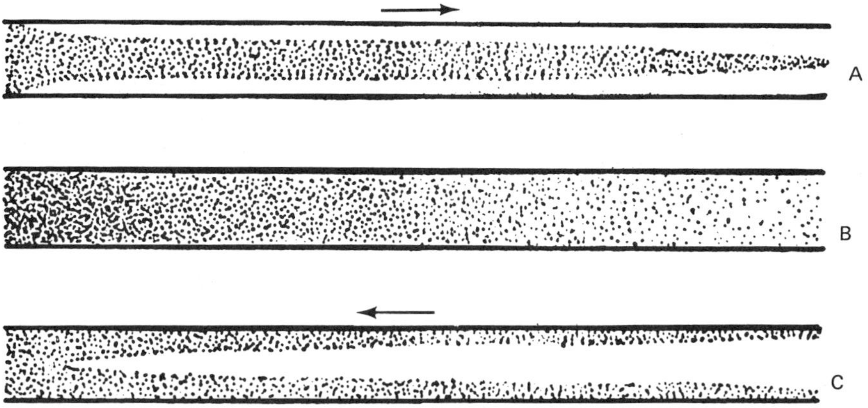

Figure 1 Results obtained by Henderson et al. (1915) from experiments in which smoke was blown through a glass tube: (A) "spike" of tobacco smoke blown from left to right through a glass tube; (B) dispersion of smoke as the flow of gas is suddenly stopped; (C) "spike" of fresh gas as flow proceeds from right to left.

lar region of their human subjects following an inhalation of 30-500 ml of 80% He-20% O_2. As shown in Figure 2, even when the tidal volume was as small as 60 ml there was some helium in the expired alveolar gas. On the basis of these observations Briscoe and colleagues concluded that "with very low tidal volumes, the formula

Alveolar ventilation = tidal volume - dead-space volume

is incorrect; it becomes correct only when the tidal volume is large." They hypothesized that this phenomenon might be due to (a) "Henderson's spike" (as described above), (2) boundary diffusion of gases, and (3) the anatomical observation of Rohrer (1915) that not all alveoli are equidistant from the carina. Although Briscoe et al. did not address the issue of HFV, if their results are valid at high frequencies, one can calculate (from their Table 1) that it would be possible to obtain eucapnia in humans at a V_T of 78 ml, applied at a frequency of just over 3 Hz.

The concept of applying high-frequency oscillations to enhance gas mixing in the lung was suggested by Emerson (1959), who obtained a patent entitled "Apparatus for vibrating portions of a patient's airway." Although the device was never fully tested, in the patent application Emerson asserted that "vibrating the column of gas doubtless causes the gas to diffuse more rapidly within the airways and therefore aids in the breathing function."

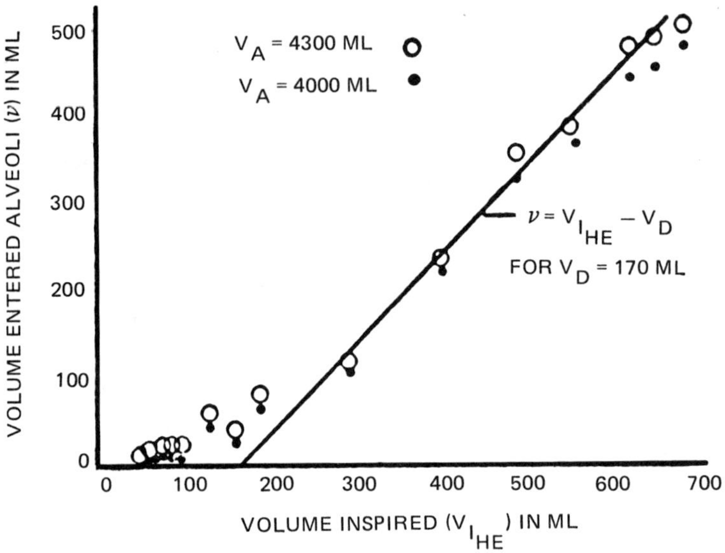

Figure 2 Volume of helium (ν) reaching the alveolar region plotted versus the inhaled volume. Note that ν is greater than zero even when the inhaled volume is less than the dead space. (From Briscoe et al., 1954.)

Emerson envisioned that this technique would be used superimposed on spontaneous or mechanical ventilation.

The first report of HFV with tidal volumes smaller than the dead space was provided by Lunkenheimer and colleagues (1972). They were developing a method for measuring cardiac performance based on the myocardial reaction to pericardial pressure oscillations generated by an "electromagnetic vibrator" at the airway opening. They employed tidal volumes of 10-20 ml and serendipitously found that after the end of an experimental run, the blood gases of the paralyzed dogs were normal (see Fig. 3).

This amazing result has subsequently been confirmed by a large number of investigators (Custer and Shannon, 1979; Bohn et al., 1980; Slutsky et al., 1980; Butler et al., 1980; Slutsky et al., 1981; Rossing et al., 1981) in animal models as well as human subjects. These data have stimulated research examining the gas mixing mechanisms that might explain these experimental results. The following section summarizes some of these concepts as applied to the lung.

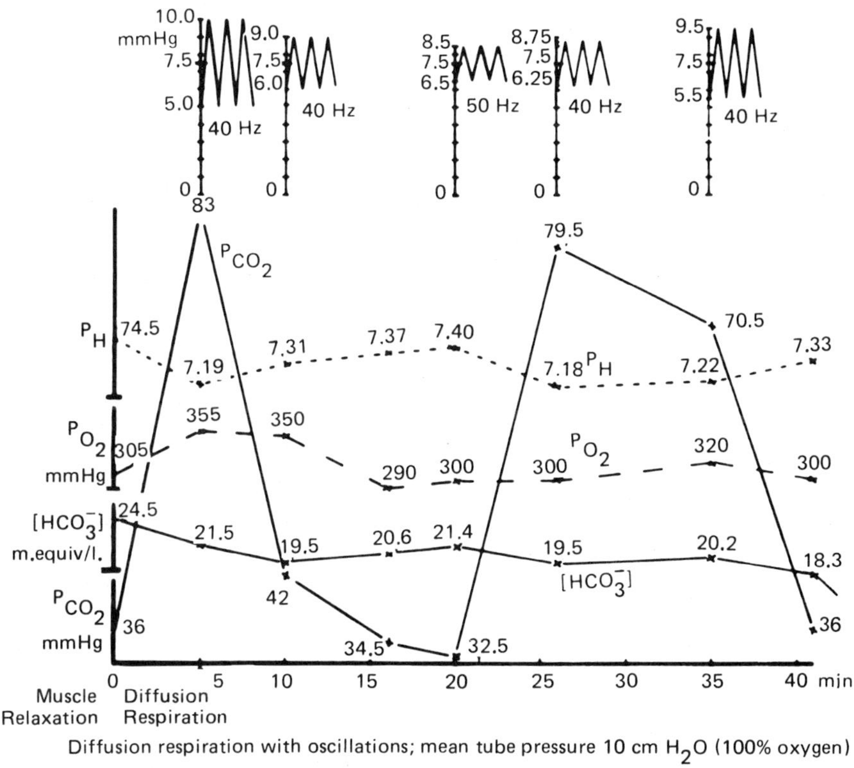

Figure 3 Arterial PO_2, PCO_2, and $[HCO_3^-]$ versus time during diffusion respiration (0-5 min) and during high-frequency oscillations of 40 or 50 Hz, as indicated at the top of the figure. (From Lunkenheimer et al., 1972.)

III. Mechanisms of Gas Transport

In the classical analysis of gas exchange, at end inspiration a certain fraction of the inhaled gas resides in the dead space (Fowler, 1948) while the rest is convected into the respiratory zone. The fraction reaching the respiratory zone, $(V_T - V_D)/V_T$ rapidly equilibrates with the gas which was there prior to inspiration (see Chap. 6 for details). Thus, during normal breathing, the dispersion that occurs as the front of fresh inspired gas traverses the airways has little effect on the rate of gas exchange. As the inspired volume is progressively reduced, however, a diminishing fraction of that volume reaches the respiratory zone and if one neglects the effects of mixing in the upper airways, alveolar ventilation will eventually fall to zero (as in the classical analysis). Consequently, in cases of low tidal volume, mechanisms that were considered unimportant when the tidal volume was large come to dominate the gas exchange process. High-frequency, low-volume ventilation lies within this regime of small tidal volume and one must therefore consider mechanisms of gas transport in addition to direct alveolar ventilation.

The different modes of gas transport that may be important during HFV are organized below in terms of fundamental mechanism. First, we discuss molecular diffusion alone. We then describe those mechanisms that involve axial (or longitudinal) convection. In the traditional description of gas flow through the conducting airways, the front of inspired gas moves into the lung retaining a distinct boundary between it and the resident gas in the lung. This represents the simplest case of axial convection, often termed "bulk flow." Next come a class of transport mechanisms that can collectively be termed "augmented dispersion," which we define as those mechanisms that involve an interaction between axial convection and radial or cross-stream mixing. The term "augmented dispersion" can be misleading when applied to steady flow since lateral mixing tends to *reduce* the rate of axial dispersion due to axial convection alone. The term is appropriate, however, in the case of purely oscillatory flow since the rate of transport is greater than would have occurred due to either axial convection or lateral transport alone.

A. Molecular Diffusion

In regions of the lung where the total cross-sectional area is very large and velocities are small, gas transport occurs primarily by means of molecular diffusion. The rate of transport ($\dot{V}$) is therefore governed by the Fick equation

$$\dot{V} = -D_{mol} \frac{A\ dC}{dx} \tag{1}$$

where D_{mol} is the molecular diffusion coefficient, A is the cross-sectional area available for exchange, and dC/dx is the local concentration gradient. The importance of molecular diffusion in gas exchange during normal breathing is discussed in Chapters 1 and 6. These same principles apply to HFV as well and will not be discussed further in this chapter.

B. Convection with No Cross-Stream Mixing

Bulk Flow Leading to Direct Alveolar Ventilation

When tidal volumes comparable to the anatomical dead-space volume are used for ventilation, some fraction of the inspired gas is likely to reach the respiratory zone due to asymmetries in path length between the longest and shortest routes to the gas exchange region (Rohrer, 1915; Ross, 1957). Under these circumstances, the regions of the lung being directly ventilated are likely to account for a significant fraction of the total gas exchange due to the high efficiency of bulk flow as a mechanism of transport. When direct alveolar ventilation occurs, gas exchange can be described by conventional methods of analysis. The rate of gas exchange is therefore proportional both to the breathing rate and to the difference between tidal volume and dead-space volume. As tidal volume increases, however, not only does the rate of gas exchange to regions that are directly ventilated increase, but the volumetric extent of the directly ventilated region also grows. Thus the gas exchange rate is a strong function of tidal volume (V_T) and aside from the increase in V_D with f, varies linearly with frequency at any given V_T.

The importance of direct alveolar ventilation can be demonstrated by the following example. According to the morphometric data of Ross (1957) the airway volumes to various bronchopulmonary segments of the dog vary considerably. If we assume, as he did, that the distribution of gas is directly proportional to the number of terminal bronchi and further, that each terminal bronchus is associated with an equal alveolar volume, the regions with the longest path lengths will cease to be directly ventilated when the tidal volume falls below about 150 ml, and the nearest regions when the tidal volume is less than 50 ml. For tidal volumes between these two limits, some variable fraction of the lung receives fresh gas directly with each inspiration. Later in this chapter (Sec. V.B, Kamm's model) estimates are made of pulmonary ventilation based on these published morphometric data and on assumptions concerning the distribution of inspired gas.

Pendelluft

At ordinary respiratory rates, the distribution of tidal volume is determined by local parenchymal compliances (Otis et al., 1956; Mead, 1969a) and all alveoli are ventilated in phase. In this circumstance it has been demonstrated that once inspired gas reaches airways about 0.5 mm in diameter [equivalent to the fifteenth generation in the model of Weibel (1963)], this gas rapidly equilibrates with the alveolar gas by molecular diffusion together with the effects of cardiogenic oscillations (Fukuchi et al., 1976). However, as respiratory frequencies and velocities increase, airway impedance exerts an increasing influence on gas flow and may result in alveoli ventilating asynchronously. This asynchronous ventilation has some important implications for alveolar gas exchange. For example, in Figure 4, a back-and-forth "sloshing" motion between two neighboring alveolar zones is shown. This convective motion will tend to make the gas contained in common airways uniform in composition.

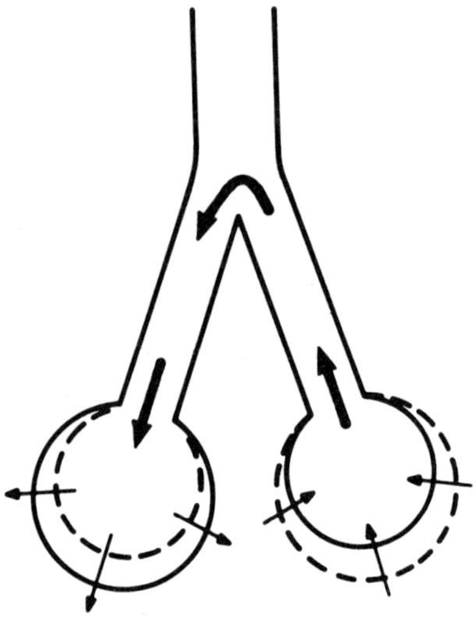

Figure 4 Schematic of asynchronous flow between two neighboring alveolar zones oscillating out of phase with each other (pendelluft) due, for example to asymmetries of input impedance. (From Kamm et al., 1984b.)

Several recent experiments have suggested that this asynchronous motion between adjacent alveolar regions might occur during high-frequency ventilation (Lehr, 1980; Lehr et al., 1982). In these experiments, an excised lung was excited at the trachea by high frequency (5-30 Hz), small-volume (<50 ml) oscillations, while the deformations of the outer surface were photographed by high-speed photography. Analysis of the films shows that different parts of the lung surface move out of phase with one another at frequencies above about 5 Hz, and that the distance decreases with increasing frequency. This motion will result in a flow of gas into neighboring alveolar regions that is also out of phase, producing the sloshing motion described above. Although the extent to which this influences the rate of gas exchange in a lung constrained by the thoracic cage cannot be easily ascertained, pendelluft will likely have a beneficial effect. However, no theoretical models have been used to predict quantitatively the effect of pendelluft on pulmonary gas transport.

Streaming

The term "streaming" is used here to denote the axial dispersion of a gas mixture that occurs in purely oscillatory flow as a result of a directionally asymmetric velocity profile—that is, the time-averaged velocity profile during inspiration differs from the time-averaged expiratory profile. For example, oscillatory flow in a diverging duct, as shown in Figure 5, would exhibit this effect. During the course of a single oscillation period, fluid particles in the

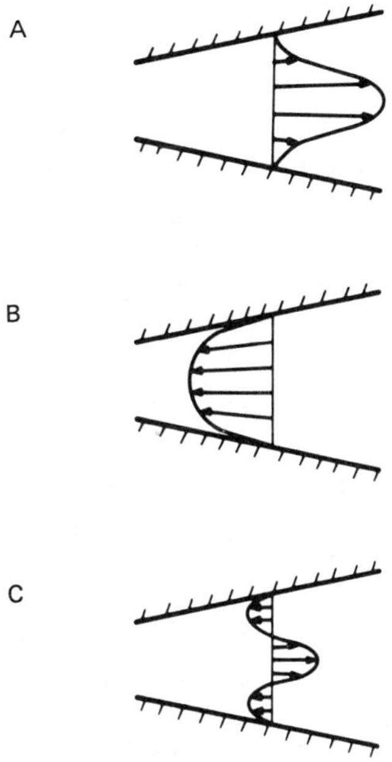

Figure 5 Velocity profiles in a tapered two-dimensional duct: (A) instantaneous profile for flow passing to the right; (B) instantaneous velocity profile when the flow direction is reversed; (C) time-averaged velocity profile for oscillatory flow. (From Kamm et al., 1983.)

core tend to move toward the right in the figure, whereas fluid near the wall moves leftward (Schlichting, 1968). Averaged over many cycles, the fluid undergoes a bidirectional flow which could result in a net exchange of fluid across a stationary reference plane as illustrated in Figure 5C. One might imagine "pure streaming" as a bidirectional flow with no mixing between streams. The net transport of a given species across any cross-sectional plane ($\dot{M}$) is simply the product of the bidirectional flow rate (Q_{bd}) and the difference in concentration between the two streams (ΔC):

$$\dot{M} = Q_{bd}\ \Delta C \tag{2}$$

From such simple expressions, the rate of exchange due to streaming could, in principle, be estimated once we know the cross-sectional velocity and concentration profiles. Although Menon et al. (1982) have recently measured velocity profiles under the appropriate conditions, we currently have no way of estimating the concentration profiles. The latter are influenced by many factors, including both the swirling motions that exist in the branching airways and the lateral exchange due to molecular diffusion that is certain to be important in the smaller airways. Because of these complexities, it may not be practical to calculate the rate of exchange due to streaming using expressions of the type given above.

In lieu of calculations based on the velocity and concentration profiles, axial exchange due to streaming can be demonstrated by experiments in which the dispersion is made visible by the use of tracers within the fluid. Haselton and Scherer (1980, 1982) have oscillated small particles suspended in a viscous liquid both within a branching network of tubes geometrically similar to the conducting airways of the lung and within a single bifurcation. Their findings clearly demonstrate (Haselton and Scherer, 1982) that particles introduced at the "mouth" will progressively penetrate throughout the entire branching network, even when tidal volumes are considerably less than the model volume.

For the purpose of comparison to transport by augmented dispersion, note that "pure streaming," as defined above, can occur in the absence of an axial concentration gradient. Moreover, it is optimized, for a particular situation, when a minimum amount of lateral or cross-stream mixing occurs. In practice, when the Reynolds number is sufficiently high, secondary swirling motions are present in the pulmonary airways and some lateral mixing will undoubtedly occur. In those circumstances, it is extremely difficult to separate streaming from augmented dispersion since the two act simultaneously. The experimental results obtained for steady or oscillatory flow in a branching network, discussed later, must therefore reflect transport due to both mechanisms.

C. Convection with Cross-Stream Mixing

Gas exchange can also occur through an interaction between axial convection and lateral or cross-stream mixing (in the plane perpendicular to the mean flow direction) which we call augmented dispersion. The lateral exchange can be due either to molecular diffusion as in laminar, unidirectional flows, or to convective mixing as in turbulent flows or flows with secondary swirling motions. The most familiar examples of augmented dispersion are those considered by Taylor for the case of steady duct flow: laminar flow in which lateral exchange is due to molecular diffusion* (Taylor, 1953), and turbulent flow in which convective mixing results from turbulent eddies (Taylor, 1954).

*This process is often referred to as "augmented diffusion" because the lateral transport is due to molecular diffusion. However, this term is somewhat misleading since in steady flow, molecular diffusion reduces the role of axial dispersion.

Straight Tube, Steady Flow

Lateral Transport by Molecular Diffusion

To illustrate augmented dispersion, consider the case of steady flow through a duct of circular cross section of a fluid mixture having a linear axial gradient in mean concentration which extends far upstream and downstream from the point of observation. If we adopt a reference frame moving with the mean speed of the fluid, the velocity profile will be as shown in Figure 6. Fluid in the core travels to the right with respect to this reference frame while fluid near the wall flows to the left. We define a bidirectional flow rate (Q_{bd}) as the volume flow integrated over the core of the tube from the centerline to the radial position where the local velocity in this moving reference frame passes through zero. Due to the concentration gradient, the core fluid coming from the region of high concentration has a higher average concentration than the fluid near the wall. As a result of this difference in mean concentration between the two streams, the net transport across this plane can be described again by Eq. (2), where ΔC now represents the difference between the mean concentration of the core fluid and the mean concentration of the wall fluid. At any instant in time, we can therefore estimate the rate of exchange given two pieces of information: (1) the velocity profile, and (2) the difference in mean concentration, ΔC.

For the simplest case of steady laminar flow through a tube of circular

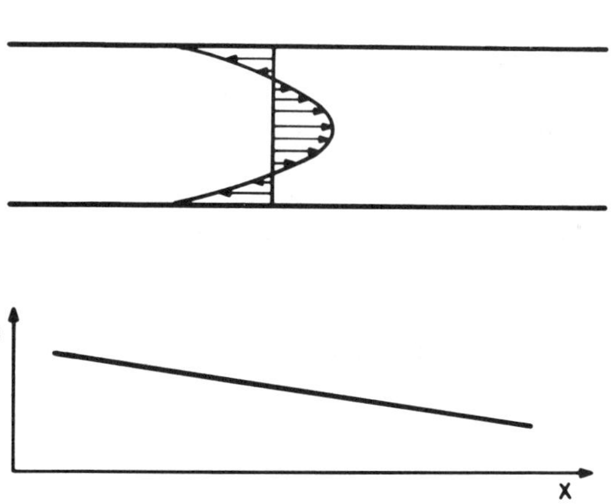

Figure 6 Top: Velocity profile during steady flow as seen by an observer traveling at the mean speed of the fluid. The bidirectional flow is computed by integrating the velocity distribution over the fraction of the tube cross-section in which the flow is to the right. Bottom: Gradient in the cross-sectional average concentration of some gas. (From Kamm et al., 1984b.)

cross section, the velocity profile in the stationary reference frame is parabolic and satisfies the relationship

$$u(r) = 2U\left[1 - \left(\frac{r}{a}\right)^2\right] \tag{3}$$

where U is the cross-sectional average velocity, a is the tube radius, and r is distance measured from the tube centerline. This corresponds to a bidirectional flow in the moving reference frame of

$$Q_{bd} = \frac{a^2 U}{4} \tag{4}$$

In general, the more nonuniform the velocity profile, the greater the bidirectional flow rate.

To determine the difference in mean concentration, we need to consider the nature of lateral transport. In the present case, because the flow is laminar and unidirectional, lateral exchange is due solely to molecular diffusion. Recognizing that the radial concentration difference is established through a balance between the mechanism that produced it–axial convection of high concentration fluid in the core–and that which dissipates it–radial molecular diffusion–we can estimate its magnitude as the product of the axial concentration gradient and the average distance a fluid particle travels in the time required for radial equilibration. The latter is approximated by the diffusion time, $K_1 a^2/D_{mol}$, where D_{mol} is the molecular diffusion coefficient and K_1 is a dimensionless coefficient. Therefore,

$$\Delta C = K_1 U \frac{a^2}{D_{mol}} \frac{dC}{dx} \tag{5}$$

When substituted into Eq. (2), we obtain

$$\dot{M} = \frac{K_1}{4} \frac{U^2 a^2}{D_{mol}} A \frac{dC}{dx} \tag{6}$$

This result can be expressed in a more familiar form if we define an effective diffusion coefficient as

$$D_{eff} = \frac{\dot{M}}{A(dC/dx)} \tag{7}$$

yielding for D_{eff}/D_{mol},

$$\frac{D_{eff}}{D_{mol}} = 1 + \frac{K_1}{4}\left(\frac{Ua}{D_{mol}}\right)^2 \tag{8}$$

where one has been added to the right-hand side to provide the correct limit as Ua/D_{mol} approaches zero. This is the general form for dispersion in steady, laminar flow (if $K_1 = 1/12$) (Aris, 1956).

Lateral Transport by Turbulent Mixing

If the flow is turbulent, the importance of molecular diffusion tends to diminish. The essential components of augmented dispersion (axial convection and lateral mixing) are, however, still present. The difference lies with the scaling of the lateral mixing process. This can be accounted for in one of two ways. First, if we continue to use the approximate method of analysis that enabled us to predict values for D_{eff} when molecular diffusion was important, we could simply replace the molecular diffusion coefficient by an appropriate form for the turbulent diffusivity (D_{turb}) (Tennekes and Lumley, 1972). Typically, the turbulent diffusivity scales with the axial velocity and the vessel radius yielding, by dimensional arguments, $D_{turb} \propto Ua$ (Pedley et al., 1977). Substituting this for D_{mol} in Eq. (8) immediately yields the expression

$$D_{eff} \propto Ua \tag{9}$$

This estimate agrees with the more rigorous prediction of Taylor (1954) for turbulent flow in pipes.*

Straight Tube, Oscillatory Flow

Dispersion in laminar oscillatory flow has recently been studied theoretically by a number of investigators (Farrell and Larson, 1973; Chatwin, 1975; Watson, 1983). Two regimes of dispersion have been identified which depend on whether the dispersion phenomenon is either quasi-steady or intrinsically unsteady. In the former case, the predictions for D_{eff} reduce to the steady flow result given above [Eq. (8)], where U is now the instantaneous cross-sectional mean velocity. In the latter, the velocity and concentration profiles are influenced by the effects of unsteadiness and gives rise to a D_{eff} that depends on the dimensionless frequency. The result for respiratory gases for which the Schmidt number ($Sc = \upsilon/D_{mol}$, where υ = kinematic viscosity) is approximately unity can be expressed as (Watson, 1983)

$$\frac{D_{eff}}{D_{mol}} = 1 + f(\alpha)\left(\frac{U_{rms}a}{D_{mol}}\right)^2 \tag{10}$$

---

*Taylor's exact expression can be written f(Re) × Ua, where f(Re) is a very weak function of Reynolds number having a value of order 1.

where U_{rms} is the root-mean-square value of the cross-sectional average velocity, α = dimensionless frequency (Womersley parameter) = $a(\omega/\upsilon)^{1/2}$, and $f(\alpha)$ ranges from a constant value of 1/48 for $\alpha < 1$ to $(\alpha + 3/\sqrt{2})/(\alpha^4 8\sqrt{2})$ for $\alpha >> 1$. This theoretical prediction has been verified for $1 < \alpha < 10$ by Joshi et al. (1983).

Although the theoretical development leading to Eq. (10) is beyond the scope of this chapter, the approximate method of analysis that led to Eq. (8) could also be used to describe oscillatory flows. In that limit, if the oscillations are sufficiently slow so that the flow is considered to be "quasi-steady" (e.g., for $\alpha < 1$ and Sc = 1), the instantaneous dispersion is described by Eq. (8) if U is taken to be the instantaneous mean velocity. The time-averaged transport is then given by Eq. (8) but with U replaced by U_{rms} as in the low-α limit of Eq. (10).

When the frequency of oscillation is high (e.g., $\alpha >> 1$ and Sc = 1) all variations in both the velocity and concentration profiles are confined to a narrow boundary layer adjacent to the vessel wall. Assuming approximately a linear velocity profile inside the boundary layer of thickness δ which varies as $\sqrt{\upsilon/\omega}$ (where ω = angular frequency = $2\pi f$), the bidirectional flow rate scales with $Ua\delta$. Since the boundary layer never penetrates to the core of the tube, the concentration difference between the wall and core fluid is approximately $(L_{st}/2)\ dC/dx$, where L_{st} is the average displacement of a fluid particle per stroke. Combining these in an expression of the form of Eq. (8), one obtains

$$D_{eff} \sim \frac{Re^2}{\alpha^3}$$

which is consistent with the high-frequency limit of Eq. (10) when Sc = 1.

Lateral Transport by a Secondary Velocity Field

The salient characteristic of turbulent flow for augmented dispersion is the cross-stream mixing produced by the turbulent eddy motion. All flows that transport fluid between streamlines of different axial velocity possess this trait and will therefore impede axial exchange. The velocities set up in the plane perpendicular to the tube axis when flow traverses a bend or bifurcation serve this purpose. The essential difference between the effect of turbulence and that of an organized secondary velocity field is that while turbulence produces random motions (when viewed over a time scale long compared to the longest time scale of the turbulence), laminar secondary flows, although often very complex, are nonrandom in character and hence deterministic (to the extent that molecular diffusion can be ignored). The most important implication of this is that while lateral transport by turbulence can be modeled as a diffusionlike process, laminar convective motions, in general, cannot.

The simplest flow in which secondary motions interact with axial transport is that in a curved tube. Tube curvature has two effects on axial transport. First, the velocity profile (at least for steady flow) is somewhat skewed toward the outside of the bend due to the convection of high-velocity fluid away from the center of curvature. As we demonstrated in the order-of-magnitude estimate of augmented dispersion in laminar flow, the velocity profile, in that it affects the value of Q_{bd}, also exerts an influence over axial transport. In general, the more nonuniform the axial velocity profile, the greater Q_{bd} and therefore the greater the rate of axial transport. Second, the secondary velocity field tends to increase the rate of lateral mixing, thereby tending to decrease ΔC and reduce axial transport. Experimental measurements (von Andel et al., 1964) and a theoretical analysis (Ergodan and Chatwin, 1967) applicable to cases of small curvature demonstrate that axial dispersion is generally reduced due to curvature. This is due to the dominance of the effects of lateral mixing. Notably, both studies indicated that axial transport behaves as a diffusive process even though the mechanism of lateral transport may not.

Unfortunately, these secondary flows are sufficiently complex even in a tube of uniform curvature that a generally applicable theoretical analysis has not been developed. Networks such as the lung with numerous bifurcations pose even greater difficulties. Although these studies in straight and curved tubes provide useful insight into the mechanisms of transport that must also prevail in the lung, the expressions derived above clearly have limited applicability. For this reason it is necessary to rely largely on empirical data in systems with lunglike geometry.

IV. Measurements of Gas Transport in Hardware Models

A. A Dimensional Analysis of Unsteady Dispersion

To provide a framework for the consideration of experimental results, it is useful first to derive a nondimensional form for the axial dispersion coefficient in a system of arbitrary geometry. We begin by recognizing that D_{eff} will, in general, depend on the following dimensional parameters:

$$D_{eff} = f_1\ (u,\omega,a,\nu,D_{mol},g) \tag{11}$$

where ω is the oscillation frequency in radians per second, and g symbolically represents all the parameters associated with airway geometry other than scale which is defined by the tube radius, a. This function can be expressed in dimensionless form as

$$\frac{D_{eff}}{D_{mol}} = f_2(Pe,\alpha,Sc,G) \tag{12}$$

where G denotes all dimensionless parameters having to do exclusively with system geometry and Pe = Péclet number = $2ua/D_{mol}$.

When dealing with gases, axial molecular diffusion by itself can be significant. Therefore, it is more convenient to separate this effect from augmented transport and write Eq. (12) as

$$D_1 = \frac{D_{eff} - D_{mol}}{D_{mol}} = f_3(Pe,\alpha,Sc,G) \tag{13}$$

In studies conducted in liquids, or for the transport of aerosols in gas, D_{mol} is generally small compared to υ. Hence the effects of molecular diffusion can be neglected and Eq. (13) can be expressed as

$$D_2 = \frac{D_{eff}}{\upsilon} = f_4(Re,\alpha,G) \tag{14}$$

Under certain circumstances, one or more of the dimensionless groups in Eq. (13) can be eliminated. Several examples are of particular interest in the following discussions. If the flow were quasi-steady, D_1 would be independent of α. If the flow were highly turbulent, convective mixing would overwhelm the effects of molecular diffusion and Sc would consequently have little effect. If the flow were both quasi-steady and highly turbulent, we would expect D_1 to be independent of α and Sc.

B. Steady Flow Experiments

In the case of steady flow through a system of fixed geometry (constant G), the dimensionless dispersion coefficient can be expressed in general form as

$$D_1 = f(Pe,Sc)$$

This is consistent with the results of Scherer et al. (1975), who studied steady flow through a five-generation network using benzene vapor. Tests were conducted for a range of conditions ($30 < Re < 2000$) typical of normal breathing. Scherer et al. found that their results could be expressed as

$$D_1 = 0.37Pe_0 \tag{15a}$$

for steady expiratory flow, and

$$D_1 = 1.08Pe_0 \tag{15b}$$

for steady inspiratory flow, where Pe_0 is the Péclet number based on the spatial mean velocity in the parent tube of the network. Haselton and Scherer (1979) later demonstrated that these results can be explained on the basis of purely convective transport.

C. Oscillatory Flow Experiments

Experiments to study transport during oscillatory flow have recently been conducted by Tarbell et al. (1982) and Kamm et al. (1984a) in similar branching geometries constructed from tubes of constant diameter. Both groups used a symmetric system of branching Y tubes with a length-to-diameter ratio of 3.5:1. Although the measurement techniques differed considerably, as did the conduct of the experiment, the results exhibited some basic similarities. The results can be summarized as

$$D_1 = \frac{0.078\ Pe^{1.66}}{(\alpha\sqrt{Sc})^{1.45}} \tag{16}$$

from Kamm et al. ($Pe = Re \cdot Sc$ and Re is the Reynolds number based on the cross-sectional mean velocity amplitude in the generation where measurements were made and on tube diameter), and

$$D_2 = \frac{0.00028 Re_0{}^{1.82}}{\alpha^{0.86}} \tag{17}$$

from Tarbell et al., where Re_0 is based on velocity amplitude and tube diameter in the "zeroth" generation. Here Eq. (16) is applicable to gases ($Sc = 0.8$)* and Eq. (17) applies to liquids with high Schmidt numbers. The experiments of Kamm et al. were conducted over a lower range of Reynolds number ($35 < Re < 1100$) than were those of Tarbell et al. ($200 < Re < 10{,}000$).

---

*While the molecular diffusivity is included in Eq. (16), the experiments were conducted with only a single gas mixture. Therefore, there could be an additional dependence on Schmidt number that was not evident in these experiments.

Due to differences in the way the two experiments were conducted, it is difficult to make a direct comparison between the two expressions given above. Equation (16) represents a local transport coefficient based on measurements across a single tube in the network, whereas Eq. (17) reflects the transport characteristics of the entire network. If, for the sake of comparison, we assume that Eq. (17) approximately represents the characteristics of the transport process near the point at which the tracer was injected, we can recast the equation in terms of the Reynolds number in the second generation, changing the numerical coefficient from 0.00028 to 0.0035. In so doing, values of the transport coefficient predicted by the two expressions are found to differ by no more than a factor of 4 within the parameter range covered in both experiments.

The extent to which the two expressions [Eqs. (16) and (17)] agree suggests that the rate of transport is independent of D_{mol} since one was obtained using a liquid mixture while the other used gases. As the expressions are somewhat different, both in terms of the numerical prediction and in the relative importance of unsteadiness, the question of the importance of molecular diffusion must remain unresolved until further experiments are completed. If D_{eff} is shown to be independent of D_{mol}, we can conclude that lateral mixing occurs largely by virtue of convective motions rather than by molecular diffusion. In that case it would be more appropriate to replace Pe by Re, and $\alpha\sqrt{Sc}$ by α, in Eq. (16). The differences between these expressions might also be due to a transition to turbulence in the range of parameters examined in the experiments of Tarbell and associates.

With regard to HFV, the rate of gas exchange is often expressed in terms of the frequency and tidal volume of oscillation. The results of Kamm et al. can therefore be expressed as

$$D_1 \propto f^{0.94} V_T{}^{1.66}$$

Tarbell's experiments yield the following proportionality:

$$D_2 \propto f^{1.39} V_T{}^{1.82}$$

The expressions given above help to identify different regimes of transport that occur in HFV. Specifically:

1. When Pe (or Re) is sufficiently small, the enhancement of axial transport due to either streaming or augmented dispersion becomes insignificant.
2. Although there appear to be some differences between the liquid and gas results, suggesting a significant influence due to molecular diffusion, these differences are rather small and therefore are not conclusive.

V. Theories of Gas Exchange During HFV

A. Assumptions Basic to All Models

Quantities that Are Not Known: Airway Geometry and Airflow Distribution

Each of the mechanisms for gas mixing described previously can be used in the prediction of gas exchange rates during HFV (i.e., in a computational model of gas exchange by HFV). In order to make these predictions, a number of characteristics of the lung and the flow of gas within it must be determined or assumed. These include airway lengths, airway diameters, airway branching angles, airway wall characteristics, the distribution of volume flow among the various airways, and the flow regime within each airway branch. Since none of this information is known with the precision needed to make quantitative predictions, various investigators have made certain specific assumptions about each of these aspects of pulmonary behavior during HFV, and have developed models based on these assumptions.

Common Assumptions

Most models are based on the assumption that the airways are relatively rigid and that their geometry is that given by Weibel (1963) for human lungs or by Horsfield and Cumming (1976) or Ross (1957) for dog lungs. Airflow is assumed to be partitioned among airways on the basis of the parenchymal volume subtended by each or on the basis of local complex impedances. With this information, it is possible to determine the character of the flow that will prevail within the airways by calculating appropriate parameters of the flow such as Re or α. Once these parameters are known, their values can be used to help determine which specific physical mechanisms may control gas transport at any given location in the lung and which of the theoretically or empirically determined equations discussed in Sections III and IV are most appropriate.

Validity of Assumptions

Although there are detailed morphometric models for both human and dog lungs which give airway lengths and diameters, information about how these airways change in size with lung volume or during an oscillatory cycle is known in substantially less detail. Similarly, the factors that influence gas flow and its distribution are not known in any great detail and their study constitutes the entire discipline of pulmonary oscillation mechanics. Further, most of the theoretical and experimental studies of oscillation mechanics assume or make use of low-amplitude oscillations (<50 ml/sec; Fulton et al., 1982) so that analysis by linear theory will be valid. However, during HFV, flow amplitudes are relatively large and can exceed 2000 ml/sec. Thus results based on studies at low flows are probably not valid. Since the gas transport predicted by any model may depend to a substantial extent on the precise values used in calculations, this is an area where assumptions can substantially influence results.

B. Gas Transport Models

A number of investigators have incorporated the various gas transport mechanisms mentioned earlier into models that can be used to predict overall gas transport rates during HFV. We will review them in the chronological order in which they appeared.

Fredberg Model

This was the first model that made specific predictions of gas transport rates during HFV (with V_T less than the dead space) under a number of physiological conditions (Fredberg, 1980). The model is based on a number of assumptions: (1) that gas flow during HFV can be considered turbulent and quasi-steady; as such, relationships for gas transport can be calculated from known steady-flow relationships; and (2) each airway generation can be considered as an independent resistance to gas exchange and that the time averaged tracer flux through it during oscillatory flow will depend only on the specific concentration difference across it (i.e., these gas transport resistors are linear).

It is worthwhile to consider the justification for these assumptions. Fredberg argued for the quasi-steady assumption on the basis that the time scale of oscillation was long compared to the lifetime of turbulent eddies in the upper airways and that α was small in the peripheral airways. For example, the time scale of oscillation is on the order of 100 msec (10 Hz), while a turbulent eddy, for flow conditions in the upper airways, has a lifetime on the order of 1 msec. Further, in the airways, where flow should be laminar, he computed α to be of order unity or less. These arguments were the basis for the steadiness assumption. Further, in the airways where laminar flow might exist, the local Pe number (= ud/D_{mol}) was near unity and he argued that augmentation due to augmented diffusion was likely to be negligible. As a result, he claimed that the relationship given by Taylor for diffusivity in turbulent flow could be applied to all airways.

The use of gas transport resistance was justified on the basis that over an integer number of cycles convective transport was negligible. With this assumption he was able to show that a resistance to gas transport could be calculated for each airway generation and that the value of the resistance would depend on the amplitude of the applied oscillatory flow, the length, and the cross-sectional area of the airway in question.

Fredberg computed gas transport rates by first determining the distribution of airflow that would prevail within the lung at a given applied oscillatory pressure gradient. From this distribution of airflow he computed the resistance to gas transport of each airway generation and summed them as one would sum electrical resistances in a network. Once the total resistance to gas transport was known, gas transport rates could easily be determined.

He made a number of specific predictions based on this analysis. First he predicted that the gas exchange rates resulting from HFV would depend only on the applied flow amplitude (product of f and V_T) and not on the specific values to achieve this flow. This prediction arises from his assumption that the turbulent dispersion relationship given by Taylor (which is proportional to flow) controls gas transport throughout the airways. He further predicted that at a given applied frequency and tidal volume, altering lung volume would not alter gas transport rates. This arises because as lung volume increases, although local flow velocities decrease, local areas increase in proportion to decreasing velocities and their product (and therefore the resistance to gas transport) remains constant. This theory has been tested in a number of experimental settings as outlined in Section VI.

Model of Slutsky and Co-Workers

Slutsky and co-workers (1980) introduced another model based on an analysis similar to the one proposed by Fredberg (1980), but it differed in a number of ways. These workers divided the lung into three gas mixing zones: the alveolar region, the small airways, and the central airways (Fig. 7). In the central airways flow was modeled as turbulent and their analysis is similar to that offered by Fredberg. The difference in the model is in the small airways. Specifically, Slutsky and colleagues argued that gas transport within the zone of laminar flow could alter overall gas transport. In the laminar zone they used the relationships developed by Chatwin (1975) and Watson (1983) to describe the local effective diffusivity, while simple molecular diffusion was assumed to apply in the alveolar zone. They used the same approach as Fredberg in that a resistance to gas transport was calculated for each airway generation and from these resistances overall transport rates were determined. In addition to predicting gas transport due to HFV, this model

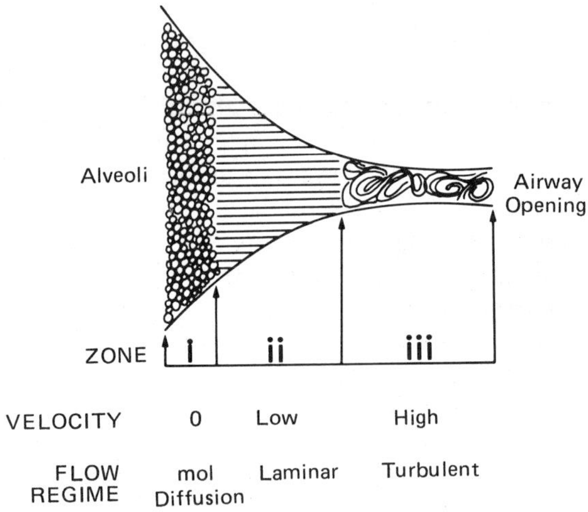

Figure 7 Schematic diagram of the cross-sectional area of the lung from the alveolar region (on the right) to the airway opening (on the left). The change in cross-sectional area is orders of magnitude greater than shown. Gas velocities and mixing regimes associated with each region are also shown. (From Slutsky and Brown, 1982.)

was also used to predict the enhanced mixing secondary to cardiogenic oscillations (Slutsky, 1981).

One additional important difference between the model offered by Fredberg and that of Slutsky and co-workers was that an allowance was made for convective gas transport near the airway opening and near the alveolar zone. Slutsky and colleagues (1981) reasoned that the resistance to gas transport in the airways near the airway opening would be reduced due to the effective removal of CO_2 from all gas that passes the bias flow location. Similarly, all gas that is convected into the alveolar zone is well mixed by molecular diffusion. Thus they set the resistance to zero in these two regions, which had the effect of introducing a tidal volume dependent decrement in overall transport resistance at a given total airway flow ($f \cdot V_T$ product).

Predictions from the theoretical model were presented in terms of the CO_2 removal rate ($\dot{V}CO_2$), for any given f and V_T, that would occur if the alveolar PCO_2 could be maintained constant at a value equal to 40 mmHg.

It is thus an index which is dependent on the efficacy of the HFV and not on the metabolic CO_2 production ($\dot{V}CO_2{}^M$). The steady-state Pa_{CO_2} can then be predicted for any $\dot{V}CO_2$ by taking the ratio of $\dot{V}CO_2{}^M/\dot{V}CO_2$ and multiplying by 40 mmHg. This approach was taken to facilitate comparisons with experimental results (see Sec. VI). The model predicts that for values of f less than about 25 Hz and V_T less than the anatomic dead space, CO_2 elimination ($\dot{V}CO_2$) varies relatively linearly with $f \cdot V_T$ and will be relatively independent of lung volume if the lung increases in size isotropically (lengths and diameters increase proportionally). The explanation for the relative unimportance of V_L is that with an increase in V_L there are two competing phenomena occurring simultaneously. First, the increasing cross-sectional area of the airway tends to increase $\dot{V}CO_2$ in the alveolar zone. However, at any fV_T the Reynolds number decreases as the diameter of the tube increases; thus regions of the lung that were originally turbulent may become laminar. Since for $Re < 100$, the calculated effective diffusivity is smaller if determined by the equations for laminar dispersion than by the equations for turbulent dispersion, altering the "extent" of a lung zone will alter transport rates. Even though there are factors that tend to enhance and inhibit transport, the net effect is very little change in $\dot{V}CO_2$ with increasing V_L,

A further feature of this model is the tidal volume dependence of gas transport introduced to account for convective purging at a given overall flow rate ($f \cdot V_T$ product). As a result of this addition, increasing V_T and decreasing f results in a lower overall resistance and increased gas transport. The predictions that arise from this model are shown in Figure 8. This model has recently been changed to incorporate the effects of convection in a more realistic fashion (Khoo et al., 1984). Predictions from this model are very close to those of the earlier model at low V_T ($\lesssim$20 ml), but the revised model also provides realistic estimates of gas transport during normal tidal ventilation, whereas the earlier model was only valid at V_T values below V_D.

Model of Permutt and Co-Workers

These investigators (Mitzner et al., 1983) modeled the airways as a series of gas exchange compartments and calculated dispersions based on an assumed gamma distribution of transit times within the airways. They argued, based on these considerations, that an effective diffusivity coefficient could be shown to depend only on the local stroke length (V_T divided by area) squared and the applied oscillatory frequency. If this concept is applied to the entire lung and if the imposed overall concentration gradient is not a

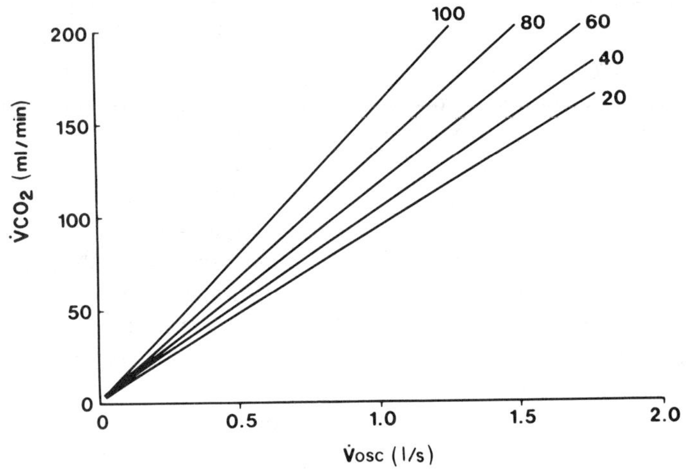

Figure 8 Theoretical results of $\dot{V}CO_2$ versus $\dot{V}OSC$ using the resistive model and the boundary conditions of zero resistance within a distance correspondign to one-half the tidal volume at the airway opening and at the alveolar region. (Adapted from Slutsky et al., 1981.)

function of f and VT, their model predicts that overall gas exchange will vary as $f \cdot VT^2$ rather than the $f \cdot VT$ predicted by the Fredberg model.

Model of Kamm and Associates

This model is a distinct departure from the previous three models in that the effects of gas mixing in the conducting airways are ignored; the effects of a variety of gas transport path lengths are considered. As such, it examines specifically the importance of direct convection to the respiratory zones made possible by the nonuniform distribution of path lengths from mouth to alveoli found in a real lung. The model is based on four assumptions: (1) no mixing occurs in the conducting airways; (2) once gas passes into the local alveolar space, it is instantaneously mixed with the local resident gas; and (3) the respiratory exchange ratio is approximately 1 (Kamm et al., 1984b).

In their description of local gas transport, both local blood flow and local ventilation were considered leading to the result shown in Figure 9. For tidal volumes less than that required to reach the closest alveolar zone (VT = 50 ml), no CO_2 transport is predicted. At each tidal volume greater than this value, CO_2 transport is at first a linear function of frequency. However, as local ventilation exceeds the ability of local blood flow to deliver CO_2

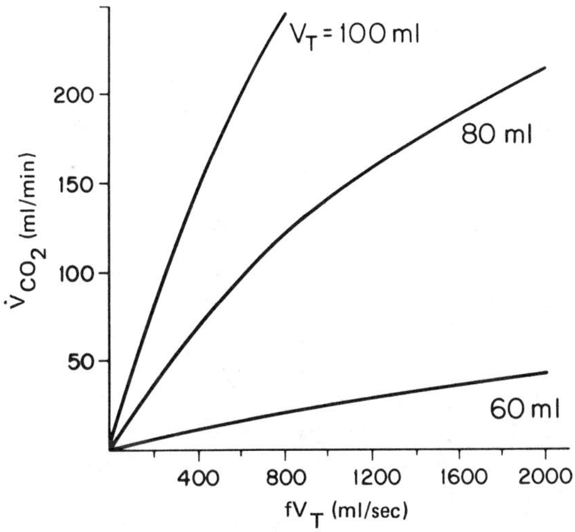

Figure 9 Predicted CO_2 elimination using the model for direct alveolar ventilation. (From Kamm et al., 1984b.)

to the alveolar zone in question (by increasing f), CO_2 removal becomes blood-flow limited and $\dot{V}CO_2$ becomes less dependent on frequency.

In these computational models various investigators have combined known physical mechanisms and lunglike geometry to predict gas transport during HFV. In the following section, we compare these model predictions to actual experimental data.

VI. Physiological Studies

Although a large number of studies have been published on the use of HFV, many have been clinically oriented and do not provide insight into the mechanisms operative during HFV. In this section we review some of the physiologic studies that allow conclusions to be drawn about the gas mixing mechanisms.

A. Animal Studies

Studies in Normal Animals

One of the original studies to present data on HFV at a number of frequencies was that by Bohn et al. (1980). They ventilated dogs using a piston pump that produced a tidal volume of about 25% of the dog's estimated dead space applied at frequencies of 5-30 Hz. They found that the lowest Pa_{CO_2} was obtained at 15 Hz (Fig. 10) and using this frequency they suc-

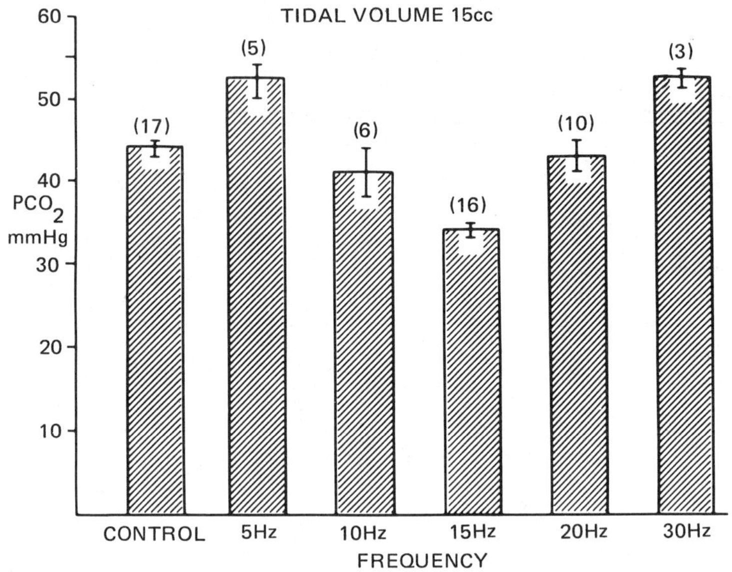

Figure 10 Arterial blood gases versus oscillatory frequency in anesthetized paralyzed dogs during conventional mechanical ventilation and high-frequency oscillation. The stroke volume of the piston pump was 15 ml. (From Bohn et al., 1980.)

cessfully ventilated a number of dogs over a 5-hr period. Although these data suggested that there was an optimum frequency (15 Hz) for CO_2 elimination, this was probably related to the specifics of their experimental setup. Although their piston pump generated a constant stroke volume, they had no independent measure of the volume actually entering the animal. This volume was a function of the ratio of the dog's impedance to the impedance of the tubing delivering gas to and removing gas from the airway opening (Froese and Bryan, 1981).

Slutsky and co-workers (1980) expanded these observations by developing an experimental circuit that allowed quantification of the tidal volume delivered to the subject (Fig. 11). The critical feature is the bias flow of gas which consists of a high-impedance fresh gas source and a vacuum source, also of high impedance. The fresh gas is bled through a needle valve from the high-pressure source and in a similar manner, a vacuum sink removes gas from the circuit into a low-pressure reservoir. Mean airway pressure is independently controlled by adjusting the vacuum pressure. There are two main advantages to this system. First, the pressure excursions at the airway open-

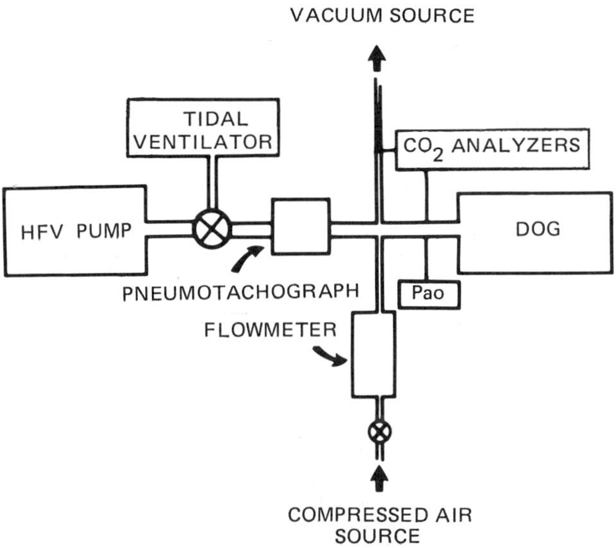

Figure 11 Schematic diagram of the experimental apparatus used to obtain the results shown in Figures 12 and 13. See the text for details. (From Slutsky et al., 1980.)

ing due to the high-frequency oscillations are a very small fraction of the pressure losses across the needle valves and thus do not significantly affect the magnitude of the bias flow. Therefore, virtually all the tidal volume generated by the pump and measured by the pneumotachygraph enters the experimental subject, with no loss to the bias flow circuit. Second, all the gas must leave the system via the vacuum sink, and thus it is possible to determine the rate of CO_2 elimination ($\dot{V}CO_2$) quickly (~30 sec) by multiplying the CO_2 concentration (after an initial transient) in the bias flow times the bias flow rate.

This experimental setup was used to quantify the effects of frequency (f), tidal volume (V_T), and lung volume (V_L) on $\dot{V}CO_2$. Results from initial studies in four anesthetized paralyzed dogs used oscillatory frequencies from 4 to 28 Hz and V_T values of 20-85% of the anatomic dead space. As shown in Figure 12, the important variable in determining $\dot{V}CO_2$ appeared to be the $f \cdot V_T$ product. In a subsequent study (Slutsky et al., 1981), the effects of increasing f at a constant V_T were determined. As shown in Figure 13, $\dot{V}CO_2$ increased roughly linearly with f at any constant V_T, with greater values of V_T producing greater values of $\dot{V}CO_2$ It was possible to achieve

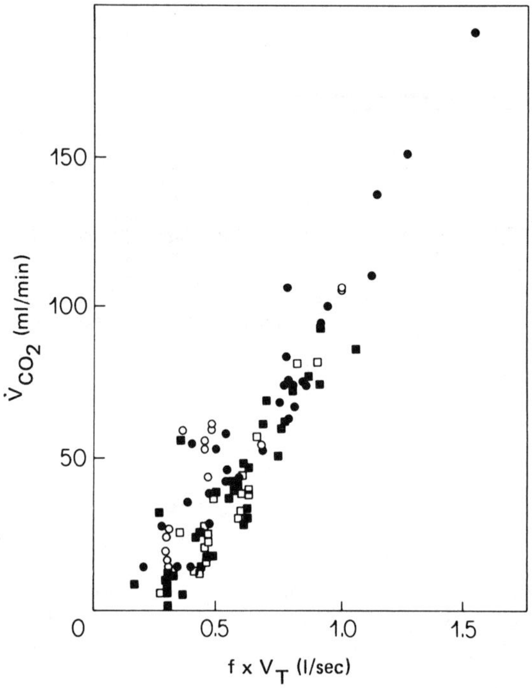

Figure 12 Experimental results for CO_2 elimination ($\dot{V}CO_2$) versus f·VT in four anesthetized paralyzed dogs. (From Slutsky et al., 1980.)

eucapnia in these dogs with VT as low as 40 ml (~40% of the anatomic plus equipment dead space) when the oscillating frequency was about 15-20 Hz. In addition, the effects of f and VT on $\dot{V}CO_2$ were quantified and it was found that at any f·VT product, the $\dot{V}CO_2$ was greater at larger VT values. The results for the 13 dogs were summarized using the equation

$$\dot{V}CO_2 = afVT\left(\frac{VT}{VTo}\right)^b\left(\frac{f}{fo}\right)^c$$

where VTo and fo were the mean values of VT and f, respectively, and a, b, and c were determined using regression techniques. The mean values of these constants were a = 2.1×10^{-3}, b = 0.49, and c = 0.076. At a constant f·VT, the $\dot{V}CO_2$ increased 35% as VT was doubled (and f decreased to one-half). $\dot{V}CO_2$ was also found to be independent of lung volume when studied at a frequency of 16 Hz and at values of f·VT < 1.5 liters/sec.

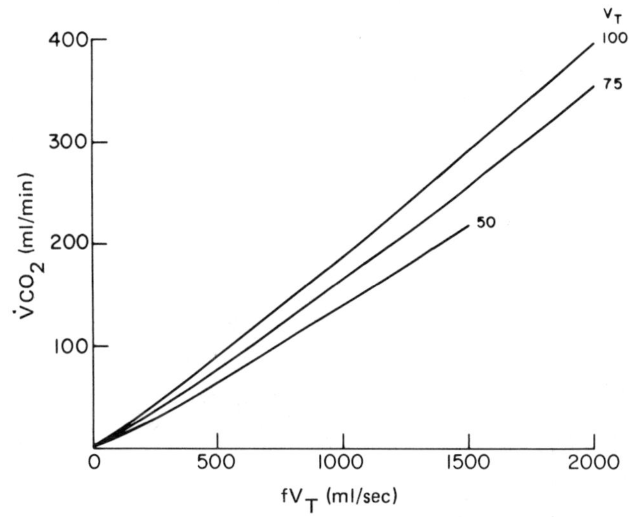

Figure 13 Summary of experimental results of $\dot{V}CO_2$ versus f•VT in 13 dogs showing the independent effect of VT in determining $\dot{V}CO_2$ (at any given f•VT). (Adapted from Slutsky et al., 1981.)

Schmid et al. (1981) used the clearance of ^{133}Xe after equilibration in the lung to examine gas mixing mechanisms during HFV. They found that interregional mixing of ^{133}Xe occurred during the oscillations (Fig. 14), where the regional concentration of Xe increased transiently after the start of HFV in nondependent regions (AND and BND), whereas in the basal dependent region (BD), ^{133}Xe cleared immediately and rapidly. Further, increasing f resulted in faster and more uniform pulmonary ^{133}Xe clearance rates. On the other hand, Robertson et al. (1982), in a study using three different density carrier gases, came to the conclusion that there appears to be extensive intraregional gas mixing during HFV.

To determine whether molecular diffusion constitutes the rate-limiting step in gas transport, during HFV, two groups have studied the effect of HFV on the gas transport of tracer gases (Knopp et al., 1983; Kaethner et al., 1984). Knopp et al. (1983) measured the washout from dogs' lungs of trace amounts of He and SF_6 (D_{mol} for He is about nine times that of SF_6) using varying stroke volumes and oscillation frequencies (10-30 Hz). They found that the washout could be described as the sum of two exponentials (see Fig. 15), and that there were no significant differences between the time constants for He and SF_6. They concluded that in the range of diffu-

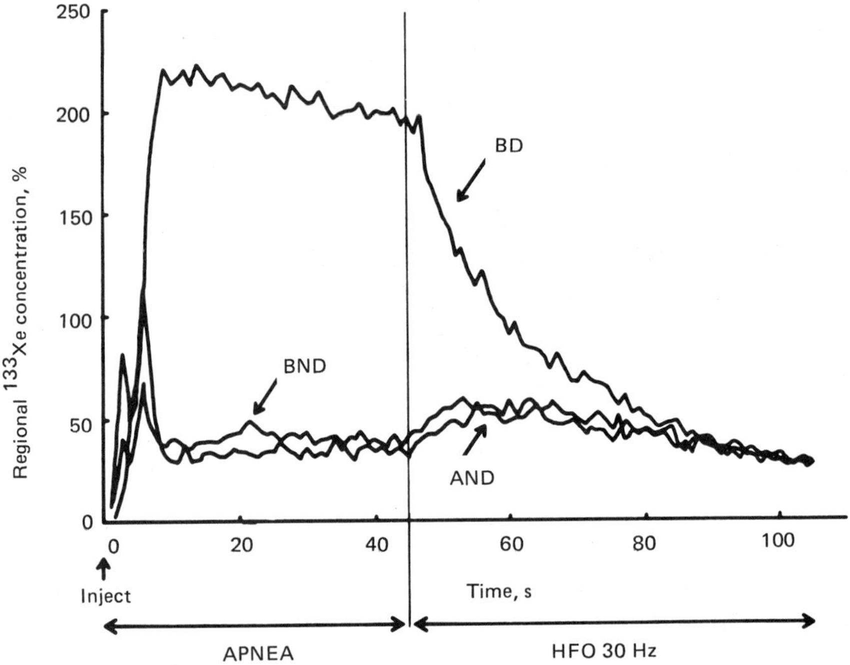

Figure 14 Plots of regional ^{133}Xe concentrations after injection into the right atrium during apnea and during high-frequency oscillations in one dog. Lung regions: AND, Apical nondependent; BND, basal nondependent; BD, basal dependent. (From Schmid et al., 1981.)

sivities studied, molecular diffusion does not constitute a rate-limiting step in the airways, during ventilation with HFV.

Kaethner et al. (1983) used a somewhat different technique to determine the importance of D_{mol} during HFV. Following equilibration with He and SF_6, dogs' lungs were partially washed out using either HFV or conventional mechanical ventilation. Immediately thereafter, expirograms of inert gas concentration versus time were obtained. The Fowler dead spaces calculated from these curves were identical for He and SF_6. Plots of concentration versus linear distance showed that most of the concentration drop (therefore, most of the resistance to gas transport) occurred along the endotracheal tube and the upper airways with no difference between He and SF_6. These data are similar to those of Knopp et al. (1983), supporting the concept that gas transport in the upper airways is not diffusion limited. However, for regions cor-

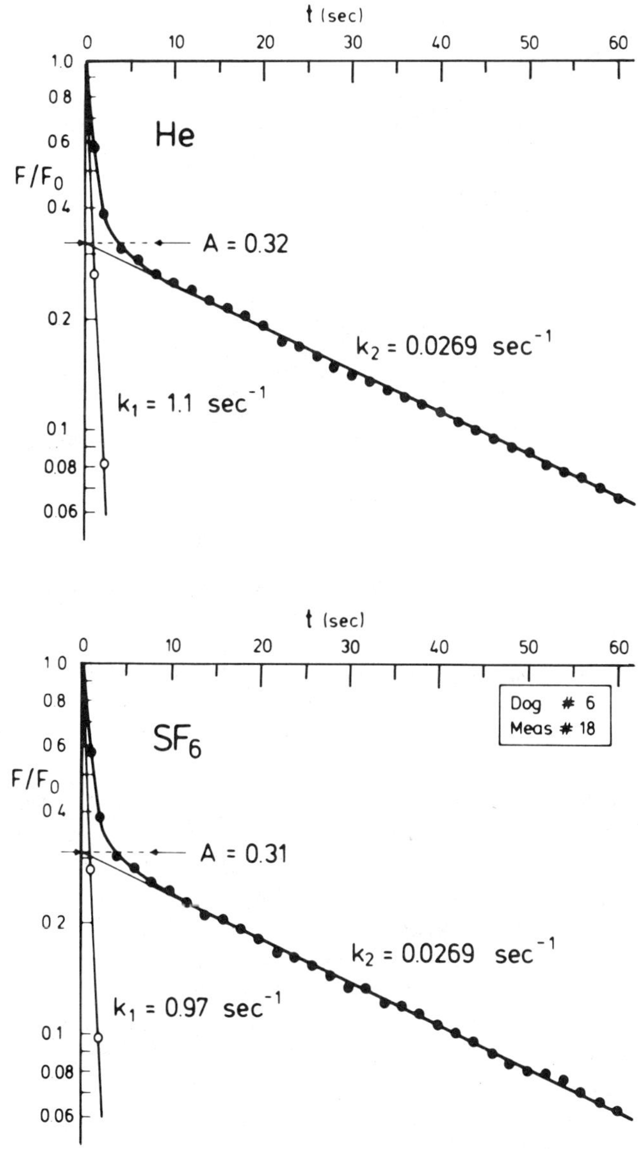

Figure 15 Semilogarithmic plots of normalized concentration versus time for He and SF_6 during high-frequency oscillations. Note that the rate constants (k_1 and k_2) for the two gases are identical. (From Knopp et al., 1983.)

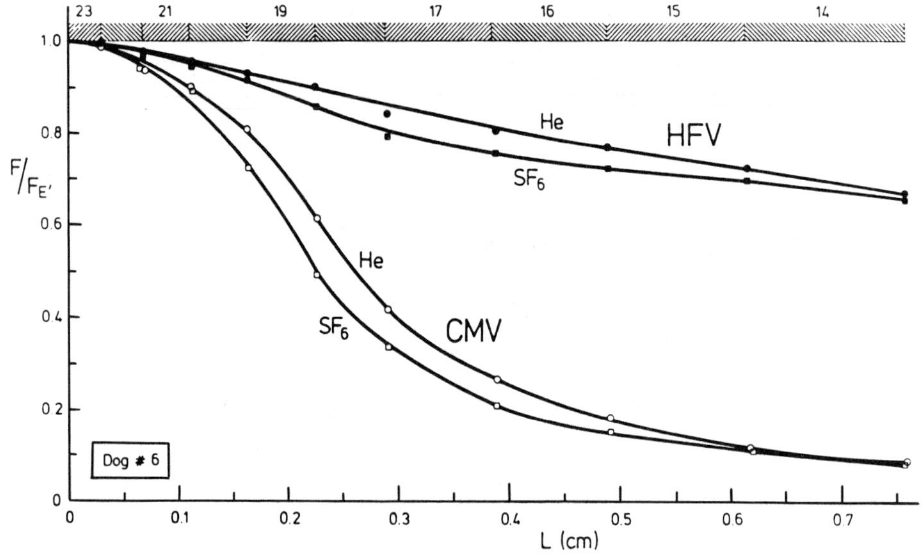

Figure 16 Concentration profiles of He and SF_6 calculated from expirograms for HFV and CMV. The concentrations are normalized to end-expired levels, FE'. The x axis has been converted from exhaled volume to linear distance using model A of Weibel (1963). Weibel generations are denoted at the top of the figure. (From Kaethner et al., 1984.)

responding to the alveolar zone, the plots of trace concentration versus linear distance into the lung showed separation of He and SF_6 (Fig. 16). These data show that gas transport in the alveolar regions is limited by diffusion, although it does not appreciably limit overall gas transport during HFV. However, under conditions in which the resistance of the endotracheal tube and upper airway is bypassed (e.g., when the bias flow is introduced at the carina) the gas transport resistance in the alveolar region may become rate limiting.

Of note, one reported study in rabbits suggested that it was not possible to provide adequate alveolar ventilation when the tidal volumes were smaller than the anatomical dead space (Fletcher and Epstein, 1982). The explanation for the discrepancy between this study and others (Bohn et al., 1980; Slutsky et al., 1980, 1981; Wright et al., 1981; Rossing et al., 1981) is not clear.

Studies in Animals with Lung Disease

The efficacy of HFV in various models of lung disease has been well documented by a number of different groups in animals with (1) oleic acid pul-

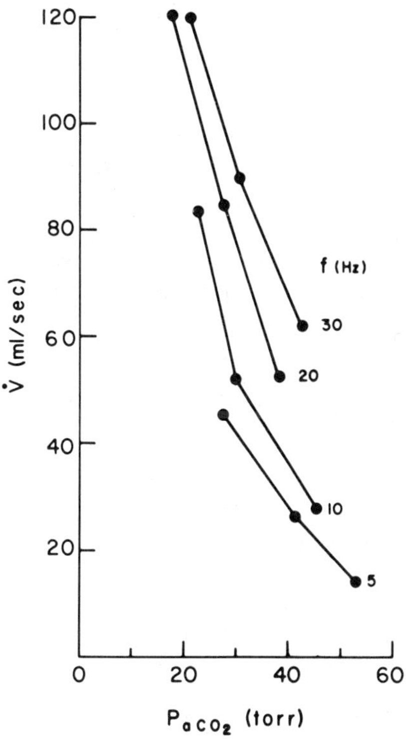

Figure 17 Arterial PCO_2 obtained at any given oscillatory flow rate ($\dot{V}$). The solid lines join points obtained at a constant frequency. (Adapted from Wright et al., 1981.)

monary edema (Wright et al., 1981; Kolton et al., 1982), (2) surfactant depletion (Kolton et al., 1982), and (3) histamine induced bronchoconstriction (Rossing et al., 1982).

Wright et al. (1981) studied the gas exchange by HFV in rabbits with oleic acid induced diffuse lung injury. They measured arterial blood gases at a number of frequencies and tidal volumes 24 hr after infusion of 0.12 mg/kg of oleic acid. Although they did not directly measure the delivered tidal volume during their experimental runs, they estimated an effective stroke volume (V_{S_e}). When they then plotted oscillatory flow rate versus Pa_{CO_2}, they obtained the graph shown in Figure 17. Note that there is a relatively good relationship between $\dot{V}$ and Pa_{CO_2}. However, on closer examination of their data it appears that greater CO_2 elimination was obtained when a given $\dot{V}$ was achieved with a lower f (and hence a higher V_{S_e}), consistent with results in healthy dogs (see Fig. 13). These authors also examined the effect of the magnitude of the fresh gas flow on gas exchange and found that in their studies using rabbits with a mean weight of 3.3 kg (and hence a metabolic CO_2 production of roughly 40 ml/min) that increasing the bias flow from 1 to 2 liters/

min resulted in a significant decrease in Pa_{CO_2} of about 18 mmHg, but further increasing it to 6 liters/min had no significant effect. Thus the boundary condition imposed by the magnitude of the bias flow is potentially quite important and has recently been modeled by Solway et al. (1982).

Rossing and colleagues (1982) studied the effect of intravenous histamine (which by this route preferentially constricts peripheral airways) on $\dot{V}CO_2$ in dogs. Prior to the initiation of the intravenous histamine, $\dot{V}CO_2$ versus f was relatively linear. However, following histamine, the shape of the curves was significantly altered, displaying an initial linear portion with respect to frequency and then approaching a plateau as frequency increased further. These authors hypothesized that this tendency to reach a plateau might be due to the nonrigid upper airways acting as a shunt compliance in parallel with the distal airways (Mead, 1969b). At higher frequencies, this would lead to a portion of the tidal volume being lost to the upper airways with each stroke. Evidence supporting this hypothesis has recently been obtained by Gavriely et al. (1984) in studies in which they obtained cineradiographic movies of the upper airways during HFV before and after injection of intravenous histamine. These results graphically demonstrate the marked expansion and contraction of the upper airways during HFV in the bronchoconstricted dogs.

B. Studies in Humans

A large number of clinical studies using HFV have been performed in patients requiring mechanical ventilatory support. Butler et al. (1980) studied 12 patients with various forms of ventilatory failure and found that they were able to maintain eucapnia with tidal volumes ranging from 50 to 150 ml at an oscillatory frequency of 15 Hz. However, they did not present data in which they varied oscillatory frequency or tidal volume and examined gas exchange.

Rossing and colleagues (1981) quantified the effects of f and V_T on $\dot{V}CO_2$ in six patients with chronic ventilatory failure due mainly to central neurological problems. All patients had tracheostomy tubes and had lung disease as demonstrated by an increased $(A\text{-}a)DO_2$. It was possible to maintain eucapnia in all subjects using V_T values ranging from 45 to 90 ml applied at 3 Hz (Fig. 18). $\dot{V}CO_2$ varied roughly linearly with $f \cdot V_T$ product for frequencies below 3 Hz with a tendency for $\dot{V}CO_2$ to be greater at higher V_T values. These data are very similar to the previously described data in healthy dogs (see Fig. 13). However, for each subject there appeared to be some critical frequency (3-6 Hz) among subjects above which $\dot{V}CO_2$ versus f (at constant V_T) reached a plateau (Fig. 19). These results were very similar to those described in dogs given intravenous histamine and suggested that these results

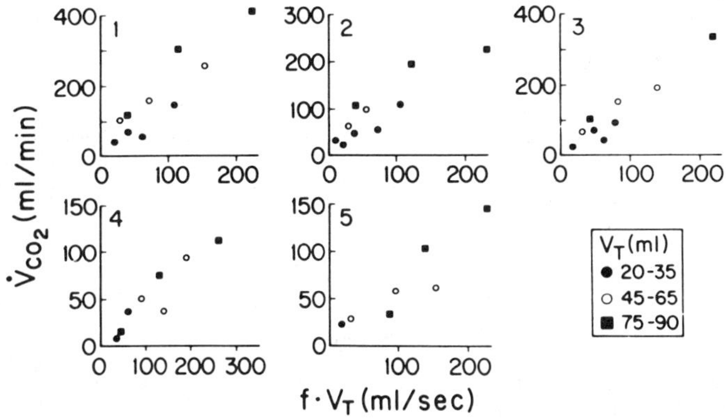

Figure 18 $\dot{V}CO_2$ versus f•VT in five human subjects. These data were obtained at oscillatory frequencies below 3 Hz. (From Rossing et al., 1981.)

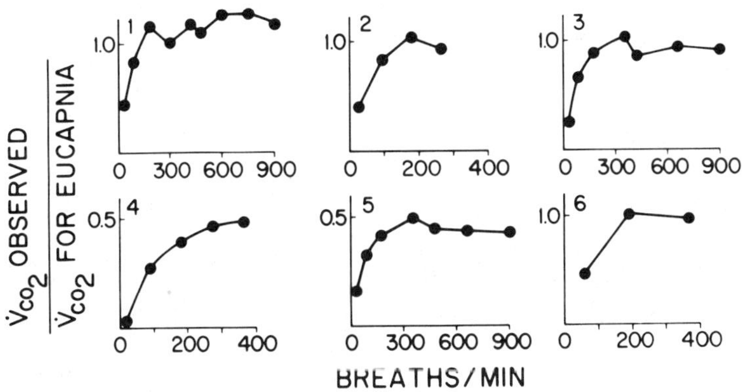

Figure 19 Normalized CO_2 elimination versus frequency at a VT of 50 ml in six human subjects. (From Rossing et al., 1982.)

might also be explained on the basis of the central airways acting as a shunt compliance in these patients with probable peripheral airways disease.

VII. Summary and Conclusions

High-frequency ventilation is a relatively new and exciting method of mechanical ventilation in which effective gas transport is possible using tidal volumes smaller than the anatomic dead space. The precise mechanisms operative during HFV are not known with certainty, but it seems likely that a number of the gas transport mechanisms discussed in Section III are important, each operating in a different region of the lung. The relative importance of each of these mechanisms is also not known, but on the basis of the available data we can draw certain conclusions. First, direct alveolar ventilation or pendelluft cannot be the sole mechanism causing the effective ventilation since gas exchange is possible even when the tidal volumes used are smaller than the equipment dead space. Second, molecular diffusion is not a rate-limiting mechanism during HFV but, as in conventional modes of ventilation, is probably important in the alveolar region (Kaethner et al., 1984). Third, in situations in which there is significant lung disease (e.g., peripheral airways obstruction) the mechanical properties of the lungs are an important determinant of gas exchange.

At the present time there remain a large number of important, unanswered questions relating to this new mode of mechanical ventilation. Further experimental and theoretical investigations are required to determine the precise gas transport mechanisms. The results of these studies, in conjunction with controlled studies, will ultimately determine the long-term utility of high-frequency ventilation.

References

Aris, R. (1956). On the dispersion of a solute flowing through a tube. *Proc. R. Soc. Lond.*, **A235**:67-77.

Bohn, D. J., Miyasaka, K., Marchak, B. E., Thompson, W. K., Froese, A. B., and Bryan, A. C. (1980). Ventilation by high frequency oscillation. *J. Appl. Physiol. Respir. Environ. Exercise Physiol.*, **48**(4):710-716.

Briscoe, W. A., Forster, R. E., and Comroe, J. H. (1954). Alveolar ventilation at very low tidal volumes. *J. Appl. Physiol.*, **7**:27-30.

Butler, W. J., Bohn, D. J., Bryan, A. C., and Froese, A. B. (1980). Ventilation by high-frequency oscillation in humans. *Anesth. Analg.*, **59**(8): 577-584.

Chatwin, P. C. (1975). On the longitudinal dispersion of passive contaminant in oscillatory flows in tubes. *J. Fluid Mech.*, **71**(3):513-527.

Collins, J. M. (1982). Dispersion of a passive contaminant in oscillatory flow within a branching network. S. M. thesis, MIT.

Comroe, J. H., Bahnson, E. R., and Coates, E. O., Jr. (1950). Mental changes occurring in chronically anoxemic patients during oxygen therapy. *JAMA*, **143**:1044-1048.

Custer, J. R., and Shannon, D. C. (1979). High frequency ventilation enhances oxygenation and alveolar ventilation at reduced airway pressures in animal model of pulmonary edema. *Am. Rev. Respir. Dis.*, **119** (Suppl.):226.

Emerson, J. H. (1959). Apparatus for vibrating portions of a patient's airway. U.S. Patent 2,918,917.

Ergodan, M. E., and Chatwin, P. C. (1967). The effects of curvature and buoyancy on the laminar dispersion of solute in a horizontal tube. *J. Fluid Mech.*, **29**(3):465-484.

Farrell, D. A., and Larson, W. E. (1973). The effect of fluctuations in fluid velocity on hydrodynamic dispersion. *Water Res.*, **9**:173-184.

Fletcher, P. R., and Epstein, R. A. (1982). Constancy of physiological dead space during high-frequency ventilation. *Respir. Physiol.*, **47**:39-49.

Fowler, W. W. (1948). Lung function studies: II. The respiratory dead space. *Am. J. Physiol.*, **154**:405-416.

Fredberg, J. J. (1980). Augmented diffusion in the airways can support pulmonary gas exchange. *J. Appl. Physiol. Respir. Environ. Exercise Physiol.*, **49**:232-238.

Froese, A. B., and Bryan, A. C. (1981). High frequency ventilation [Editorial]. *Am. Rev. Respir. Dis.*, **123**(3):249-250.

Fukuchi, Y., Roussos, C. S., Macklem, P. T., and Engel, L. A. (1976). Convection, diffusion and cardiogenic mixing of inspired gas in the lung; an experimental approach. *Respir. Physiol.*, **26**:77-90.

Fulton, J. M., Hayes, D. A., and Pimmel, R. L. (1982). Pulmonary impedance in dogs measured by forced random noise with a retrograde catheter. *J. Appl. Physiol. Respir. Environ. Exercise Physiol.*, **53**(2): 725-733.

Gavriely, N., Solway, J., Drazen, J. M., Slutsky, A. S., Brown, R., Loring, S. H., and Ingram, R. H., Jr. (1984). Radiographic visualization of airway wall movement during oscillatory flow in dogs. *J. Appl. Physiol. Respir. Environ. Exercise Physiol.* (in press).

Haselton, F. R., and Scherer, P. W. (1979). Convective mixing in tube networks. *AIChE J.*, **25**:542-549.

Haselton, F. R., and Scherer, P. W. (1980). Bronchial bifurcations and respiratory mass transport. *Science*, **208**:69-71.

Henderson, Y., Chillingsworth, F. P., and Whitney, J. L. (1915). The respiratory dead space. *Am. J. Physiol.*, **38**(1):1-19.

Horsfield, K., and Cumming, G. (1976). Morphology of the bronchial tree in the dog. *Respir. Physiol.*, **26**:176-182.

Joshi, C. H., Kamm, R. D., Drazen, J. M., and Slutsky, A. S. (1983). An experimental study of gas exchange in laminar oscillatory flow. *J. Fluid Mech.*, **133**:245-254.

Kaethner, T., Kohl, J., and Scheid, P. (1984). Gas concentration profiles along airways of dog lungs during high-frequency ventilation. *J. Appl. Physiol. Respirat. Environ. Exercise Physiol.*, **56**(6):1491-1499.

Kamm, R. D., Collins, J. M., Whang, J., Slutsky, A. S., and Greiner, M. (1984a). Gas transport during oscillatory flow in a network of branching tubes. *J. Biomech. Eng.* (in press).

Kamm, R. K., Slutsky, A. S., and Drazen, J. M. (1984b). High frequency ventilation. *CRC Reviews in Biomed. Eng.*, **9**(4):347-379.

Khoo, M. C. K., Slutsky, A. S., Drazen, J. M., Solway, J., Gafriely, N., and Kamm, R. D. (1984). Gas mixing during high frequency ventilation: an improved model. *J. Appl. Physiol. Respir. Environ. Exercise Physiol.*, **57**(2):493-506.

Knopp, T. J., Kaethner, T., Meyer, M., Rehder, K., and Scheid, P. (1983). Gas mixing in the airways of dog lungs during high frequency ventilation. *J. Appl. Physiol. Respir. Environ. Exercise Physiol.*, **55**(4):1141-1146.

Kolton, M., Cattran, C. B., Kent, G., Volgyesi, G., Froese, A. B., and Bryan, A. C. (1982). Oxygenation during high-frequency ventilation compared with conventional mechanical ventilation is two models of lung injury. *Anesth. Analg.*, **61**:323-332.

Lehr, J. (1980). Circulating currents during high frequency ventilation. [Abstract]. *Fed. Proc.*, **39**:576A.

Lehr, J., Drazen, J. M., Westerman, P. A., and Zatz, S. L. (1982). Regional expansion of excised dog lung during high frequency ventilation. [Abstract]. *Fed. Proc.*, **41**:1747.

Lunkenheimer, P. P., Frank, I., Ising, H., Keller, H., and Dickhut, H. H. (1972). Intrapulmonaler Gaswechsel unter simultierter Apnoe durch transtrachealen, periodishen intrathorakealen Druckweechsel. *Anesthetist*, **22**:232-238.

Mead, J. (1969a). The distribution of gas flow in the lungs. In *Ciba Foundation Symposium on Circulatory Mass Transport.* Edited by G. E. W. Wolstenholme and J. Knight. London, J. & A. Churchill, pp. 204-209.

Mead, J. (1969b). Contribution of compliance of airways to frequency dependent behavior of the lungs. *J. Appl. Physiol.*, **26**:670-673.

Menon, A. S., Weber, M. E., and Chang, H. K. (1982). A model study of flow dynamics in the human central airways. Part III. Oscillatory velocity profiles. *Respir. Physiol.*, **55**:1-21.

Mitzner, W., Permutt, S., and Weinmann, G. (1983). A model of airway gas transport during high frequency ventilation. [Abstract]. *Ann. Biomed. Eng.*, **11**(1):61.

Otis, A. B., McKerrow, C. B., Bartlett, R. A., Mead, J., McIlroy, M. B., Selverstone, N. J., and Radford, E. P. (1956). Mechanical factors in distribution of pulmonary ventilation. *J. Appl. Physiol.*, **8**:427-433.

Pedley, T. J., Schroter, R. C., and Sudlow, M. F. (1977). Gas flow and mixing in airways. In *Bioengineering Aspects of the Lung.* Edited by J. B. West. New York, Marcel Dekker.

Robertson, H. T., Coffey, R. L., and Hlastala, M. P. (1982). Influence of carrier gas density on gas exchange during high frequency ventilation. *Bull. Eur. Physiopathol. Respir.*, **18**:381-387.

Rohrer, F. (1915). Der Strömungswiderstand in den menschlichen Antenwegen und der Einfluss der unregelmassigen Verzweigung des Bronchialsystems auf den Atmungsverlauf verschiedenen Lungenbezirken. *Arch. Gesamte Physiol.*, **162**:225-299.

Ross, B. B. (1957). Influence of bronchial tree structure on ventilation in the dog's lung as inferred from measurements of a plastic cast. *J. Appl. Physiol.*, **10**(1):1-14.

Rossing, T. H., Slutsky, A. S., Lehr, J., Drinker, P., Kamm, R. D., and Drazen, J. M. (1981). Tidal volume and frequency dependence of carbon dioxide elimination by high-frequency ventilation. *N. Engl. J. Med.*, **305**:1375-1397.

Rossing, T. H., Slutsky, A. S., Ingram, R. H., Jr., Kamm, R. D., Shapiro, A. H., and Drazen, J. M. (1982). CO_2 elimination by high frequency oscillations in dogs–effects of histamine infusion. *J. Appl. Physiol. Respir. Environ. Exercise Physiol.*, **53**:1256-1262.

Scherer, P. W., and Haselton, F. R. (1982). Convective exchange in oscillatory flow through bronchial-tree models. *J. Appl. Physiol. Respir. Environ. Exercise Physiol.*, **53**(4):1023-1033.

Scherer, P. W., Schendalman, L. H., Greene, N. M., and Bouhuys, A. (1975). Measurement of axial diffusivities in a model of the bronchial airways. *J. Appl. Physiol.*, **38**:719-723.

Schlichting, H. (1968). *Boundary Layer Theory.* New York, McGraw-Hill, pp. 99-100.

Schmid, E. R., Knopp, T. J., and Rehder, K. (1981). Intrapulmonary gas transport and perfusion during high-frequency oscillation. *J. Appl. Physiol. Respir. Environ. Exercise Physiol.*, **51**(6):1507-1514.

Slutsky, A. S. (1981). Gas mixing by cardiogenic oscillations: a theoretical quantitative analysis. *J. Appl. Physiol. Respir. Environ. Exercise Physiol.*, **51**(5):1287-1293.

Slutsky, A. S., and Brown, R. (1982). Cardiogenic oscillations: a potential mechanism enhancing oxygenation during apneic respiration. *Med. Hypotheses,* **8**:393-400.

Slutsky, A. S., Drazen, J. M., Ingram, R. H., Jr., Kamm, R. D., Shapiro, A. H., Fredberg, J. J., Loring, S. H., and Lehr, J. (1980). Effective pulmonary ventilation with small volume oscillations at high frequency. *Science,* **209**:609-611.

Slutsky, A. S., Kamm, R. D., Rossing, T. H., Loring, S. H., Lehr, J., Shapiro, A. H., Ingram, R. H., Jr., and Drazen, J. M. (1981). Effects of frequency, tidal volume and lung volume on CO_2 elimination in dogs by high frequency (2-30 Hz), low tidal volume ventilation. *J. Clin. Invest.*, **68**:1475-1484.

Solway, J., Gavriely, N., Drazen, J. M., Slutsky, A. S., Lehr, J. L., Drinker, P. A., Saari, A., Rossing, T. H. (1982). Effect of bias flow rate on CO_2 removal during high frequency ventilation in human subjects. [Abstract]. *Physiologist,* **25**:283.

Tarbell, J. M., Ultman, J. S., and Durlofsky, L. (1982). Oscillatory dispersion in a branching tube network. *J. Biomed. Eng.*, **104**:338-345.

Taylor, G. I. (1953). Dispersion of soluble matter in solvent flowing slowing through a tube. *Proc. R. Soc. Lond.*, **A219**:186.

Taylor, G. I. (1954). The dispersion of matter in turbulent flow through a pipe. *Proc. R. Soc. Lond.*, [Biol.] **A223**:446.

Tennekes, H., and Lumley, J. L. (1972). *A First Course in Turbulence.* MIT Press, Cambridge, Mass., pp. 2, 8.

von Andel, E., Kramers, H., and de Voogd, A. (1964). The residence time distribution of laminar flow in curved tubes. *Chem. Eng. Sci.*, **19**:77-79.

Watson, E. J. (1983). Diffusion in oscillatory pipe flow. *J. Fluid Mech.* **133**:233-244.

Weibel, E. (1963). *Morphometry of the Human Lung.* New York, Academic Press Heidelberg, Springer-Verlag.

Wright, K., Lyrene, R. K., Truog, W. E., Standaert, T. A., Murphy, J., and Woodrum, D. E. (1981). Ventilation by high-frequency oscillation in rabbits with oleic acid lung disease. *J. Appl. Physiol. Respir. Environ. Exercise Physiol.*, **50**(5):1056-1060.

5

Regional Ventilation Distribution

J. M. B. HUGHES

Royal Postgraduate Medical School
and Hammersmith Hospital
London, England

TERENCE C. AMIS

School of Veterinary Medicine
University of California at Davis
Davis, California

I. Introduction

This chapter will concentrate on the inhalation of radioactive gases, detected externally over the chest with an array of scintillation counters or a gamma camera, as a means of measuring the topographic distribution of ventilation and regional lung expansion. The nonradioactive methods, mainly bronchospirometric, which preceded the introduction of radioactive gas techniques, have been reviewed by West (1977a).

The first use of radioactive gases to measure regional ventilation was by Knipping et al. (1955) in Cologne, initially with methyl ^{131}I vapor, and later with an insoluble radioactive gas, ^{133}Xe. Sixteen Geiger counters were positioned over the posterior aspect of the chest. The production of ^{15}O, a short-lived ($t_{1/2}$ 2.1 min) cyclotron-produced isotope, at Hammersmith Hospital in 1957 was a stimulus to further research and the inhalation of ^{15}O, $C^{15}O$, and $C^{15}O_2$ was extensively investigated. The apex-base distribu-

Table 1 Radioactive Gases Used for Studies of Regional Ventilation

Radionuclide	$t_{1/2}$	γ energy (keV)	Solubility in blood at 37°C ($ml\ ml^{-1}\ atm^{-1}$)
^{133}Xe	5.3 days	80	0.14
^{127}Xe	38.4 days	203 and 170	0.14
^{135}Xe	9.2 hr	250	0.14
^{85m}Kr	4.4 hr	150	0.046[a]
^{13}N	10 min	511	0.015[b]
^{19}Ne	17 sec	511	0.0097[c] (water)
^{81m}Kr	13 sec	190	0.046

[a]Yeh and Peterson (1965).
[b]Van Slyke et al. (1934).
[c]Seeman (1972).

tion of ventilation in erect normal subjects was described by West and Dollery (1960) using inhalations of $C^{15}O_2$. Subsequently, ^{133}Xe became the radionuclide of choice for most investigations. Other radionuclides which have been used more recently include ^{127}Xe, ^{13}N, ^{19}Ne, ^{81m}Kr, ^{85m}Kr, and radioactive aerosols (Hughes, 1979). Some properties of these gases are summarized in Table 1.

II. Theory and Methods

A. Long or Medium Half-Life Gases

Properties

1. Xenon is relatively insoluble (0.085 ml gas STPD/ml H_2O per mmHg at 37°C), but it is more soluble in fat than in water and can combine with hemoglobin; its solubility in blood, in the same units, is 0.16 (Yeh and Peterson, 1965). Thus, if xenon is breathed in a closed circuit, a significant amount of radioactivity enters the blood and finds its way to the tissues of the chest wall. Xenon washout curves, after prolonged rebreathing, are subject to error because of the accumulation of the radionuclide in extrapulmonary tissues (Matthews and Dollery, 1965; Ronchetti et al., 1980). In practice, if prolonged rebreathing times (>2 min) are avoided, the error is small (<10%). Nevertheless, the tail of the xenon washout curves, when activity has fallen to 30% of initial, should be interpreted with caution (Fig. 1).

^{133}Xe has a convenient half-life (5.3 days), but it emits 81-keV γ rays

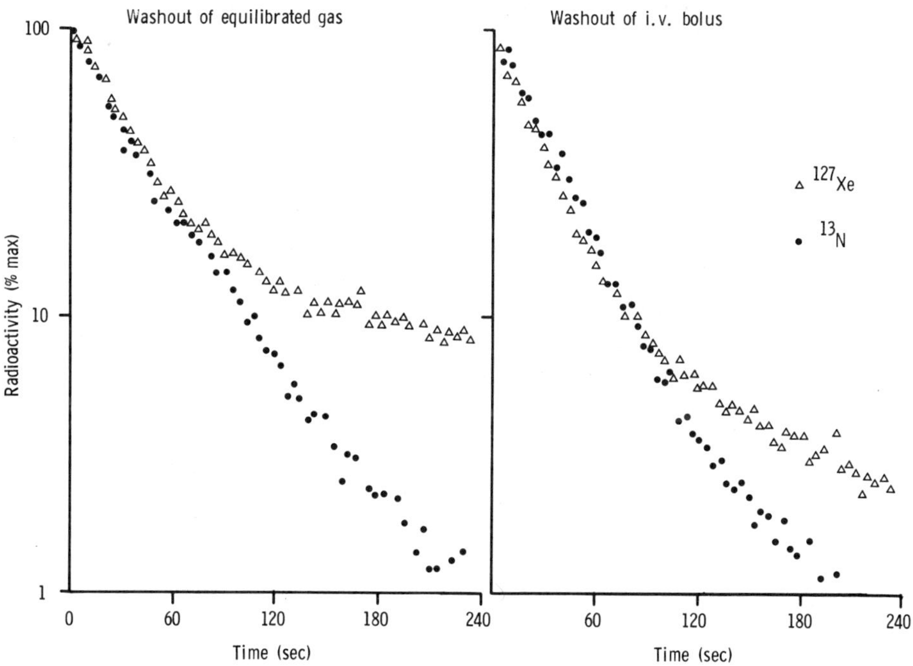

Figure 1 Radioactivity on log scale against time (sec) in a normal subject following equilibration in closed circuit (washout of equilibrated gas) or after intravenous bolus injection. There is good agreement down to at least 70% elimination, but note the clearance delay for ^{127}Xe compared to ^{13}N because of its higher solubility (Table 1). (From Ronchetti et al., 1980.)

which are rather low for detection. The soft tissues of a chest wall, 3.9 cm thick, will attenuate 81-keV radiation by one-half. Thus a larger radiation dose must be administered to obtain adequate counting statistics. ^{127}Xe has a longer half-life (36.4 days) and higher γ-energy emission (Table 1), which makes it more suitable for the Anger gamma camera. The cost is greater than for ^{133}Xe and it has not come into general use.

2. ^{13}N. Nitrogen 13 is a cyclotron-produced radioisotope (Clark and Buckingham, 1975) with a solubility in blood which is approximately one-tenth of that of xenon. It decays by emitting positrons each of which give rise to two 511-keV γ rays at 180° to each other. The high-energy "gammas" can be counted conventionally or in coincidence mode. With coincidence counting and a positron scanner, tomographic reconstructions can be made, as

with computerized tomographic scanning and x rays, termed "emission computer-assisted tomography" (ECAT).

3. ^{85m}Kr. Krypton 85m has been used only in combination with ^{81m}Kr (Amis et al., 1984; Amis et al., 1977).

Theory

1. Single breath. Except near the hilum, lung regions seen by external counters consist in the main (>90%) of alveolar units. Following a single inhalation of a radioactive gas, the regional external count rate (N_r) reflects the product of the regional (r) alveolar (A) concentration (C) and regional alveolar volume (V_A) times a geometric counting factor which includes attenuation of counts by lung and chest wall tissues (k).

$$N_r = CA_r VA_r k \tag{1}$$

CA_r, the regional alveolar concentration, is proportional to radioactive counts per unit volume or the regional inspired volume (ΔVI) (minus regional dead space) times the inspired concentration (CI) per unit regional alveolar volume:

$$CA_r = \Delta VI_r \frac{CI}{VA_r} \tag{2}$$

Combining Eqs. (1) and (2) yields

$$N_r = \Delta VI_r CIk \tag{3}$$

During a breath hold, the count rate from insoluble gases with a reasonably long half-life will remain steady. A second measurement is usually made after rebreathing the radioactive tracer in closed circuit to equilibrium when $CI = CA_r$ in all regions. Therefore, from Eq. (1),

$$N_{r(eq)} = CI_{(eq)} VA_r K \tag{4}$$

By relating the count rates for a single inhalation (N_r) and for equilibration ($N_{r(eq)}$), assuming that both measurements are made at the same VA_r:

$$\frac{N_r}{N_{r(eq)}} = \frac{\Delta VI_r}{VA_r} \frac{CI_{(eq)}}{CI} \tag{5}$$

where $\Delta VI_r/VA_r$ is regional alveolar ventilation per unit alveolar volume. $CI_{(eq)}$ and CI can be measured directly, but if the whole lung is included in the counting fields, N_r and $N_{r(eq)}$ can be normalized, that is, expressed as a fraction of the total counts (N_{tot}).

Inspiring a single breath of ^{133}Xe from functional residual capacity

(FRC) to total lung capacity (TLC) and relating the counts to the equilibrium ($N_{r(eq)}$) counts at TLC yields

$$\frac{N_r}{N_{r(eq)}} = \frac{IC_r}{TLC_r} \frac{C_{I(eq)}}{C_I} \tag{6}$$

where IC is the inspiratory capacity. I - (IC_r/TLC_r) equals FRC_r/TLC_r. If an inspiration is made from residual volume to TLC, $N_r/N_{r(eq)}$ equals VC_r/TLC_r, from which RV_r/TLC_r can be calculated. The ability to measure regional lung expansion at any overall lung volume, as well as quasi-static regional ventilation, was pointed out by Milic-Emili et al. (1966). C_I and C_{eq} have to be measured to obtain an absolute value of these ratios.

2. Multibreath (washin and washout). During prolonged breathing of a radioactive gas in a closed circuit, N_r will increase in a quasi-exponential fashion until a plateau is reached. A washout phase follows after switching out of closed circuit to inactive room air. The time course of the approach to the equilibrium (washin) or of its subsequent decay represents the turnover of the tracer gas within each lung region. The principles of analysis of washin and washout curves are approximately the same, but washout analysis has been used much more frequently. In a single lung compartment, the fall in N with a constant tidal volume will be linear on a semilog plot against breath number or time (t). The slope (N/t) of this exponential represents the ventilation rate constant with units of min^{-1} or, in respiratory terms, ventilation (liters/min) per unit volume (liters). The time for activity to fall to 50% ($t_{1/2}$) is often measured. A $t_{1/2}$ of 0.5 min represents a turnover of 1.4 min^{-1}, which, for the lung as a whole, would be compatible with an alveolar ventilation of 4.2 liters/min and an alveolar volume of 3.0 liters.

With xenon, the washout curves, even in normal subjects, are never straight on a semilog plot but have a pronounced tail. The tail is caused mainly by the solubility of xenon in tissue since ^{13}N washout curves are almost linear in normal subjects (Rosenzweig et al., 1969), the solubility of ^{13}N being about one-tenth of xenon (Table 1). In normal subjects the $^{13}N/^{127}Xe$ ratio for 50% washout time (averaging all lung zones) following equilibration was 0.97, falling to 0.7 for 90% elimination and 0.47 for 95% elimination (Ronchetti et al., 1980). ^{133}Xe or ^{127}Xe washouts are acceptable down to 70% elimination (see Fig. 1).

The estimation of $t_{1/2}$ or, if the curve is very alinear, of the initial slope of the washout curve after equilibration represents the mean turnover of the well and poorly ventilated units in the counting region, weighted by their respective volumes, that is, the mean total specific ventilation for that region [$\Delta V_{I(tot)}/V_{A(tot)}$]. The washout slope after a single breath of a radioactive tracer represents a ventilation-weighted regional specific ventilation; after an intravenous injection of tracer, a perfusion-weighted mean ventilatory turnover is measured. The time for 50% or 90% elimination is affected by the overall ventilation and some authors prefer to calculate the total expired volume for 90% regional elimination (VE_{90}) (Ewan et al., 1978; Eiser et al., 1977) or the total expired alveolar volume (assuming 200 ml of instrumental and anatomic dead space) for 50% elimination (Forkert et al., 1978).

The efficiency of regional ventilation in terms of number of turnovers of volume for 90% elimination (Cumming and Jones, 1966) cannot be estimated until regional gas volumes (VA_r) can be defined in terms of absolute volume. This is now possible with the positron scanner.

B. Ultra-Short Half-Life Gases

Properties

1. ^{81m}Kr. This 13-sec half-life (Table 1) radionuclide is produced continuously from its "parent," ^{81}Ru, whose half-life is 4.58 hr.
2. ^{19}Ne. Neon 19 is a positron emitter, emitting 511-keV γ rays. The half-life (17.4 sec) is similar to that of ^{81m}Kr. It is produced by bombarding ^{16}O with α particles (Crouzel et al., 1980).

Theory

With ultra-short half-life radionuclides, regional ventilation is measured by a steady-state technique. The radioactive gas is added, at a fixed flow rate, to the inspired gas and N_r is recorded while the subject continues to breathe. After 30 sec, counting begins and continues until sufficient counts have accumulated. In the steady state, the input [inspired ventilation (ΔVI) × inspired concentration (CI) equals the output (expired ventilation (ΔVE) × alveolar concentration (CA) *plus* alveolar concentration × alveolar volume × the radioactive decay constant (λ)]. Thus

$$\Delta VI_r CI = \Delta VE_r CA_r + CA_r VA_r \lambda \qquad (7)$$

Equation (7) can be solved for $\Delta VI/VA_r$ (regional ventilation per unit alveolar volume), assuming that ΔVI_r and ΔVE_r are equal:

$$\frac{\Delta VI_r}{VA_r} = \frac{\lambda}{CI/CA_r - I} \qquad (8)$$

In practice, how is CA_r measured? For ^{81m}Kr, Amis and Jones (1980) proposed a solution which is similar in principle to the single breath and equilibration method outlined in Eqs. (1) to (5). Since $CA_r = N_r/VA_r$, N_r is estimated from the count rate of the short-life tracer (^{81m}Kr) and VA_r

after equilibration in closed circuit with a long-life tracer with a similar γ-energy emission (^{85m}Kr).

For the positron emitter, ^{19}Ne, Valind et al. (1983) have estimated CA_r in a novel way. With the positron camera, lung density (δ) can be estimated in grams per cubic centimeter of thoracic volume by positron transmission scanning (Rhodes et al., 1981) and VA_r as $1 - \delta/\rho$ where ρ is mean tissue density (1.04 g/ml). Thus, for ^{19}Ne, $CA_r = N_r(1 - \delta/\rho)$.

Tomographic reconstruction with positron cameras, or rotating gamma cameras for single photons, will in the future extend our knowledge of the topography of ventilation into three dimensions. For technical reasons, tomographic lung scanning will take a long time (>2 min) and ultrashort half-life radioisotopes (^{19}Ne, ^{81m}Kr) and steady-state techniques will have to be used.

The spatial resolution of detection systems depends on many factors: collimator design, γ-energy emission, distance from the point source, and so on. At a distance of 10 cm from the collimator aperture, a spatial resolution (full width at 50% isocount rate) varying from 2.5 to 3.5 cm can be achieved in relation to a point source. With gamma cameras 1.5 to 2.0-cm resolution can be expected. The resolution of the Ortec positron camera at Hammersmith Hospital (Rhodes et al., 1981) is 1.7 cm^3, independent of distance. Measurements of washout or those with ultrashort half-life radioisotopes are made during normal breathing. Apart from the lung edges, where there are major problems, respiratory movement will worsen spatial resolution in proportion to the dimensional changes in each lung region. As a rough estimate, during quiet breathing up to 1 cm (or 1 cm^3 for the positron camera) should be added to the calculation of spatial resolution (and more during hyperventilation) toward the periphery of the lung; near the center of the lung, the artifact will be negligible (~0.1 cm, or 0.1 cm^3).

III. Distribution of Ventilation in Normal Subjects

This section concentrates on the distribution of ventilation per unit volume when inspiration starts from the normal end-expiratory position (FRC). The important effects introduced by varying preinspiratory lung volume or shape will be discussed in Sections IV and V.

A. Postural Influences

In the erect position, a tidal inspiration is distributed preferentially to the lower (dependent) zones. The results, using a variety of methods and radioisotopes, summarized in Table 2, are remarkably consistent with a mean upper/lower zone ventilation ratio of 0.72, especially since "upper" and "lower" are

Table 2 Vertical Gradient of Ventilation (Superior/Inferior Lung Zone Ratio) in Erect and Supine Lung in Normal Subjects Inspiring from FRC

Reference	Radionuclide	Method	Posture	Superior/ inferior zone ratio
West and Dollery (1960)	$C^{15}O_2$	1-liter inspiration	Erect	0.72
Ball et al. (1962)	^{133}Xe	Tidal breath	Erect	0.64
		Deep inspiration	Erect	0.72
Dollery et al. (1962)	^{133}Xe	Washout (t_{50})	Erect	0.82
Bryan et al. (1964)	^{133}Xe	Tidal breath	Erect	0.62
		Inspiratory capacity	Erect	0.69
		Washin (t_{90})	Erect	0.58
Rosenzweig et al. (1969)	^{13}N	Washout	Erect	0.8
Ewan et al. (1978)	^{13}N	Washout	Erect	0.73
Amis et al. (1984)	$^{81m}Kr/^{85m}Kr$	Tidal breathing	Supine	0.4
	^{85m}Kr	Washout (t_{50})	Supine	0.5
Prefaut and Engel (1981)	^{133}Xe	Bolus	Supine	1.45 (FRC)
			Supine	0.93 (40% VC)
			Supine	0.78 (60% VC)
Valind et al. (1983)	^{19}Ne	Tidal breathing	Supine	0.37

not precisely defined. In the horizontal direction (medial to lateral) at a given vertical height, no differences have been found (Newhouse et al., 1968). In the vertical direction in the supine posture (upper = ventral, lower = dorsal) there is a larger upper/lower gradient of ventilation in spite of a 30% reduction in vertical lung height (Table 2). The study of Prefaut and Engel (1981) is an exception in that a gravity-dependent gradient was seen only when pre-inspiratory lung volume was raised above the normal FRC. Somewhat surprisingly, the closing capacity in their subjects exceeded FRC by 150 ml. Since the bolus technique labels the first part of inspiration only, it is reasonable that the tracer went to the nondependent zones. Their subjects were relatively young (37 ± 6 years), but they were selected to be slightly obese (Engel and Prefaut, 1981).

In the craniocaudal, or nongravity dependent axis, ventilation has long been thought to be unformly distributed in supine subjects (Kaneko et al., 1966). However, recently, evidence has emerged which suggests that, under some circumstances, cranial-to-caudal ventilation gradients may exist in decubitus postures (see Table 3). Bynum et al. (1976) demonstrated decreased ventilation to caudal lung zones in supine subjects using ^{133}Xe. Amis et al. (1984) placed a gamma camera to the side of supine subjects and studied ventilation distribution for superior and inferior horizontal lung strips using ^{81m}Kr during tidal breathing. Decreased ventilation was found in caudal (paradiaphragmatic) zones compared to cranial lung zones. Recently, Engel and Prefaut (1981) found large craniocaudal gradients (craniocaudal ratio $>$1.5) in supine subjects whose closing capacity exceeded FRC. Increasing lung volume to 40% of vital capacity resulted in a more uniform distribution, while at 60% of vital capacity caudal lung zones were better ventilated than cranial zones.

There are relatively few studies in other postures. In the prone posture, ventilation is uniformly distributed in the vertical direction (Amis et al., 1984), although Kaneko et al. (1966) predicted from quasi-static measurements a vertical gradient similar to the erect posture. Amis et al. (1984) found a craniocaudal ratio of 0.72. In the prone suspended position with shoulder and pelvic girdles supported and abdomen protruding, ventilation appears to be greater in the dependent zones (Rehder et al., 1978). Interestingly, no gradient was found in conscious standing greyhound dogs (Amis et al., 1982). There are large vertical gradients in the lateral decubitus posture with a ventilation ratio between the upper and lower lung of about 0.5 (Kaneko et al., 1966; Roussos et al., 1977; Amis et al., 1984). Demedts (1978), using xenon-133, found a craniocaudal ratio for regional ventilation in young healthy subjects in right lateral decubitus of about 1.26. Amis et al. (1984), studying both right and left lateral decubitus, found craniocaudal ratios of 1.21 in the upper lung and 1.28 in the lower lung. In the inverted position, the lung apex, which is now dependent, has a larger ventilation (X 1.66) than the base (Glaister, 1967).

It is clear that gravity is playing a major role in determining the distribution of ventilation per unit volume because the dependent zones in all postures except prone receive more ventilation. In support of this concept, Bryan et al. (1966) found that the upper-lower ventilation gradient increased in subjects exposed to positive acceleration on a human centrifuge. Extrapolating that data to the "weightless" condition, they suggested that regional

Table 3 Horizontal Gradient (Cranial/Caudal Ratio) of Ventilation in Decubitus Lung in Normal Subjects Inspiring from FRC

References	Radionuclide	Method	Posture	Cranial/caudal ratio[a]
Glazier and DeNardo (1966)	^{133}Xe	1-liter inspiration	Supine	0.95
Glaister (1967)	^{133}Xe	Washin	Supine	1.11
Sybrecht et al. (1976)	^{133}Xe	Bolus (4 ml)	Supine	0.8 ($\dot{V}I$ 0.25 liter/sec)
				1.1 ($\dot{V}I$ 1.5 liters/sec)
Engel and Prefaut (1981)	^{133}Xe	Bolus (4 ml)	Supine	1.0 (CC < FRC)
				1.46 (CC > FRC)
Amis et al. (1984)	$^{81m}Kr/^{85m}Kr$	Tidal breathing	Supine (superior)	1.74
			Supine (inferior)	1.27
			Prone	0.72
			Prone suspended	1.25
			Lat. decubitus (upper lung)	1.21
			Lat. decubitus (lower lung)	1.28

[a]CC, closing capacity.

lung expansion and ventilation should be uniform. Work by Michels and West (1978) under weightless conditions has shown a marked diminution in uneven ventilation as judged by the slope of the alveolar plateau in single-breath nitrogen washout tests.

The origin of ventilation gradients at the same lung height in decubitus postures remains speculative. In some subjects airway closure may be responsible (Engel and Prefaut, 1981). Sybrecht et al. (1976) have shown an effect of inspiratory flow rate on horizontal ventilation gradients in the supine posture, suggesting that the origin of these gradients might lie in regional variations in pleural pressure change associated with the pattern of respiratory muscle action (Roussos et al., 1976a).

B. Effect of Inspiratory Flow Rate

Several studies have shown that the upper-lower gradient of ventilation (from a bolus inhalation) in the erect posture decreases, and may even reverse, as inspiratory flow rate increases (Table 4). An attractive explanation for these findings is the time constant theory, as originally outlined by Otis et al. (1956) and later applied to regional gas distribution (Pedley et al., 1972). The greater expansion of the upper zones in the upright lung (Glazier et al., 1966; Milic-Emili et al., 1966) and the associated smaller compliance and larger bronchial dimensions (Wilson et al., 1974), leading to a lower apical time constant (resistance × compliance), supports this notion. To the extent that the apex-base bolus distribution at a very low inspiratory flow rate is determined by the distribution of local compliance, and at high flow rates by the distribution of local resistances, the slow/fast ratio of ventilation will be proportional to the local time constant. Granted this assumption, the ratio of upper to lower time constants (Table 4) varies from 0.55 to 0.79, which is in good agreement with the value of 0.5 predicted by Sybrecht et al. (1976) by deriving upper and lower zone airway resistances from regional lung expansion data.

Nevertheless, theory demanded that the distribution of applied pleural pressure (ΔP_{PL}) was uniform throughout the lung. Sybrecht et al. (1976) looked at the flow dependence of bolus distribution in the erect and supine postures. As shown in Figure 2, for the same change of inspiratory flow, there was more redistribution in the supine posture, although the calculated apex-base time constant ratio was somewhat closer to unity (0.7) in that posture. Their model suggested that differences of ΔP_{pl} between apex and base of less than 1 cm H_2O could explain most of the flow dependence in the erect lung.

Increasing the frequency of breathing from 10 min^{-1} to 60 min^{-1}, at constant tidal volume, has very little effect on the apex-base gradient of in-

Table 4 Distribution of a ^{133}Xe Bolus Inhaled from FRC in Erect Posture at Slow and Fast Inspiratory Flow Rates ($\dot{V}_I$) with Upper/Lower (U/L) Zone Ventilation ($\dot{V}/V_A$) Ratios at Each Flow and Slow/Fast $\dot{V}/V_A$ Ratios for Upper and Lower Zones[a]

Reference	$\dot{V}_1$ (liters/min)	$\dot{V}/V_A$ (U/L)	$\dot{V}_I$ (liters/min)	$\dot{V}/V_A$ (U/L)	Slow/fast $\dot{V}/V_A$ ratio			Bolus volume (ml)
					Upper	Lower	U/L	
Martin et al. (1972)	0.25	—	5-7.5	—	0.83	1.25	0.66	4
Hughes et al. (1972)	<0.3	0.7	>5.0	1.4	0.8	1.45	0.55	5
Bake et al. (1974)	0.2	0.65	4.0	0.9	0.8	1.21	0.66	4
	0.2	0.65	1.0	0.9	0.93	1.17	0.79	4
Grant et al. (1974)	0.1	0.75	1.0	1.1	0.87	1.2	0.73	5
Sybrecht et al. (1976)	0.2	0.74	1.0	0.8	—	—	—	4
	0.2	0.72[b]	1.0	1.01[b]				4
Connolly et al. (1975)	0.2	0.74	4.0	0.9	0.89	1.09	0.82	480

[a] $\dot{V}/V_A$ ratios are in arbitrary units normalized to 1.
[b] Supine but at equal lung volume to erect.

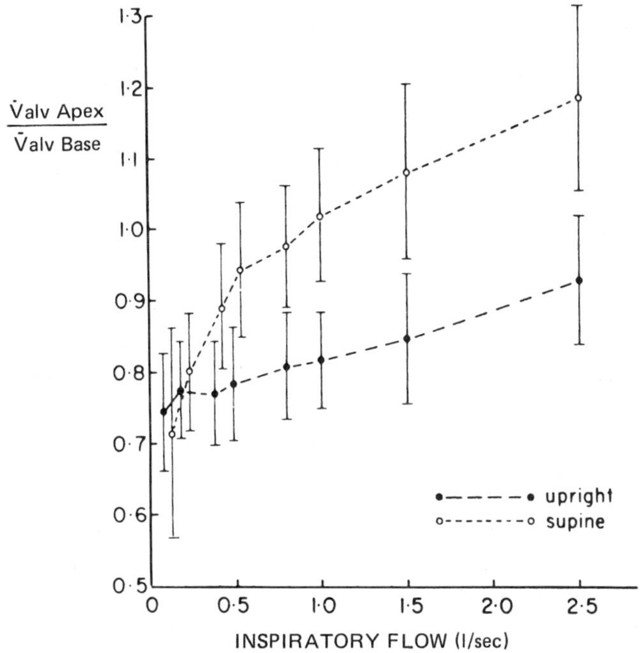

Figure 2 Apex/base (cranial/caudal) distribution ratio of ^{133}Xe bolus (100 ml) inhaled from FRC at different flow rates in seven subjects (bars ± 1 SE). (From Sybrecht et al., 1976.)

spired gas (Jones et al., 1977) or of the washout of an inhaled bolus (Forkert et al., 1978). These results are somewhat surprising in view of the changing apex-base distribution following the inhalation of single boluses at different flow rates (Table 4). Taking a time constant ratio of about 0.5 in a two-compartment model, Forkert et al. (1978) showed that distribution was independent of frequency up to 45 min^{-1} as long as there were no differences in applied pressure (ΔP_{pl}). Kronenberg et al. (1976) found a small decrease in basal clearance relative to apical at 50 min^{-1}. They used a gamma camera and may have looked lower down in the lung; in addition, the washout followed equilibration with ^{133}Xe so that units were weighted initially according to volume rather than ventilation.

The frequency dependence of the distribution is also influenced by the portion of the inspirate which is labeled with tracer (Grant et al., 1974), being most flow dependent for the earliest gas inspired (from the upper airways) and almost independent of flow during the last part of a 500-ml inspiration.

Interestingly, at normal inspiratory flow rates (0.4 liter/sec) the common dead-space gas is reinspired preferentially to the less-perfused upper zones. When the whole tidal volume is labeled there is, as expected, somewhat less flow dependence (Connolly et al., 1975), as shown in Table 4.

C. Intraregional Inhomogeneity

Forkert et al. (1978) showed that when the breathing frequency, at constant V_T, was increased fourfold the regional washout times did not decrease correspondingly, as judged by washout times measured at the mouth with a scintillation counter. In fact, the regional/mouth retention ratio increased from about 0.9 to 1.2 in the lower zones and from 1.3 to 2.1 in the upper zones. In other words, regional clearance corrected for overall ventilation was less effective at higher frequencies, as found also by Kronenberg et al. (1976). If there is a wide dispersion of lung time constants, the *output* of tracer (as seen by the mouth counter) at higher frequencies will reflect chiefly those units with short time constants, but the *retention* of the tracer gas (reflected in counts over the chest) will be dominated by the slower time constant units. Hence the delay in lung clearance in relation to clearance recorded at the mouth. For similar reasons, dynamic compliance (C_{dyn}) was frequency dependent, and there was a correlation between the fall in C_{dyn} and the regional washout delay with frequency. A tenfold dispersion of time constants within lung regions would account for their results. Interestingly, frequency dependence was not affected by breathing 80% SF_6-20% O_2, indicating that the intraregional inhomogeneity was not diffusion dependent.

Exponential analysis of regional washout curves during normal breathing is another way of looking for intraregional inhomogeneity. It is necessary to use a very insoluble gas such as ^{13}N (Table 1) in order to define washout curves precisely beyond 20% elimination (Fig. 1). Rosenzweig et al. (1969) measured regional clearance after equilibration with ^{13}N, following the count rate over two decades. In six out of eight subjects two components (fast and slow) were recognized. The fast/slow ventilation ratio was 4 and 2.8 for upper and lower zones, respectively. The amount of inhomogeneity was relatively trivial since the slow component comprised 86% (lower) and 95% (upper) of total compartmental volume.

Ewan et al. (1978) compared ^{13}N washout after equilibration with that after intravenous injection. The blood-flow weighted clearance after intravenous injection of ^{13}N was 19% faster in the lower zones and 4% in the upper. These results imply uneven intraregional distribution of perfusion and ventilation in relation to volume, with the better perfused alveoli also being the better ventilated. The inspiration of hyperoxic or hypoxic gas mixtures did not alter this relationship. Similar results, using ^{133}Xe, were reported by Devos et al. (1978).

IV. Regional Lung Expansion in Normal Subjects

A. Relationship Between Regional and Overall Volume

The effective ventilation of a lung is given by $\Delta V_r/VA_r$, where V_r is the local tidal volume and VA_r is the time-averaged local alveolar volume. Therefore, for the same ΔV_r, regions with a high VA_r will be less effectively ventilated. In addition, because the elastic properties of lungs [transpulmonary pressure-lung volume (PV) curve] are alinear, local specific compliance ($\Delta V_r/\Delta P \cdot VA_r$) varies at different overall lung volumes, so that, for a given ΔPpl, ΔV_r will be less if compliance as predicted from the PV curve is low. Regional VA cannot be measured in absolute terms but is expressed as a fraction of VA_r(max) (i.e., TLC_r) using gas-dilution principles and external counting, as outlined in Section II. If VA_r as a fraction of TLC_r is measured at different states of total lung expansion, usually expressed as the VA/TLC ratio, the change of VA_r/TLC_r (= $\Delta V_r/VA_r$) for any tidal volume (ΔV) starting from any lung volume (VA) can be plotted. Thus, for quasi-static conditions, a single diagram can predict in a given posture all possible interregional distributions of ventilation for any combination of overall tidal and lung volume (Fig. 3). This brilliant concept was introduced by Milic-Emili et al. (1966) and several succinct reviews can be consulted (Milic-Emili, 1974, 1977, 1980). A brief description only can be given in this section.

From the "onionskin" diagram (Fig. 3) many inferences have been drawn concerning regional expansion of the lung under quasi-static conditions (Milic-Emili, 1981). They rest on certain assumptions: (1) homogeneous elastic properties of all lung parenchyma with a monoexponential pressure-volume curve for all regions, and (2) a constant vertical gradient, except at low lung volumes, of pleural surface pressure; there is now good experimental support for these assumptions (Milic-Emili, 1981, 1982) in upright humans under normal conditions. Figure 3 shows that at FRC the upper zone expansion equals 60% TLC_r compared with 40% for the lower zones. Since all alveoli are probably of equal size at TLC, apical alveoli must be 50% larger in volume than basal alveoli at FRC; there is direct experimental evidence for this in dogs (Glazier et al., 1966) and rabbits (D'Angelo, 1972). The slopes ($\Delta V_r/\Delta VA$) for the upper and lower zones reflect the rate of filling or emptying of alveoli as lung volume changes from FRC to TLC, or vice versa [there is no discernible effect of volume history (Sutherland et al., 1968)]. The ratio (U/L) of the slopes (0.66) shows that ventilation distribution under quasi-static conditions is similar to that during breathing at normal frequencies (Table 2, tidal breathing). From FRC to TLC the upper and lower zone slopes are linear, implying a constant filling and emptying ratio (i.e., no sequential behavior). On the other hand, Anthonisen et al. (1970) and Demedts (1978) found that during a slow expiration from TLC the upper/lower emptying ratio steadily increased instead of remaining constant. Demedts et al.

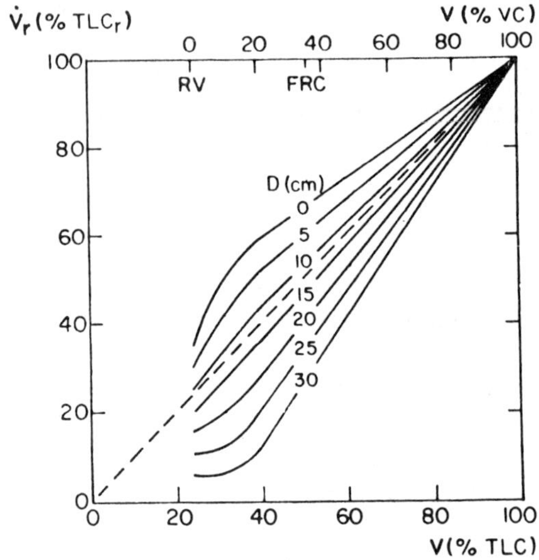

Figure 3 Regional lung volume ($\dot{V}_r$) as percent maximum (TLC_r) plotted against overall lung volume (V) as percent maximum (TLC) in an erect normal subject. Vertical distance (D) from lung top is indicated on each curve. Dashed line (of identity) indicates equal expansion of a region with overall lung. (From Milic-Emili et al., 1966.)

(1980) showed some curvilinearity in upper and lower zone slopes (see Fig. 3) consistent with some sequential behavior.

B. Postural Effects

As with ventilation, gravity plays a major role in determining the distribution of lung expansion. Table 5 shows that in all postures the superior zones are more expanded than the inferior ones. The gradient of expansion (ΔFRC_r/ Δvertical distance) is greatest in the supine and lateral decubitus postures and least in the prone and prone suspended postures. The vertical gradients found by Amis et al. (1984) are less than those found by Kaneko et al. (1966), possibly because of different placing of counters or a different overall FRC. Rhodes et al. (1981) measured the vertical distribution of lung density during quiet breathing in the supine posture for a transaxial (cross-sectional) slice of lung 1.7 cm thick. They used a positron camera and ^{68}Ga transmission from a ring source around the thorax. The mean alveolar gas volume was 0.78 ml/ml of lung in the superior (ventral) part and 0.64 ml/ml in the inferior (dorsal) portion. Unfortunately, measurements cannot be made at TLC to compare with the data in Table 5.

Table 5 Upper and Lower (Superior and Inferior) Regional Expansion at FRC (as Percent Regional TLC) in Different Postures and Change of Regional Expansion Per Centimeter of Vertical Distance of Lung

Reference	Posture	FRC_r/TLC_r (%) Upper zone	Lower zone	Lower/upper ratio	Vertical distance: (cm) upper-lower	$\Delta FRC_r/\Delta$ distance (%/cm)
Milic-Emili et al. (1966)	Erect	65	28	0.43	30	1.23
Amis et al. (1984)	Erect	55	42	0.76		
Kaneko et al. (1966)	Supine	57	30	0.53	19	1.42
Amis et al. (1984)	Supine	60	41	0.68		
Kaneko et al. (1966)	Lateral decubitus	65	23	0.35	27	1.55
Amis et al. (1984)	Lateral decubitus	65	40	0.62		
Rehder et al. (1977)	Lateral decubitus					
	Normal	55	35	0.5		
	Paralyzed	60	30	0.58		
Roussos et al. (1977)	Lateral decubitus					
	Low PDI[a]	56	37	0.66		
	High PDI	51	45	0.88		
Kaneko et al. (1966)	Prone	52	30	0.58	19	1.15
Amis et al. (1984)	Prone	41	36	0.88		
Amis et al. (1984)	Prone suspended	65	62	0.95		
Rehder et al. (1978)	Prone suspended	49	38	0.78		
Demedts et al. (1983)	Inverted	56	38	0.68		

[a]PDI, transdiaphragmatic pressure.

Table 6 Cranial and Caudal Regional Lung Expansion at FRC (as Percent Regional TLC) at Same Horizontal Level and Horizontal Gradient (Cranial/Caudal Ratio) in Decubitus Postures

		FRC_r/TLC_r (%)		
Reference	Posture	Cranial	Caudal	Cranial/caudal
Bake et al. (1967)[a]	Supine	40	25	1.63
Grassino et al. (1975)[b]	Supine	60	48	1.25
Sybrecht et al. (1976)[b]	Supine	55	45	1.22
Amis et al. (1984)[c]	Supine (superior)	53	53	1.0
	Supine (inferior)	54	41	1.32
	Prone	34	38	0.9
	Prone suspended	64	69	0.93
	Lat. decubitus (upper lung)	65	62	1.05
	Lat. decubitus (lower lung)	50	43	1.16

[a]Counters over ventral aspect only.
[b]Counters over dorsal aspect only.
[c]Gamma camera over lateral aspect.

Although differences in elastic properties between or within lobes must always be borne in mind, regional differences in expansion are linked primarily to local differences in distending pressure, and under normal circumstances reflect the vertical gradient of pleural pressure. In humans the main determinant of the vertical gradient of pleural pressure is the weight of the lung itself (Vawter et al., 1975; West, 1977b). The nature of the pleural pressure gradient will be discussed in a later section.

Differences in expansion between the cranial and caudal parts of the lung at the same horizontal level are small compared to the vertical gradient of expansion (Amis et al., 1984) (Table 6). Some decrease of expansion of caudal regions relative to cranial exists in the supine (Bake et al., 1967; Grassino et al., 1975; Sybrecht et al., 1976) and lateral decubitus postures (Demedts, 1978), but Amis et al. (1984), using a gamma camera over the lateral aspect of the thorax, found that gradients were restricted to the inferior part (or lower lung in lateral decubitus), with the upper regions being uniformly expanded in the craniocaudal direction in supine and lateral decubitus postures (Table 6). While the reasons for these gradients remain obscure, their occurrence in more dependent zones suggests that in decubitus postures the weight of the caudal mediastinum, transmission of abdominal hydrostatic pressure gradients through the diaphragm, and distortion of the dependent rib cage (particularly in lateral decubitus postures) may play a role individually or in combination.

C. Effect of Shape Changes

Since the shape of the lung conforms to that of the chest wall, changes in thoracic configuration should be accompanied by alterations in the distribution of alveolar expansion (VA_r), pleural pressure, and possibly ventilation ($\Delta V_r/VA_r$). Data in animals confirm that this is so (Agostoni, 1977), but it has proved much harder in humans to introduce significant chest wall distortions. Neither voluntarily induced changes of abdominal wall configuration (Grassino et al., 1975) nor strapping of the chest (Sybrecht et al., 1975) sufficient to increase lung recoil pressure by 4.3 cm H_2O had any effect on the distribution of expansion. Nevertheless, powerful contraction of the inspiratory muscles at FRC with a pressure gradient across the chest wall or diaphragm exceeding 35 cm H_2O reduces or abolishes the vertical gradient of expansion in erect (Grassino and Anthonisen, 1975) and lateral decubitus postures (Roussos et al., 1977). Lateral compression of the rib cage in the erect posture had a similar effect. Lung emptying during a slow expiration following helium bolus inhalation was more uniform when transdiaphragmatic pressure (PDI) exceeded 30 cm H_2O (Roussos et al., 1976b). In horizontal postures, the contracted or tense diaphragm may isolate the caudal surface of the lung from the larger (1 cm H_2O/cm of distance) vertical gradient of abdominal pressure. In the opposite sense, diaphragm shape changes markedly during anaesthesia with muscle paralysis (Froese and Bryan, 1974), leading to greater expansion of the lung superiorly and relative deflation and cephalad movement inferiorly (Rehder et al., 1977).

On the other hand, neither removal of the weight of the abdominal contents (by water immersion) (Greene et al., 1974) nor passive inflation of the respiratory system (Lemelin et al., 1972) affected the vertical gradient of expansion in the erect posture, nor did negative pressure applied to the abdomen in relaxed supine subjects (Grassino et al., 1975). The most deformable part of the chest wall is its diaphragmatic boundary and a greater potential for distortion exists in decubitus postures because of the abdominal pressure gradient. Therefore, it is not surprising that changes in the distribution of regional expansion occur in horizontal postures, either when the stiffness of the diaphragm is increased (by voluntary contraction) or decreased (by muscle paralysis). In addition, tensing the diaphragm displaces the mediastinum upward (Roussos et al., 1976b).

D. Effect of Voluntary Muscle Contraction

Roussos et al. (1976b) have investigated the effects of three patterns of inspiration on the distribution of inspired gas: (1) natural inspiration, (2) intercostal and accessory muscle inspiration with distortion of the rib cage from its relaxation characteristics, and (3) abdominal inspiration with contraction of the diaphragm and outward movement of the abdominal wall together with contraction of expiratory intercostals so that the anteroposterior rib cage diameter remains unchanged. Transdiaphragmatic pressure change (PDI) is low in the case of intercostal breathing and high for abdominal inspiration. In the lateral decubitus, erect, and supine postures (Roussos et al., 1976) a bolus of ^{133}Xe inhaled at FRC was more evenly distributed in the vertical direction than with natural breathing, while abdominal breathing exaggerated the normal upper-lower difference. Similar differences were found using tidal inspirations of ^{133}Xe in the lateral decubitus posture (Chevrolet et al., 1979) (Fig. 4). Fixley et al. (1978) inhaled ^{133}Xe boluses at 0.25, 0.75, and 1.5 liters/sec constant inspiratory flow with the three inspiratory patterns. The U/L distribution in seated subjects was more uniform with intercostal pattern (2) but increased by a roughly similar amount in all cases with increasing flow; at lower flows natural inspiration (pattern 1) was closer to the abdominal pattern and tended to move toward the intercostal pattern at high flows. Following abdominal inspirations, the subsequent alveolar plateau was independent of expiratory flow rate, while it increased with increasing expiratory flow after natural or intercostal inspirations.

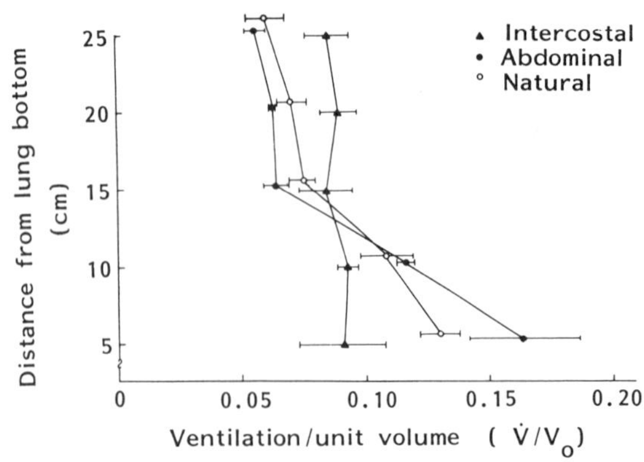

Figure 4 Influence of different breathing patterns on vertical distribution of ventilation during ^{133}Xe washout (after equilibration) in four subjects in lateral decubitus posture. (From Chevrolet et al., 1979.)

Evidence that the flow dependence of ^{133}Xe boli inhaled at FRC is linked to the pattern of inspiratory muscle activity comes from other sources. During a slow expiration in the single-breath nitrogen maneuver, transient increases in expiratory flow ($\dot{V}_E$) resulted in transient increases in expired nitrogen concentration (F_{EN_2}) only if associated with transient increases in transdiaphragmatic pressure (P_{DI}). Conversely, a sudden increase in P_{DI} during expiration without a change in flow resulted in a fluctuation of F_{EN_2} similar to that produced by a transient increase in flow (Roussos et al., 1976a). In addition, increases of P_{DI} throughout expiration reduce the slope of the single-breath alveolar plateau. Studies with magnetometers have shown that rapid inspirations and expirations are associated with rib cage (RC) deformation. At progressively faster inspirations RC expansion is greater relative to that of the abdomen (Sharp et al., 1975; Grimby et al., 1976). D'Angelo (1981) showed that for fast inspirations the cranial part of the rib cage expanded relatively more than the caudal part. Deformation of the rib cage during forced expiration has also been found (Melissinos et al., 1981).

V. Residual Volume

A. Regional Expansion at RV

It is clear from Figure 3 that at low lung volumes (<40% TLC or <20% VC) the relationship between regional and overall lung volumes becomes curvilinear except at midlung levels. The most dependent zone tends toward a minimum volume where further deflation ceases although continuing in the upper and middle zones. This curvilinear behavior of upper and lower zones can be seen for superior and inferior lung zones in other postures (Kaneko et al., 1960). The explanation is that the dependent zones became very stiff due to closure of their airways, as elegantly demonstrated by Engel et al. (1975). These authors showed that by breathing nitrous oxide (N_2O) a ^{133}Xe bolus, injected at the mouth during a breath hold at residual volume (RV), was carried into all of the lung as N_2O was absorbed except to the most dependent zones. Intravenous injections of ^{133}Xe confirmed that the most dependent zones were still perfused at RV. A visual display of the N_2O technique at RV using ^{13}N and a positron camera from the work of Hales et al. (1976) is shown in Figure 5.

In the erect position the volume of lung trapped behind closed airways at RV increases linearly with age, from 1.5% TLC at 20 years to 6% TLC at age 65 years (Hales et al., 1976). Because of the vertical gradient of pleural pressure, local transpulmonary pressures are least in the most dependent parts of the lung; in these regions the parenchymal forces holding open intrapulmonary airways are lowest. At a given overall lung volume, airway closure is

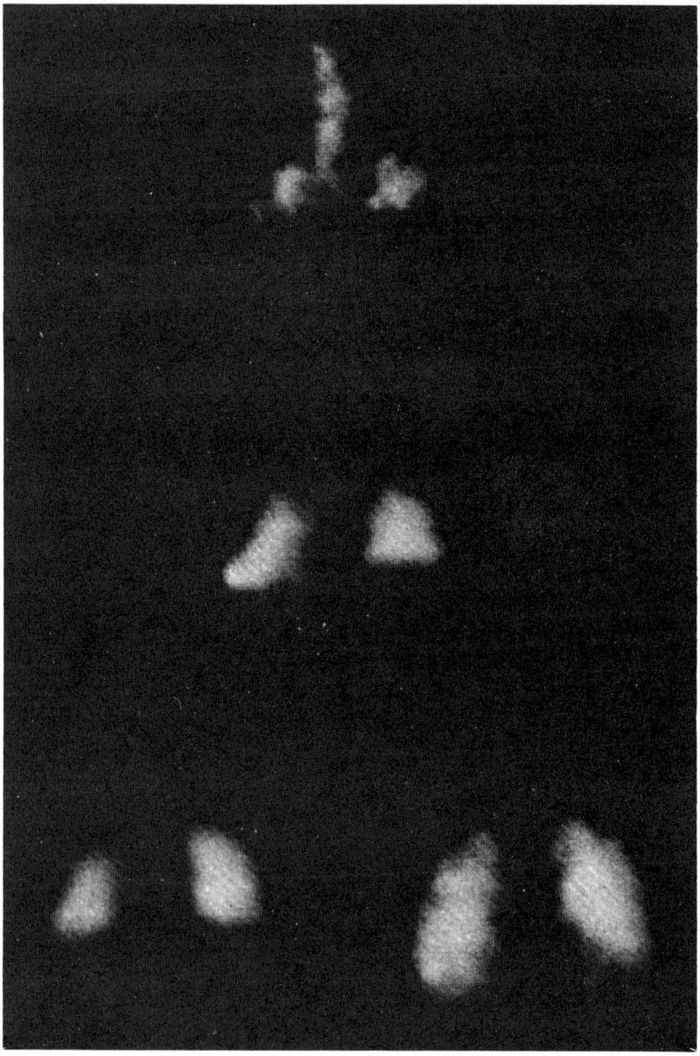

Figure 5 Scintigrams in an erect subject, using ^{13}N and a positron camera, breath holding at residual volume (RV) after prior inhalation of ^{13}N bolus at RV (bottom left), equilibration with ^{13}N gas, and exhalation to RV (bottom right). Upper two scintigrams obtained 8 sec and 24 sec after injection of 4 ml of ^{13}N gas at mouth in presence of nitrous oxide (N_2O), showing ^{13}N carried into lung through all patent airways as N_2O is absorbed by pulmonary tissue and blood. Distribution in middle is similar to bottom left, indicating dependent zone airway closure at RV. (From Hales et al., 1976.)

likely to extend further up the lung if (1) overall or local transpulmonary pressures are less, or (2) bronchomotor tone is increased. Old age (Holland et al., 1968) and obesity (Holley et al., 1967) are associated with increases in dependent zone closure because of decreased lung parenchymal recoil forces. A bronchoconstrictor, such as mecholyl, in creases dependent zone residual volume and reduces the upper-lower gradient of alveolar expansion at RV (Engel et al., 1976).

B. Regional Ventilation at RV

Dollfuss et al. (1967) were the first to correlate the concentration changes of a tracer gas measured at the mouth throughout expiration with the regional distribution of that tracer before the start of the expiration. A small (2-4 ml) bolus of tracer gas (^{133}Xe) was introduced into the inspiratory line at the onset of inspirations, starting from a variety of lung volumes and continuing up to TLC. The regional concentrations, calculated after a second equilibrium measurement at TLC, were similar to predictions made from the slopes ($\Delta V_r/VA_r$) of the onionskin diagram (Fig. 3). Interest was centered on the distribution of a bolus inhaled at RV, because upper zone concentration exceeded that in the lower zone by 2.5 times. During the subsequent expiration from TLC, concentration at the mouth, after dead-space washout, remained fairly uniform as all lung regions emptied nearly synchronously (as predicted by the linear slopes for all regions in Fig. 3) until about 35% TLC (or 18% VC), when the expired concentration changed because of airway closure in the most dependent zones, accompanied by a relatively greater contribution to expiration from the upper zones, where ^{133}Xe concentration was highest. The overall lung volume at which this occurred was called closing capacity. Inspection of Figure 2 shows that it occurs at about 40% TLC. In older subjects, the curvilinearity of the upper and lower zones in the onionskin diagram below FRC extends farther up and down the lung in erect (Demedts, 1980) and supine (Bake et al., 1967) postures, so that closing capacity increases with age.

The apex-base concentration gradient after bolus inhalation at RV was reduced (from 10:1 to 2:1) if a fast instead of a slow inspiration was made (Robertson et al., 1969). It is thought that the large ΔP_{pl}, associated with the muscular effort required for a fast inspiration when airway resistance is relatively high, and the high transpulmonary pressure in the trapped regions, is sufficient to open airways earlier in inspiration.

A further point of interest is that as dependent airways close as RV is approached, local alveolar pressure must initially be considerably higher than atmospheric pressure, so that during a breath hold at RV trapped gas in the dependent zones should escape via collateral ventilation (Milic-Emili,

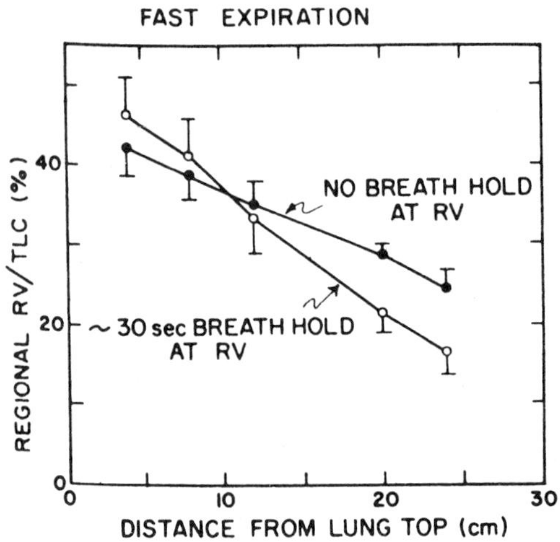

Figure 6 Regional distribution of residual volume as percent maximum [RV/TLC (%)] against vertical distance in six subjects in erect posture following a fast expiration to RV. Redistribution of gas occurs via collateral pathways during breath holding. (From Ruff et al., 1981.)

1980). In fact, the distribution of RV_r/TLC_r changes during a 30-sec breath hold at RV (Fig. 6) from that predicted from Figure 3 to the distribution that would be expected assuming the same pleural pressure gradient at RV as at higher lung volumes (Ruff et al., 1982).

VI. Anesthesia and Muscle Paralysis

A. Normal Subjects

In anaesthetized paralyzed subjects with mechanical ventilation the respiratory system is being expanded in accordance with its passive characteristics. Studies of the distribution of ventilation have clarified the role of the respiratory muscles, especially in the diaphragm, in stabilizing and expanding it.

By partitioning the lungs with a Carlens tube, Rehder et al. (1972) showed that the difference in N_2 elimination between the dependent and nondependent lung in the lateral decubitus position was virtually abolished by anesthesia with paralysis and mechanical ventilation (APMV). Froese and Bryan (1974), in a classic study, sought an explanation for these findings in terms of the mechanics of the diaphragm. In the nonparalyzed state, in lateral decubitus and supine postures, the dependent part of the diaphragm

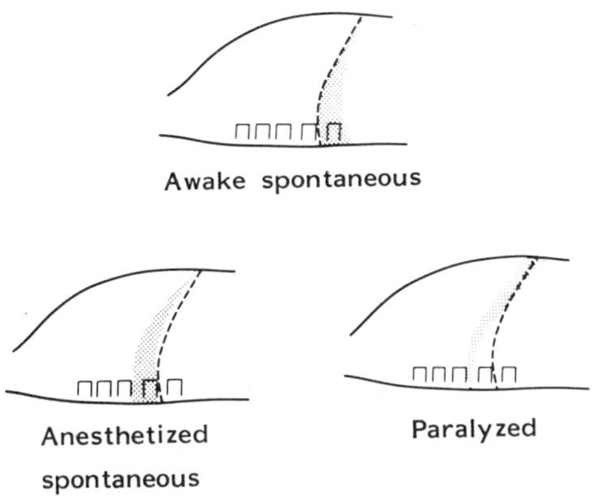

Figure 7 Diaphragm position and displacement (from radiographs) during tidal breathing in a supine subject. Dashed line: FRC position (awake, spontaneous); stippled area: diaphragmatic excursion. (From Froese and Bryan, 1974.)

had the greatest tidal excursion, but with APMV there was a pronounced cephalad shift of the lower portion of the diaphragm where abdominal pressure was greatest, with a shift of the region of maximum tidal excursion to the nondependent part (Fig. 7). Clearly, in horizontal postures, the diaphragm acts as a stabilizing influence because the vertical gradient of pleural pressure (0.25 cm H_2O/cm of distance) is opposed by a fourfold greater gradient of abdominal pressure. On the other hand, APMV has less effect on the distribution of ventilation in the supine or seated postures (Rehder et al., 1977) and no effect in the prone (suspended) position (Fig. 8) because abdominal pressure is no longer compressing the lung. Chevrolet et al. (1978) trained conscious subjects to relax during intermittent positive pressure ventilation (IPPB) [P_{DI}(max) being -3.5 cm H_2O compared to +9.4 cm H_2O during natural breathing]. In the lateral decubitus posture, the U/L ventilation ratio during IPPB was 0.95 compared to 0.61 with normal breathing, a result similar to studies in paralyzed subjects.

If FRC falls in the dependent lung with APMV, a decrease in compliance, rise in resistance, and airway closure may also contribute to the shift of ventilation from dependent to nondependent lung (Bindslev et al., 1981; Hedenstierna et al., 1981). On the other hand, no frequency dependence of ^{133}Xe washout after equilibration was shown in APMV or awake subjects in the lateral decubitus posture (Rehder et al., 1981). Inspiratory flow was increased from 0.1 liter/sec to 1.6 liters/sec, but the respiratory cycle duration was kept constant by increasing inspiratory or expiratory pauses.

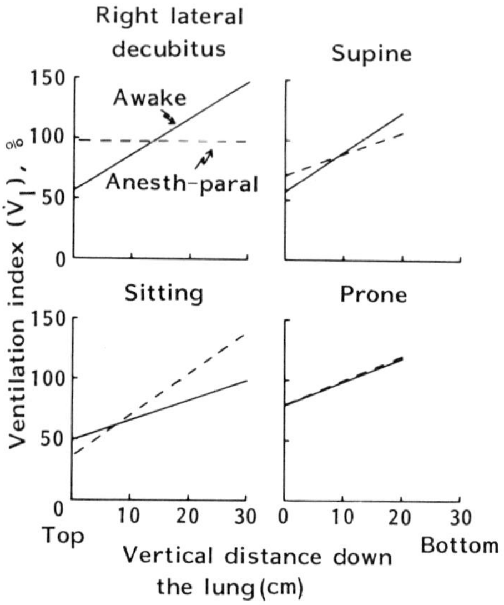

Figure 8 Vertical distribution of tidal volume per unit alveolar volume ($\dot{V}_1$), as a function of body position, in awake and anesthetized-paralyzed subjects. (From Rehder et al., 1978.)

The effect of APMV on the regional distribution of expansion at FRC was investigated by Rehder et al. (1977). An increase in the vertical gradient was found in the lateral decubitus posture (Table 5) but not in the sitting or suping positions.

B. Patients with Respiratory Muscle Paralysis

Ventilation distribution was measured with a combination of ^{81m}Kr and ^{85m}Kr in six patients with bilateral diaphragm paralysis by Amis et al. (1980); none of the patients could generate a significant transdiaphragmatic pressure. The distribution of ventilation, shown in Figure 9, shows similar postural effects to those observed in anesthetized paralyzed subjects (Rehder et al., 1977) but with a more marked reduction in the dependent zones in the supine and lateral decubitus postures. Presumably, similar mechanisms are operating in each case, as discussed in Section VI.A. The paralyzed diaphragm cannot raise the mediastinum away from the dependent lung on inspiration, nor can it oppose the compressing force coming from the gradient of abdominal pressure. Local compression may also lead to a reduction of compliance from an increase in surface tension or airway closure. Measurements of regional volumes have not been made in such patients.

In hemidiaphragmatic paralysis, the study of Arborelius et al. (1975) in 11 subjects is of particular interest because ventilation and FRC were measured in each lung in the lateral decubitus posture. Ventilation (as per-

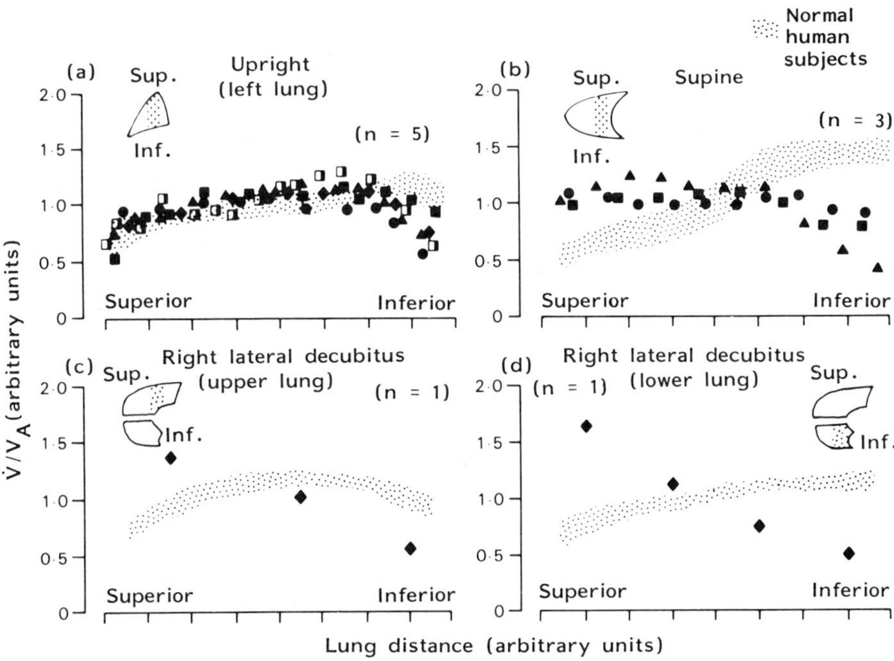

Figure 9 Vertical distribution of tidal volume (V̇/VA) per unit alveolar volume measured with ^{81m}Kr and ^{85m}Kr in bilateral diaphragmatic paralysis in different postures, compared with distributions found in normal subjects (stippled region). Shaded areas within lung diagrams indicate lung regions analyzed; n, number of subjects. (From Amis et al., 1980.)

cent total) to the paralyzed side was 34% when dependent and 26% when nondependent; alveolar volume increased from 34% (dependent) to 43% (nondependent). It is strange that ventilation to the paralyzed side increased when in the dependent position. There was little effect on ventilation distribution in the sitting position, as expected from the studies in bilateral paralysis or in APMV subjects. Ridyard and Stewart (1976) found a 50% reduction in ventilation in the caudal part of the affected lung in five patients in the supine posture, but the ventrodorsal gradient was not measured.

Bake et al. (1972) studied six patients with cervical cord transection with normal diaphragm function but paralyzed intercostal and accessory muscles. In the erect posture, regional FRC was normally distributed but basal ventilation was decreased. It is probable that this change is secondary to mucus retention and infection, because of an impaired ability to cough. Studies in decubitus postures might settle the issue.

VII. Distribution of Ventilation in Lung Disease

In this section we concentrate on a few common conditions. More comprehensive reviews have appeared (Milic-Emili, 1977; Fazio and Wollmer, 1981). The limitations of radioactive gas studies in diffuse pulmonary disease are well known. Considerable inhomogeneity exists within each counting zone, however small, and the dispersion rather than the mean is the index of interest. For this reason, many investigators have turned to multibreath wash-in and washout techniques. Not only are these easier for patients, for whom breath-holding maneuvers may be difficult, but the shape of the washout curve itself may reveal additional inhomogeneity. The most interesting aspect of the use of radioactive gas washout has been the comparison of perfusion-weighted clearances (regional washout after intravenous injection of ^{133}Xe or ^{13}N) and volume or ventilation-weighted clearances (washout after a single inhalation or equilibration).

At the same time, the advent of gamma cameras and a new steady-state technique for measuring regional ventilation, using the 13-sec half-life radionuclide, ^{81m}Kr (Fazio and Jones, 1975), has produced images of ventilation of high quality with much more detail apparent than was possible previously.

A. Emphysema

Bentivoglio et al. (1963a) showed that the regional clearance of ^{133}Xe after equilibration was very delayed both in relation to normal subjects and in comparison to the clearance after intravenous injection. This suggested that poorly ventilated alveoli were also poorly perfused. The perfusion-weighted clearance was also abnormal, showing that well-perfused areas were also poorly ventilated. By dividing the lungs into six zones, gross differences in zonal function correlated in most instances with the amount of destruction shown by radiographic techniques. Nevertheless, newer imaging techniques have showsn widespread abnormalities of ventilation, using ^{81m}Kr, in the presence of a normal chest x-ray (Fazio et al., 1978). Large bullae visible in the radiographs appear virtually unventilated.

B. Chronic Bronchitis

Anthonisen et al. (1968) pointed out that ^{133}Xe clearances in some regions could be very abnormal, especially in the lower zones, even though overall function was minimally impaired. In contrast to the emphysematous patients, clearance after equilibration was faster than after intravenous ^{133}Xe, suggesting a mixture of well-ventilated, poorly perfused units, and well-perfused, poorly ventilated units—a bad combination for pulmonary gas exchange and probably related to the more severe hypoxemia in chronic bronchitis compared to emphysema. Basal impairment of ventilation in patients with normal forced expired volumes was noted by Hughes et al. (1972). Eiser et al. (1977) compared the washout of ^{13}N after intravenous injection in patients breathing air or 30% oxygen. The clearances were followed for one decade (90% elimination); all curves were multiexponential in shape, indicating intraregional inhomogeneity, although large zones (20% of lung) were studied. Hyperoxic breathing delayed the clearance of intravenous ^{13}N by 38% (corrected for total ventilation) but had no effect on the clearance of equilibrated ^{13}N. Interestingly, intravenous clearance was faster than equilibrium clearance breathing air but slower when 30% oxygen was breathed. Eiser et al. (1977) concluded that a significant delay in intravenous ^{13}N clearance occurred during oxygen breathing in 23 out of 64 zones and in 6 of the 16 patients, suggesting inhibition of local hypoxic vasoconstriction and diversion of blood flow from better to more poorly ventilated units.

C. Asthma

The first study of regional ventilation in asthma in clinical remission, using ^{133}Xe (Bentivoglio et al., 1963b), showed abnormal washin curves, although static distributions (slow inspiration from FRC to TLC) were normal. The ventilatory abnormalities were patchy, at segmental or even lobar level, rather than diffuse, as shown later by Fazio et al. (1979) using ^{81m}Kr imaging. With five counters at the back of each lung, no difference between the clearance of equilibrated ^{133}Xe and after intravenous injection was seen (Heckscher et al., 1968), unlike patients with chronic bronchitis. Hughes et al. (1978) induced bronchoconstriction in an asthmatic subject with a nebulized solution of acetylcholine (1 g in 20 ml of saline) to which 50 mg of hexamethonium had been added as an antitussive agent. The development of bronchoconstriction in this subject (Fig. 10) was accompanied by a fall in FEV_1 from 3.2 liters to 1.1 liters. Note the patchy appearance of the scan and the improvement after bronchodilator inhalation, and the increase in lung length after acetylcholine, after only 5 min of inhalation, corresponding roughly to a 70% increase in lung volume during tidal breathing.

^{81m}Kr images are not a quantitative index of ventilation: (1) the relationship between the count rate and ventilation per unit volume is not linear (Fazio and Jones, 1975); (2) no account is taken of the volume of lung seen, and (3) only relative differences are revealed. In Figure 10, the left lung

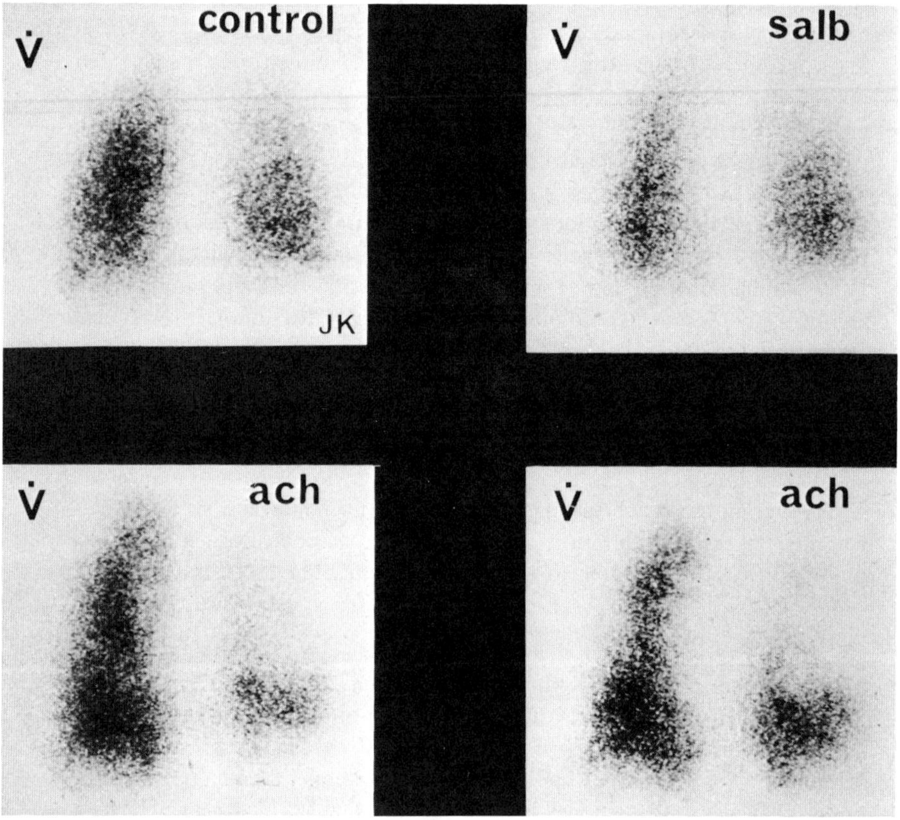

Figure 10 Posterior view of distribution of ^{81m}Kr given by continuous inhalation in an asthmatic subject before (control) and after 2 min (ach, lower left) and 4 min (ach, lower right) inhalation of nebulized acetylcholine, and subsequently (top right) after the inhalation of a bronchodilator (salbutamol). (From Hughes et al., 1978.)

(posterior view) appears spared in relation to the right lung, but in absolute terms its clearance efficiency may have declined compared to control. On the other hand, the patchy nature of regional ventilatory abnormalities in conditions associated with airflow obstruction means that all severe abnormalities will be revealed.

VIII. Mechanisms

A. Equation of Motion

Regional inspiratory flow, $\dot{V}I_r$, is achieved by means of a change in transpulmonary pressure (ΔP_r) which overcomes the local elastic recoil forces or regional compliance (C_r), the local resistance, mainly the frictional resistance of the airways (R_r) and the local inertance (I_r). Ignoring inertial forces, the equation of motion (Otis et al., 1956) is

$$\Delta P_r = \frac{\Delta V_r}{C_r} + \dot{V}_r R_r \qquad (9)$$

In seeking explanations for the distribution of ventilation ($\Delta V_r/VA_r$) the factors influencing the distribution of the applied pressure, compliance, and instantaneous flow and resistance must be taken into account. In addition, during a tidal breath, the values of all four variables may be changing continuously in a nonlinear manner (Shykoff et al., 1982). The magnitude of VA_r will also influence the effectiveness of any given ΔV_r in renewing alveolar gas.

B. Distribution of Compliance and Gradient of Pleural Pressure

The intrinsic elastic properties of the human lung are considered to be uniform (Berend et al., 1980). Therefore, differences in C_r ($\Delta V_r/\Delta P_r$) will depend on the position of any region on the pressure-volume curve. This, in turn, depends on the local transpulmonary pressure or, if alveolar pressure is zero, on pleural pressure (PPL). VA_r (as percent TLC_r) will be determined by PPL_r and the exponential shape of the PV curve. The determinants of the gradient of pleural surface pressure have been the subject of much investigation in the last 20 years. Agostoni (1977) states: "It now seems established that the transpulmonary pressure at the resting volume of the respiratory system decreases from top to bottom in all postures, but does not change markedly along the craniocaudal or dorsoventral axes at a given height and in a given posture, at least on the costal side." Clearly, gravity is playing a major role in determining the gradient of PPL_r, and the associated gradient of VA_r (Table 5, Fig. 3). The simplest and oldest explanation is that the respiratory system is being distorted by its own weight (Glazier et al., 1967). Agostoni (1977) has reasoned that the abdomen should be an important determinant of the gradient of PPL in horizontal postures since the abdomen is four times more dense than the lung, but its influence will depend on the amount of active tension in the diaphragm. Agostoni and his colleagues have estimated that 50% of the pleural pressure gradient is contributed by the weight of the abdomen, 30% by the weight of the chest wall (a gravity-dependent interaction between rib cage and diaphragm), and 20% by the weight of the lung.

On the basis of experimental and theoretical studies (West, 1977b) it is felt that in humans the weight of the lung itself is probably more important. It is interesting that under conditions of zero gravity (0 *g*), the human rib cage does not alter its shape, as judged by radiographs (Michels et al., 1979). Therefore, the return to the 1 *g* situation with the appearance of a gradient in VA_r must be accompanied by internal distortion of elastic tissue with preservation of overall lung shape.

The experimental data outlined in Sections IV.D and V support the notion that the lung is distorted in the erect position, principally by its own weight, with distortions of the chest wall (including the diaphragm) having relatively little influence on the gradient of PPL_r and VA_r. Nevertheless, in horizontal postures the vertical gradient of abdominal pressure exerts an important influence depending on the rigidity of the diaphragm. The vertical gradient of FRC_r (and by implication PPL_r) in the lateral decubitus posture diminishes progressively from approximately 1.2 FRC/cm of distance with a paralyzed diaphragm to 0.8 under normal conditions to 0.24 with a tense diaphragm (from Table 5). Table 5 also shows that the vertical gradient of lung expansion (ΔFRC_r/cm distance) is greater in the supine and lateral decubitus postures than in the erect or prone. There is some support for this notion from direct measurements of surface pressure made in animals (see Agostoni, 1977), but there is some scatter in the data.

Milic-Emili et al. (1966) analyzed the distribution of ventilation in terms of the vertical gradient of pleural pressure, the relationship between regional and overall lung volumes, and a uniform PV curve for each lung region (Fig. 11). Regions in the upper part of the lung were exposed to a more negative pleural (and transpulmonary) pressure and had a higher end-expiratory volume. Since the shape of the PV curve approximates a monoexponential function, the tangent to the curve ($\Delta V/\Delta P$) will have a less steep slope when local lung volume (FRC_r) is higher. Therefore, the more expanded upper zones are stiffer and receive less ventilation. In fact, if tracer gas concentrations are measured at TLC (as is usually done with "bolus" inhalations or techniques which involve breath holding), the upper/lower zone ventilation ratio, if it is determined by the ratio of compliances, should equal the lower/upper zone expansion (FRC_r/TLC_r) ratio (assuming that upper and lower zone alveoli are of equal size at TLC). For measurements made in the erect position with the bolus technique (with breath holding at TLC) at slow flow rates, there is good agreement between the U/L ventilation ratio (Table

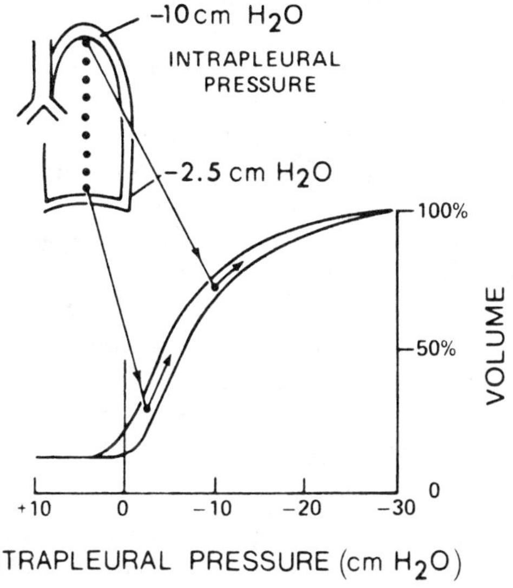

Figure 11 Effect of vertical gradient of pleural surface pressure on distribution of a tidal inspiration from FRC. Regional volume (as percent max) plotted against transpulmonary pressure (PV curve). Lower regions are on a steeper part of the compliance curve of the lungs than are apical zones. For the same transpulmonary pressure change (ΔP), the tidal volume is greater in the lower zones, as indicated by the arrows.

4) and the lower/upper zone expansion ratio of Amis et al. (1984) in Table 5. Measurements made at higher flow rates cannot be explained on this basis.

If measurements are made during tidal breathing or from the washout or washin analysis, ventilation distribution according to the model of Milic-Emili et al. (1966) should be proportional to the ratio of *specific* compliance ($\Delta V_r / \Delta P_r \cdot VA_r$). For 20 cm of vertical distance with a pleural pressure gradient of 0.2 cm H_2O/cm of distance, the upper/lower compliance ratio is about 0.65 (Pedley et al., 1972) and the ratio of I/VA_r in the erect position is 0.76, which gives a specific compliance ratio (U/L) of 0.5. Again, there is reasonable agreement with the U/L ventilation ratio (0.72) measured during tidal breathing in the erect position by steady-state or washout techniques (Table 2).

C. Distribution of Applied Pressure (ΔP)

The first models of interregional ventilation distribution (Milic-Emili et al., 1966; Pedley et al., 1972) assumed that the pleural pressure *change* during inspiration was the same for all regions. Bake et al. (1974) investigated this possibility with upper and lower esophageal balloons and found the ΔP of the lower balloon was 2.3 cm H_2O greater during rapid inspirations. Similar findings were reported by Dosman et al. (1981). In model studies, the distribution of ventilation has been extraordinarily sensitive to variations of ΔP between lung regions (Sybrecht et al., 1976; Shykoff et al., 1982). Baydur et al. (1982) compared mouth occlusion pressure changes with ΔP in the esophagus at various levels and concluded that in spontaneously breathing normal subjects, ΔPPL was uniform in sitting and decubitus postures. During tidal breathing this seems a reasonable notion, but with selective use of inspiratory muscles (Sec. IV.D), in diaphragm paralysis (Sec. V) or lung disease, ΔPPL distribution may not be uniform.

D. Distribution of Airway Resistance

The flow dependence of the distribution of inhaled gas (Table 4) raised the possibility that lower airway resistances were influencing gas distribution at medium and high flow rates. The U/L distribution ratio for boli inhaled at 1 liter/sec (Table 4) of approximately 0.93 was quite different from the distribution of compliances (0.65), implying either an uneven distribution of ΔP at different flow rates, or an uneven distribution of time constants, or both. Assuming equal ΔPPL for upper and lower zones, Bake et al. (1974) felt that the U/L flow dependence of bolus distribution (Table 4) could be explained by the known distribution of compliance and two equal but nonlinear resistances. Sybrecht et al. (1976) felt that the distribution of compliance and resistance could not explain the flow dependence of bolus distribution in the supine posture (Fig. 2) and proposed an uneven distribution of ΔPPL.

There are no measurements of the distribution of regional resistances in vivo, but the lack of effect of helium (Connolly et al., 1975) or SF_6 breathing (Bake et al., 1975) on the distribution of a ^{133}Xe bolus or tidal volume, over a wide range of inspiratory flow rates, argues in favor of a relatively even distribution of lower airway resistances and is consistent with unequal distribution of ΔPPL.

Wilson et al. (1974) measured airway dimensions in dogs using tantalum bronchograms. In the erect position the upper/lower diameter ratio was 1.16; it did not change after 1.5 mg of atropine, although absolute diameters increased by 45%. There was no craniocaudal diameter difference at the same horizontal level in the supine animal. This gives (at low flows) an upper/lower resistance ratio of 0.62, which is the same as that computed by Sybrecht et al. (1976) on the basis of regional expansion data, assuming a linear relationship between local airway conductance and regional lung volume. Clearly, more information is required in this area.

E. Flow and Frequency Dependence

It is difficult to reconcile the frequency dependence of the U/L ratio shown in Table 4 with the lack of frequency dependence of distribution found during tidal breathing at frequencies up to 60 min^{-1} (Forkert et al., 1978; Jones et al., 1978; Kronenberg et al., 1978). Nevertheless, during cyclic breathing inspiratory flow within a breath is not held constant as it was for the experiments reported in Table 4. In this respect, the recent theoretical study of Shykoff et al. (1982) is pertinent. They used a two (upper and lower)-compartment model with nonlinear resistance and compliance which differed from earlier model studies (Pedley et al., 1972; Sybrecht et al., 1976) in using sinusoidal and triangular waveforms for ΔP_{PL} rather than just a square wave. With a vertical gradient of P_{PL} of 4 cm H_2O (= 20 cm distance) but with equal ΔP_{PL_T} for each compartment, their model predicted a ratio (U/L) of tidal volumes of 0.80 for ΔP_{PL} of 1.0 cm H_2O and 0.75 at a ΔP_{PL} of 10 cm H_2O. Frequency was constant (15 min^{-1}) but the increase of ΔP_{PL} was associated with larger tidal volumes and *mean* inspiratory flows (from 0.4 to 3.5 liters, and 0.2 to 1.75 liters/sec, respectively). In terms of $\dot{V}/V_A$, upper/lower ratio at a low mean inspiratory flow was approximately 0.53 *decreasing* to 0.5 at the higher mean flow. This lack of distributional change, from low to higher flow, is very different from the experimental results for *steady* flow quoted in Table 4, but it is more in keeping with the clearance measurements of Forkert et al. (1978) and others. In the model, tidal volume was increased at constant frequency while the experimental data were obtained by changing frequency at constant tidal volume.

F. Conclusions

1. In all postures at FRC, regional lung expansion and transpulmonary pressure decreases from superior to inferior. The human lung distorts primarily under the influence of its own weight, but in horizontal postures the weight of the mediastinum and of the abdominal contents interacting with active tension in the diaphragm also play a part. In decubitus postures, the vertical gradient of alveolar expansion increases when the diaphragm is paralyzed and diminishes when it is tensed.
2. Like regional lung expansion, the distribution of ventilation follows a gravitational pattern. Upper parts of the lung are relatively overexpanded and less compliant; for a given applied pressure (ΔP) ΔV is less. In addition, the higher resting volume (V_A) diminishes the effective ventilation ($\Delta V/V_A$).

3. During tidal breathing, the vertical gradient of $\Delta V/V_A$ is relatively unaffected by increases of respiratory frequency and mean inspiratory flow.
4. Selective use of respiratory muscle groups or diaphragm paralysis can alter the gravity-determined gradients of regional ventilation and expansion especially in the lateral decubitus position.
5. With normal tidal breathing, the distributions of expansion and compliance (which are interrelated) can account for most of the inter-regional differences in ventilation. Other factors, which are not easily measured in humans, such as the distribution of applied pressure on the pleural surface (ΔP) and differences in regional airway resistance, may play a modifying role.

References

Agostoni, E. (1977). Transpulmonary pressure. In *Regional Differences in the Lung.* Edited by J. B. West. New York, Academic Press, pp. 245-280.

Amis, T. C., and Jones, T. (1980). Krypton-81m as a flow tracer in the lung: theory and quantitation. *Bull. Eur. Physiopathol. Respir.,* **16**: 245-259.

Amis, T. C., Ciofetta, G., Clark, J. C., Hughes, J. M. B., Jones, H. A., and Pratt, T. A. (1977). Use of krypton-81m and 85m for measurement of ventilation and perfusion distribution within the lungs. In *Clinical and Experimental Applications of Krypton-81m.* Edited by J. P. Lavender. Br. J. Radiol. Spec. Rep. 15, pp. 52-58.

Amis, T. C., Ciofetta, G., Hughes, J. M. B., and Loh, L. (1980). Regional lung function in bilateral diaphragmatic paralysis. *Clin. Sci.,* **59**:485-492.

Amis, T. C., Jones, H. A., Rhodes, C. G., Heather, J. D., and Hughes, J. M. B. (1982). Regional distribution of ventilation and perfusion in the conscious dog. *Am. J. Vet. Res.,* **43**:1972-1977.

Amis, T. C., Jones, H. A., and Hughes, J. M. B. (1984). Effect of posture on interregional distribution of pulmonary ventilation in man. *Respir. Physiol.,* **56**:145-167.

Anthonisen, N. R., Bass, H., Oriol., A., Place, R. E. G., and Bates, D. V. (1968). Regional lung function in patients with chronic bronchitis. *Clin. Sci.,* **35**:495-512.

Anthonisen, N. R., Robertson, P. C., and Ross, W. R. D. (1970). Gravity-dependent sequential emptying of lung regions. *J. Appl. Physiol.,* **28**: 589-595.

Anthonisen, N. R., Heckscher, T., Bass, H., Oriol, A., and Bates, D. V.

(1973). Studies of regional lung function in chronic bronchitis with emphysema. *Bull. Physiopathol. Respir.,* **9**:1025-1044.

Arborelius, M., Lilja, B., and Senyk, J. (1975). Regional and total lung function studies in patients with hemidiaphragmatic paralysis. *Respiration,* **32**:253-264.

Bake, B., Bjure, J., Grimby, E., Milic-Emili, J., and Nilsson, N. J. (1967). Regional distribution of inspired gas in supine man. *Scand. J. Respir. Dis.,* **48**:189-196.

Bake, B., Fugl-Meyer, A. R., and Grimby, G. (1972). Breathing patterns and regional ventilation distribution in tetraplegic patients and in notmal subjects. *Clin. Sci.,* **42**:117-128.

Bake, B., Wood, L., Murphy, B., Macklem, P. T., and Milic-Emili, J. (1974). Effect of inspiratory flow rate on regional distribution of inspired gas. *J. Appl. Physiol.,* **37**:8-17.

Ball, W. C., Stewart, P. B., Newsham, L. G. S., and Bates, D. V. (1962). Regional pulmonary function studied with xenon^{133}. J. Clin. Invest., **41**:519-531.

Baydur, A., Behrakis, P. K., Zin, W. A., Jager, M., and Milic-Emili, J. (1982). A simple method for assessing the validity of the esophageal balloon technique. *Am. Rev. Respir. Dis.,* **126**:788-791.

Bentivoglio, L. G., Beerel, F., Stewart, P. B., Bryan, A. C., Ball, W. C., and Bates, D. V. (1963a). Studies of regional ventilation and perfusion in pulmonary emphysema using xenon^{133}. *Am. Rev. Respir. Dis.* **88**:315-329.

Bentivoglio, L. G., Beerel, F., Bryan, A. C., Stewart, P. B., Rose, B., and Bates, D. V. (1963b). Regional pulmonary function studied with xenon^{133} in patients with bronchial asthma. *J. Clin. Invest.,* **42**:1193-1200.

Berend, N., Skoog, C., and Thurlbeck, W. M. (1980). Pressure-volume characteristics of excised human lungs: effects of sex, age and emphysema. *J. Appl. Physiol. Respir. Environ. Exercise Physiol.,* **49**:558-565.

Bindslev, L., Santesson, J., and Hedenstierna, G. (1981). Distribution of inspired gas to each lung in anesthetized human subjects. *Acta Anaesth. Scand.,* **25**:297-302.

Bryan, A. C., Bentivoglio, L. G., Beerel, F., MacLeish, H., Zidulka, A., and Bates, D. V. (1964). Factors affecting regional distribution of ventilation and perfusion in the lung. *J. Appl. Physiol.,* **19**:395-402.

Bryan, A. C., Milic-Emili, J., and Pengelly, D. (1966). Effect of gravity on the distribution of pulmonary ventilation. *J. Appl. Physiol.,* **22**:778-784.

Bynum, L. J., Wilson, J. E., and Pierce, A. K. (1976). Comparison of spontaneous and positive pressure breathing in supine normal subjects. *J. Appl. Physiol.*, **41**:341-347.

Chevrolet, J. C., Martin, J. G., Flood, R., Martin, R. R., and Engel, L. A. (1978). Topographical ventilation and perfusion distribution during IPPB in the lateral posture. *Am. Rev. Respir. Dis.*, **118**:847-854.

Chevrolet, J. C., Emrich, J., Martin, R. R., and Engel, L. A. (1979). Voluntary changes in ventilation distribution in the lateral posture. *Respir. Physiol.*, **38**:313-323.

Clark, J. C., and Buckingham, P. D. (1975). *Short-Lived Radioactive Gases for Clinical Use.* London, Butterworth.

Connolly, T., Bake, B., Wood, L., and Milic-Emili, J. (1975). Regional distribution of a ^{133}Xe labelled gas volume inspired at constant flow rate. *Scand. J. Respir. Dis.*, **56**:150-159.

Crouzel, C., Guenard, H., Comar, D., Soussaline, F., Loch, C., and Plummer, D. (1980). A new radioisotope for lung ventilation studies: 19-neon. *Eur. J. Nucl. Med.*, **5**:431-434.

Cumming, G., and Jones, J. G. (1966). The construction and repeatability of lung nitrogen clearance curves. *Respir. Physiol.*, **1**:238-248.

D'Angelo, E. (1972). Local alveolar size and transpulmonary pressure in situ and in isolated lungs. *Respir. Physiol.*, **14**:251-266.

D'Angelo, E. (1981). Cranio-caudal rib cage distortion with increasing inspiratory airflow in man. *Respir. Physiol.*, **44**:215-237.

Demedts, M. (1978). Regional distribution of lung volumes, ventilation and transpulmonary pressures. Thesis, Departement Pathofysiologie, Faculteit der Geneeskunde, Katholieke Universiteit Leuven.

Demedts, M. (1980). Regional distribution of lung volumes and of gas inspired at residual volume: influence of age, weight and body posture. *Bull. Eur. Physiopathol. Respir.*, **16**:271-285.

Demedts, M., Clarysse, I., Verhamme, M., Marq, M., and de Roo, M. (1983). Regional gas distributions and single-breath washout curves in head-down position. *J. Appl. Physiol. Respir. Environ. Exercise Physiol.*, **54**:361-365.

Devos, P., Demedts, M., Vandecruys, A., Cosemamf, J., and de Roo, M. (1978). Comparison of ^{133}Xe washout curves after bolus inhalation perfusion and equilibration. *Respiration*, **35**:115-121.

Dollery, C. T., Hugh-Jones, P., and Matthews, C. M. E. (1962). Use of radioactive xenon for studies of regional lung function. *Br. Med. J.*, **ii**:1006-1016.

Dollfuss, R. E., Milic-Emili, J., and Bates, D. V. (1967). Regional ventilation of the lung studied with boluses of 133 xenon. *Respir. Physiol.*, **2**:234-246.

Dosman, J. A., Hodgson, W., Edearson, C., Graham, B. L., Cotton, D. J., and Stirling, D. (1981). Effect of inspiratory flow rate on the esophageal pressure gradient in upright humans. *Respir. Physiol.,* **46**:105-112.

Eiser, N. M., Jones, H. A., and Hughes, J. M. B. (1977). Effect of 30% oxygen on local matching of perfusion and ventilation in chronic airways obstruction. *Clin. Sci. Mol. Med.,* **53**:387-395.

Engel, L. A., and Prefaut, C. (1981). Cranio-caudal distribution of inspired gas and perfusion in supine man. *Respir. Physiol.,* **45**:43-53.

Engel, L., Grassino, A. E., and Anthonisen, N. R. (1975). Demonstration of airway closure in man. *J. Appl. Physiol.,* **38**:1117-1125.

Engel, L., Landau, L., Taussig, L., Martin, R. R., and Sybrecht, G. (1976). Influence of bronchomotor tone on regional ventilation distribution at residual volume. *J. Appl. Physiol.,* **40**:411-416.

Ewan, P. W., Jones, H. A., Nosil, J., Obdrzalek, J., and Hughes, J. M. B. (1978). Uneven perfusion and ventilation within lung regions studied with nitrogen-13. *Respir. Physiol.,* **34**:45-59.

Fazio, F., and Jones, T. (1975). Assessment of regional ventilation by continuous inhalation of radioactive krypton-81m. *Br. Med. J.,* **3**:673-676.

Fazio, F., and Wollmer, P. (1981). Clinical ventilation-perfusion scintigraphy. *Clin. Physiol.,* **1**:323-337.

Fazio, F., Lavender, J. P., and Steiner, R. E. (1978). ^{81m}Kr ventilation and ^{99m}Tc perfusion scans in chest disease: comparison with standard radiographs. *Am. J. Roentgenol.,* **130**:421-428.

Fazio, F., Palla, A., Santolicandro, A., Solfanelli, S., Fornai, E., and Giuntini, C. (1979). Studies of regional ventilation in asthma using ^{81m}Kr. *Lung,* **156**:185-194.

Fixley, M. S., Roussos, C. S., Murphy, B., Martin, R. R., and Engel, L. A. (1978). Flow dependence of gas distribution and the pattern of inspiratory muscle contraction. *J. Appl. Physiol. Respir. Environ. Exercise Physiol.,* **45**:733-741.

Forkert, L. (1980). Effect of regional chest wall restriction on regional lung function. *J. Appl. Physiol. Respir. Environ. Exercise Physiol.,* **49**:655-662.

Forkert, L., Anthonisen, N. R., and Wood, L. D. H. (1978). Frequency dependence of regional lung washout. *J. Appl. Physiol. Respir. Environ. Exercise Physiol.,* **45**:161-170.

Froese, A., and Bryan, A. C. (1974). Effects of anesthesia and paralysis on diaphragmatic mechanics in man. *Anesthesiology,* **41**:242-255.

Glaister, D. H. (1967). The effect of posture on the distribution of ventilation and blood flow in the normal lung. *Clin. Sci.,* **33**:391-398.

Glazier, J. B., and DeNardo, G. L. (1966). Pulmonary function studies with the xenon-133 scanning technique. Normal values and a postural study. *Am. Rev. Respir. Dis.*, **94**:188-194.

Glazier, J. B., Hughes, J. M. B., Maloney, J. E., and West, J. B. (1967). Vertical gradient of alveolar size in lungs of dogs frozen intact. *J. Appl. Physiol.*, **23**:694-705.

Grant, B. J. B., Jones, H. A., and Hughes, J. M. B. (1974). Sequence of regional filling during a tidal breath in man. *J. Appl. Physiol.*, **37**:158-165.

Grassino, A. E., and Anthonisen, N. R. (1975). Chest wall distortion and regional lung volume distribution in erect humans. *J. Appl. Physiol.*, **39**:1004-1007.

Grassino, A. E., Bake, B., Martin, R. R., and Anthonisen, N. R. (1975). Voluntary changes of thoracoabdominal shape and regional lung volumes in humans. *J. Appl. Physiol.*, **39**:997-1003.

Greene, R., Hughes, J. M. B., Sudlow, M. F., and Milic-Emili, J. (1974). Regional lung volumes during water immersion to the xiphoid in seated man. *J. Appl. Physiol.*, **36**:734-736.

Grimby, G., Goldman, M., and Mead, J. (1976). Respiratory muscle action inferred from rib cage and abdominal V-P partitioning. *J. Appl. Physiol.*, **41**:739-751.

Hales, C. A., Gibbons, R., Burnham, C., and Kazemi, H. (1976). Determinants of regional distribution of a bolus inhaled from residual volume. *J. Appl. Physiol.*, **41**:400-408.

Heckscher, T., Bass, H., Oriol, O., Rose, B., Anthonisen, N. R., and Bates, D. V. (1968). Regional lung function in patients with bronchial asthma. *J. Clin. Invest.*, **47**:1063-1070.

Hedenstierna, G., Bindslev, L., Santesson, J., and Norlander, O. P. (1981). Airway closure in each lung of anesthetized subjects. *J. Appl. Physiol. Respir. Environ. Exercise Physiol.*, **50**:55-64.

Holland, J., Milic-Emili, J., Macklem, P. T., and Bates, D. V. (1968). Regional distribution of pulmonary ventilation and perfusion in elderly subjects. *J. Clin. Invest.*, **47**:81-92.

Holley, H. S., Milic-Emili, J., Becklake, M. R., and Bates, D. V. (1967). Regional distribution of pulmonary ventilation and perfusion in obesity. *J. Clin. Invest.*, **46**:475-481.

Hughes, J. M. B. (1979). Review article: Short-life radionuclides and regional lung function. *Br. J. Radiol.*, **52**:353-370.

Hughes, J. M. B., Grant, B. J. B., Greene, R. E., Iliff, L. D., and Milic-Emili, J. (1972). Inspiratory flow rate and ventilation distribution in normal subjects and in simple chronic bronchitis. *Clin. Sci.*, **43**:583-595.

Hughes, J. M. B., Gardiner, I. G., and Ciofetta, G. (1978). Induced bronchoconstriction. In *Clinical and Experimental Applications of Krypton-81m.* Edited by J. P. Lavender. Br. J. Radiol. Spec. Rep. 15, pp. 125-127.

Jones, R. L., Overton, T. R., and Sproule, B. J. (1977). Frequency dependence of ventilation distribution in normal and obstructed lungs. *J. Appl. Physiol. Respir. Environ. Exercise Physiol.*, **42**:548-553.

Kaneko, K., Milic-Emili, J., Dolovich, M. B., Dawson, A., and Bates, D. V. (1966). Regional distribution of ventilation and perfusion as a function of body position. *J. Appl. Physiol.*, **21**:767-777.

Knipping, H. W., Bolt, W., Venrath, H., Valentin, H., Ludes, H., and Endler, P. (1955). Eine neue Methode zur Prufung der Herz-und Lungenfunktion. *Dtsch. med. Wschr.*, **80**:1146-1147.

Kronenberg, R. S., Wangensteen, O. D., and Ponto, R. A. (1976). Frequency dependence of regional lung clearance of ^{133}Xe in normal men. *Respir. Physiol.*, **27**:293-303.

Lemelin, J., Ross, W. R. O., Martin, R. R., and Anthonisen, N. R. (1972). Regional lung volumes with positive pressure inflation in erect humans. *Respir. Physiol.*, **16**:273-281.

Martin, R. R., Anthonisen, N. R., and Zutter, M. (1972). Flow dependence of the intrapulmonary distribution of inspired boluses of ^{133}Xe in smokers and non-smokers. *Clin. Sci.*, **43**:319-329.

Matthews, C. M. E., and Dollery, C. T. (1965). Interpretation of ^{133}Xe lung wash-in and wash-out curves using an analogue computer. *Clin. Sci.*, **28**:573-590.

Melissinos, C. G., Goldman, M., Bruce, E., Elliot, E., and Mead, J. (1981). Chest wall shape during forced expiratory maneuvers. *J. Appl. Physiol. Respir. Environ. Exercise Physiol.*, **50**:84-93.

Michels, D. B., and West, J. B. (1978). Distribution of pulmonary ventilation and perfusion during short periods of weightlessness. *J. Appl. Physiol.*, **45**:987-998.

Michels, D. B., Friedman, P. J., and West, J. B. (1979). Radiographic comparison of human lung shape during normal gravity and weightlessness. *J. Appl. Physiol. Respir. Environ. Exercise Physiol.*, **47**:851-857.

Milic-Emili, J. (1974). Pulmonary statics. In *MTP International Reviews of Science: Respiratory Physiology*, Vol. 1. Edited by J. G. Widdicombe. London, Butterworth, pp. 105-137.

Milic-Emili, J. (1977). Ventilation. In *Regional Differences in the Lung*. Edited by J. B. West. New York, Academic Press, pp. 167-199.

Milic-Emili, J. (1980). Interregional distribution of inspired bas. In *Gas Exchange Function of Normal and Diseased Lungs*. Edited by J. Piiper and P. Scheid. Prog. Resp. Res., Vol. 16. Basel, S. Karger, pp. 33-43.

Milic-Emili, J. (1982). Interregional distribution of ventilation. *Bull. Eur. Physiopathol. Respir.*, **18**:325-327.

Milic-Emili, J., Henderson, J. A. M., Dolovich, M. B., Trop, D., and Kaneko, K. (1966). Regional distribution of inspired gas in the lung. *J. Appl. Physiol.*, **21**:749-759.

Newhouse, M. T., Wright, F. J., Ingham, C. K., Archer, N. P., Hughes, L. B., and Hopkins, O. L. (1968). Use of scintillation camera and ^{135}xenon for the study of topographic pulmonary function. *Respir. Physiol.,* **4**: 141-153.

Otis, A. B., McKerrow, C. B., Bartlett, R. A., Mead, J., McIlroy, M. B., Selverstone, N. J., and Radford, E. P. (1956). Mechanical factors in distribution of pulmonary ventilation. *J. Appl. Physiol.,* **8**:427-443.

Pedley, T. J., Sudlow, M. F., and Milic-Emili, J. (1972). A non-linear theory of the distribution of pulmonary ventilation. *Respir. Physiol.,* **15**:1-38.

Prefaut, C., and Engel, L. A. (1981). Vertical distribution of perfusion and inspired gas in supine man. *Respir. Physiol.,* **43**:209-219.

Rehder, K., Hatch, D. J., Sessler, A. D., and Fowler, W. S. (1972). The function of each lung of anesthetized and paralyzed man during mechanical ventilation. *Anesthesiology,* **37**:16-26.

Rehder, K., Sessler, A. D., and Rodarte, J. R. (1977). Regional intrapulmonary gas distribution in awake and anesthetized paralyzed man. *J. Appl. Physiol. Respir. Enciron. Exercise Physiol.,* **42**:391-402.

Rehder, K., Knopp, T. J., and Sessler, A. D. (1978). Regional intrapulmonary gas distribution in awake and anesthetized paralyzed prone man. *J. Appl. Physiol.,* **45**:528-535.

Rehder, K., Knopp, T. J., Brusasco, V., and Didier, E. P. (1981). Inspiratory flow and intrapulmonary gas distribution. *Am. Rev. Respir. Dis.,* **124**:392-296.

Rhodes, C. G., Wollmer, P., Fazio, F., and Jones, T. (1981). Quantitative measurement of regional extravascular lung density using positron emission and transmission tomography. *J. Comput. Assist. Tomogr.,* **5**:783-791.

Ridyard, J. B., and Stewart, R. M. (1976). Regional lung function in unilateral diaphragmatic paralysis. *Thorax,* **31**:438-442.

Robertson, P. C., Anthonisen, N. R., and Ross, D. (1969). Effect of inspiratory flow rate on regional distribution of inspired gas. *J. Appl. Physiol.,* **26**:438-443.

Ronchetti, R., Jones, H. A., Rhodes, C. G., Herring, A., Eiser, N. M., Renci, S., and Hughes, J. M. B. (1980). Clearance of radioactive nitrogen and xenon from the lungs of anaesthetized dogs and human subjects. *Bull. Eur. Physiopathol. Respir.,* **16**:395-409.

Rosenzweig, D. Y., Hughes, J. M. B., and Jones, T. (1969). Uneven ventilation within and between regions of the normal lung measured with nitrogen-13. *Respir. Physiol.,* **8**:86-97.

Roussos, C. S., Siegler, D. I. M., and Engel, L. A. (1976a). Influence of diaphragmatic contraction and expiratory flow on the pattern of lung emptying. *Respir. Physiol.,* **27**:157-167.

Roussos, C. S., Fukuchi, Y., Macklem, P. T., and Engel, L. A. (1976b). Influence of diaphragmatic contraction on ventilation distribution in horizontal man. *J. Appl. Physiol.,* **40**:417-424.

Roussos, C. S., Fixley, M., Genest, J., Cosio, M., Kelly, S., Martin, R. R., and Engel, L. A. (1977). Voluntary factors influencing the distribution of inspired gas. *Am. Rev. Respir. Dis.,* **116**:457-467.

Ruff, F., Martin, R. R., and Milic-Emili, J. (1981). Previous volume history of the lung and regional distribution of residual volume. *J. Appl. Physiol. Respir. Environ. Exercise Physiol.,* **51**:313-316.

Seeman, P. (1972). Membrane actions of anesthetics and tranquillizers. *Pharmacol. Rev.,* **24**:583-655.

Sharp, J. T., Goldberg, N. B., Druz, W. S., and Danon, J. (1975). Relative contributions of rib cage and abdomen to breathing in normal subjects. *J. Appl. Physiol.,* **39**:608-618.

Shykoff, B. E., Grondelle, A. Van, and Chang, H. K. (1982). Effects of unequal pressure swings and different waveforms on distribution of ventilation: a non-linear model study. *Respir. Physiol.,* **48**:157-168.

Sutherland, P. W., Katsura, T., and Milic-Emili, J. (1968). Previous volume history of the lung and regional distribution of gas. *J. Appl. Physiol.,* **25**:566-574.

Sybrecht, G. W., Garrett, L., and Anthonisen, N. R. (1975). Effect of chest strapping on regional lung function. *J. Appl. Physiol.,* **39**:707-713.

Sybrecht, G., Landau, L., Murphy, B. G., Engel, L. A., Martin, R. R., and Macklem, P. T. (1976). Influence of posture on flow dependence of distribution of inhaled ^{133}Xe boli. *J. Appl. Physiol.,* **41**:489-496.

Valind, S., Rhodes, C. G., Clarke, J., Burke, P., and Hughes, J. M. B. (1983). Quantitative measurements of regional ventilation using positron computed tomography (PCT) and a short-lived inert gas–Neon-19. *Nucl. Med. Commun.,* **4**:149.

Van Slyke, D. D., Dillon, R. T., and Margaria, R. (1934). Studies of gas and electrolyte equilibria in blood: XVIII. Solubility and physical state of atmospheric nitrogen in blood cells and plasma. *J. Biol. Chem.,* **105**:571-596.

Vawter, D. L., Matthews, F. L., and West, J. B. (1975). Effect of shape and size of lung and chest wall on stresses in the lung. *J. Appl. Physiol.,* **39**:9-17.

West, J. B., ed. (1977a). *Regional Differences in the Lung.* New York, Academic Press.

West, J. B. (1977b). Stresses. In *Regional Differences in the Lung.* Edited by J. B. West. New York, Academic Press, pp. 281-322.

West, J. B., and Dollery, C. T. (1960). Distribution of blood flow and ventilation-perfusion ratio in the lung, measured with radioactive CO_2. *J. Appl. Physiol.,* **15**:405-410.

Wilson, A. G., Jones, H. A., and Hughes, J. M. B. (1974). Effect of posture on airway length and diameter. *Respir. Physiol.,* **22**:381-397.

Yeh, S., and Peterson, R. E. (1965). Solubility of krypton and xenon in blood, protein solutions, and tissue homogenates. *J. Appl. Physiol.,* **20**:1041-1047.

6

Theoretical Studies of Gas Mixing in the Lung

MANUEL PAIVA

Institute of Interdisciplinary Research
and Respiratory Research Unit
Free University of Brussels
Brussels, Belgium

Remember that a model is a convenient artifice that may help us understand a small facet of a large and intricate machinery.

E. Weibel

I. Introduction

Although the qualitative behavior of gas mixing in the lung can be understood without mathematics, its use cannot be avoided when quantitative aspects become important. This chapter thus aims at providing those who have little mathematical background with a basis for understanding the literature in this field. We do not expect to offer readers the pleasure of studying biomathematical papers. We want only to give them the possibility of understanding the meaning of the assumptions, the main lines in the elaboration of the equations, and the search for their solutions. The aim of this chapter is not to review the literature; this has been done by others (Scheid and Piiper, 1980). It therefore necessarily deals principally with the author's own theoretical analysis.

As in any physical system, the knowledge of gas mixing in the lung

This work was partly supported by a contract of the Ministère Belge de la Politique Scientifique (Actions Concertées).

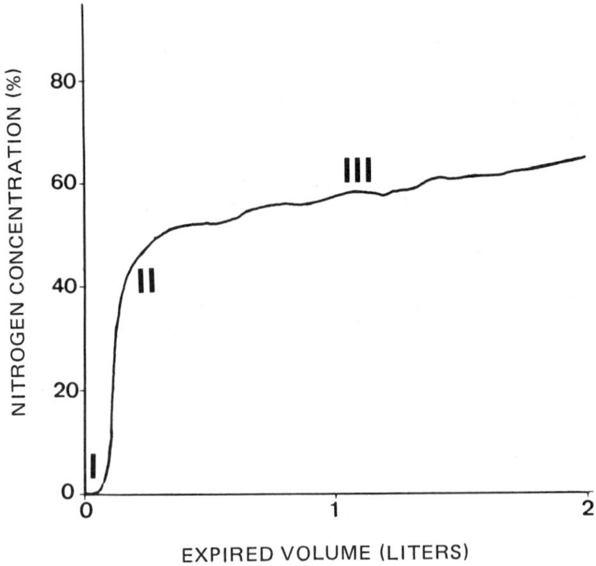

Figure 1 Single-breath N_2 washout. After an inspiration of an O_2 breath, the N_2 concentration measured at the mouth during the next expiration presents at least the three characteristic phases: phase I, with zero N_2 concentration; phase II, corresponding to a rapid concentration rise; and phase III or alveolar plateau, where the concentration increases steadily.

must rely on experimental measurements. The simplest and probably the commonest method consists of using tracer gases and the simplest gas is N_2, which is already present in the lung. After inspiration of an O_2 breath, the N_2 concentration measured at the mouth during the next expiration always presents at least the three characteristic zones or phases shown in Figure 1. After a phase I with zero N_2 concentration and a rapid rise (phase II), the N_2 concentration increases steadily during most of the expiration (phase III). This is the alveolar plateau, representing alveolar gas concentration. The recording of Figure 1 was obtained from a young subject without closing volume after a 1-liter inspiration from the functional residual capacity. If the lung behaved as a well-ventilated bellows, phase III would have been horizontal and the bellows volume could be very simply calculated using the dilution principle. Furthermore, the expired N_2 concentration would have been equal to the alveolar concentration.

A major reason for the difficulty in understanding gas transport and mixing in the alveolar zone of the lung is related to the impossibility of performing direct measurements of gas concentrations. Among others, two independent approaches were attempted in the early 1970s: a physiological approach, consisting of measuring gas concentration as peripherally as is possible in the bronchial tree of experimental animals (Engel et al., 1973); and a theoretical approach consisting of simulating the real system with a mathematical model (Paiva, 1972, 1973). A large part of this chapter is a result of the subsequent collaboration between those workers.

There are several ways to determine the concentration of alveolar gas and of gas distribution in the lung from inert gas measurements at the mouth. Some of them will be discussed in more detail in Chapter 7. We focus here on the single-breath N_2 test because the interpretation of the slope of the alveolar plateau stimulated discussions over the last decades. Furthermore, there are several advantages in using this test to study alveolar gas mixing: It is easy to perform, it is of clinical and epidemiological interest (Buist and Ross, 1973), and there are extensive published data. Yet although several explanations have been offered, an accepted interpretation of the single-breath N_2 test does not yet exist.

The two explanations of the slope of the alveolar plateau which have been alternatively accepted and rejected were clearly explained by Sikand et al. (1966) in one diagram, shown in Figure 2. The lung is represented

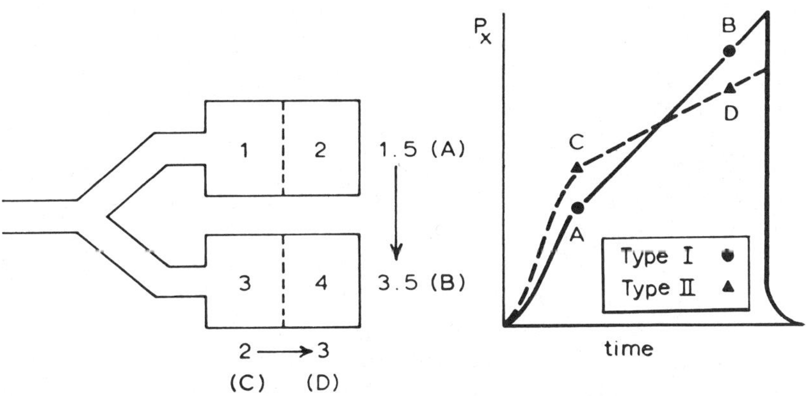

Figure 2 Possible types of uneven distribution of alveolar ventilation. The figure on the left depicts two elements in parallel. In each, the concentration of an inert gas, shown by an arbitrary figure, is higher near the bronchial opening. If the top element contributes more to the initial part of expiration and less to the terminal part (type I) the expired gas composition could move from A to B. If, on the other hand, the elements near the dead space empty first (type II), the expired gas could change from C to D. In both cases, the expiratory fraction could increase as shown on the right-hand tracing. (From Sikand et al., 1966.)

by two elements in parallel; in type II explanation each element is divided into two zones, the peripheral one being N_2 enriched. In type I explanation each element has a uniform concentration. The type I explanation assumes that the top element contributes more to the initial part of expiration and less to the terminal part, the expired gas composition moving from A to B. In type II explanation, the expired gas changes from C to D due to a series concentration gradient, called stratification by Rauwerda (1946). It simply expresses that less inspired O_2 reaches the more peripheral lung generations, producing a gradient of N_2 concentration along the airways. This explanation was first proposed by Krogh and Lindhard (1917), who suggested that the inspired gas did not have time to diffuse to the most distal part of the acinus during a respiratory cycle and that the persistent concentration gradient, on expiration, resulted in a sloping plateau. This would occur even if the two parallel elements emptied synchronously. Fowler (1949), based on continuous recording of expired N_2, considered stratification to be negligible.

The type I explanation (Fig. 2) considers that in each parallel unit the gases have enough time to homogenize but that (1) their relative expansions (from their resting volume) are different, and (2) that the unit with the small relative expansion (larger N_2 concentration) contributes more toward the end of the expiration. The type I explanation received support from the work of Rauwerda, who developed the first mathematical model of gas mixing in the lung (Rauwerda, 1946).

Although each parallel unit did not receive a precise anatomical characterization, two different mechanisms have been considered as contributing to the slope. One, proposed by Otis et al. (1956), is based on the RC (resistance-capacitance) electrical analogy, which predicts different time constants and consequently out-of-phase filling and emptying of the parallel units. Another mechanism is related to differences in pressure-volume curves of the two parallel units. The first mechanism is a time-dependent one, the second a volume-dependent one.

A major advance came from the demonstration by Milic-Emili et al. (1966) of the gravity-dependent ventilation inhomogeneity and by Anthonisen et al. (1970) of the gravity-dependent sequential emptying of units with different $\Delta V/V_0$ producing a sloping alveolar plateau. However, Engel et al. (1974) found that, in the dog, a major proportion of the slope of the alveolar plateau measured in the trachea is present in airways 2-3 mm in diameter. The volume subtended by those airways corresponds roughly to a sphere 20 mm in diameter and contains 35 terminal bronchioles and therefore 35 acini (Horsfield and Cumming, 1968). This shows that there is a component of the slope of the alveolar plateau due to the inhomogeneities between units less than a few centimeters apart (see Chap. 7). This was confirmed by single-breath N_2 tests performed at zero gravity where a sloping alveolar plateau was always present, although the interregional gravity-dependent component was eliminated (Michels and West, 1978).

It appeared clear to Rauwerda (1946), 40 years ago, that the modeling approach was an alternative possibility for obtaining information on the mechanisms of mixing within the lung. He represented the terminal lung generations by a cone and concluded that molecular diffusion was rapid enough to ensure concentration homogeneization during the time of a breath. In 1963 Weibel published the first simple morphometric description of the human lung (Weibel, 1963) which chould be applied to a mathematical analysis. This opened the way for modeling the gas transport and mixing in the human lung.

II. Diffusion Equation

Whatever the quantitative description of gas mixing in the lung, molecular diffusion necessarily plays an important role. Indeed, the net O_2-CO_2 flow across the alveolocapillary membrane is three orders of magnitude smaller than the bulk flow in the airways and the bronchial tree has a cul-de-sac structure. Therefore, the molecules that are close to the alveolocapillary membrane have an almost zero convective velocity with respect to that membrane. Molecular diffusion thus is the main mechanism of transport for the O_2 molecules to reach the blood. It is then not surprising that a diffusion equation is the central mathematical tool for a quantitative description of gas transport in the lung. The bronchial tree being a network of ducts, we take as a starting point the diffusion equation in one duct of constant cross section.

We shall restrict our mathematical formulation to the diffusion in a duct, where, due to its small cross section, the molecular diffusion in the radial direction can be considered as being instantaneous. This assumption will be justified below. Our problem, then, is to describe quantitatively the molecular diffusion of two different types of molecules, characterized by the binary diffusion molecular coefficient D (Chap. 1) in a duct of constant cross section.

At the beginning of the nineteenth century, Fourier discovered the equation of heat conduction. Half a century later, Fick (1855) recognized that the random molecular movement would lead to the same equation to describe the concentration of diffusible matter instead of temperature. Its one-dimensional form, which applies to a duct of constant cross section, is

$$\frac{\partial F}{\partial t} = D \frac{\partial^2 F}{\partial x^2} \qquad (1)$$

where F is the concentration, D the diffusion coefficient, and x the distance to a fixed point at time t. This equation expresses only two things in mathematical terms: the matter balance (the rate of concentration variation in an element of volume is given by the difference between what arrives and what leaves per unit of time and unit of volume of the element considered) and Fick's law of diffusion, expressing the matter flow in terms of the gradient of the concentration:

$$\text{Diffusion flow} = -DS\frac{\partial F}{\partial x} \tag{2}$$

If F is expressed in moles per cubic centimeter, the number of moles crossing the section S of the tube per second is obtained by multiplying the diffusion coefficient (D) by the cross section (S) and by minus the concentration gradient $\partial F/\partial x$. Minus, because matter always flows from regions of high concentration to regions of low concentration. The symbol ∂ is traditionally used (instead of d) to represent a derivative of F with respect to one variable, keeping the other constant (it is called partial derivative). Here, the concentration depends on t and x. Because of the appearance of several partial derivatives in Eq. (1), it is called a partial differential equation.

A. Analytical Solutions

In this section we shall restrict ourselves to the diffusion of O_2 in N_2 at 37°C and for P = 1 atm: $D = 0.225\ cm^2/sec$. The solutions of Eq. (1) describe the mixing of O_2 and N_2 molecules in a duct of constant cross section. However, a unique solution can be obtained only if two conditions are specified: the initial and the boundary conditions. We shall consider here the case where all the O_2 molecules are situated in x = 0 at t = 0 (Fig. 3), which is mathematically expressed as $C(x, t = 0) = M\delta(x)$. $\delta(x)$ is the Dirac function, equal to zero everywhere except for x = 0, where it is infinity. M is the molar fraction at x = 0 and t = 0. This represents an infinitely thin slice of O_2 molecules situated at x = 0. The boundary condition $C(x = \pm\infty, t) = 0$ (∞ is the symbol for infinity) only expresses the fact that the molecules cannot travel infinite distances at finite times.

With the previous initial and boundary conditions, the unique solution of Eq. (1) is

$$F(x, t) = \frac{M}{2\sqrt{\pi Dt}}\, e^{-x^2/4Dt} \tag{3}$$

It is a fortunate coincidence that the previous solution of the diffusion equation is a function for which nonmathematicians acquired an intuitive feeling. Indeed, Eq. (3) is no more than the error or gaussian distribution

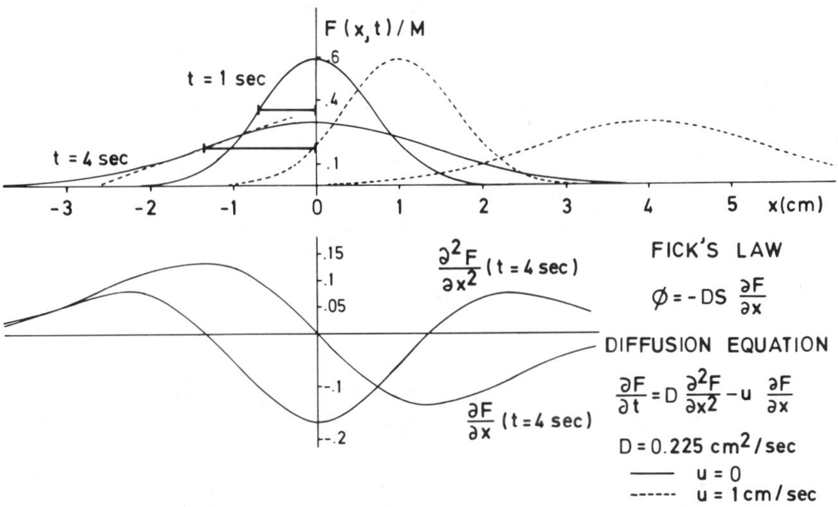

Figure 3 Solutions of the diffusion equation. See the text for details.

(solid lines in the upper panel of Fig. 3) with a mean value of zero and a standard deviation (SD) of $\sqrt{2Dt}$ (horizontal bars). This means that the square root of the mean-squared displacement (definition of the standard deviation of a distribution) of one O_2 molecule is equal to $\sqrt{2Dt}$. For t = 1 sec and D = 0.225 cm^2/sec we have SD = 0.67 cm (upper horizontal bar).

A simple exercise to prove that F given by Eq. (3) is a solution of Eq. (1) would consist of calculating the time derivative of F and checking that it is equal to the second derivative of F multiplied by D. For those who have forgotten the rules of differentiation, an intuitive feeling of their mathematical meaning can be grasped from Figure 3. We have represented Eq. (3) with D = 0.225 cm^2/sec for t = 1 sec and t = 4 sec (solid lines). The standard deviation (⊢⊣) is also represented and gives an idea of the distances covered by diffusion. It is noteworthy that the human acinus length is close to 0.67 cm (Chap. 2). It is clear that the mean distance is zero because the mean displacement to the right (positive) is equal to the mean displacement to the left (negative). If we consider the curve F(x, t = 4 sec), we can calculate $\partial F/\partial x$, which is the slope of the tangent to that curve at any point (dashed straight line for x = −1.34 cm). This slope is zero for F = 0 and for F = $\pm\infty$ and it is represented with the same scale in the lower panel. This slope multiplied by D and S gives the flow of diffusion ϕ (Fick's law). For t = 4 sec, its absolute value is maximal at points distant 1.34 cm from the origin of the coordinates (the inflection point of the error function corresponds to $x = \pm 1$ standard deviation). $\partial^2 F/\partial x^2$ is the derivative of $\partial F/\partial x$ and presents the bimodal shape with a minimum for $F = 0$. If we multiply $\partial^2 F/\partial x^2$ by D we obtain $\partial F/\partial t$ [see Eq. (1)], that is, the rate of F variation (for $t = 4$ sec) for any value of x. For example, the minimal value of $\partial^2 F/\partial x^2$ (or $\partial F/\partial t$) is at $x = 0$, which means that it is at the origin of the coordinates that the concentration decreases more rapidly (this is also true for any value of t). The two maximal values of $\partial^2 F/\partial x^2$ indicate that for $t = 4$ sec those are the two points where the concentration increases more rapidly. The two zero points indicate that for $t = 4$ sec there is a constant concentration therein. This is true because at those points the amount of O_2 coming from the origin of the coordinates equals the amount leaving in the opposite direction.

From the two solutions represented—$F(x, t = 1$ sec) and $F(x, t = 4$ sec)—it is also clear that the diffusion process is a slow one. It varies with the square root of time. To double the spread of molecules we have to wait four times longer. The diffusion coefficient has exactly the same effect: the molecular spread doubles when D quadruples.

The previous simple example, which can be understood with an elementary mathematical background, points to the limitations of the direct transposition of physics to physiology. Indeed, Eq. (3) is the exact solution of the diffusion equation for a system that does not exist (infinite length cylinder) and an initial condition—$\delta(x)$—which is impossible to obtain. The limitations of the necessary finite length (l) of real tubes implies that the comparisons between experiments and Eq. (3) are valid only for times much smaller than $2Dl^2$, the order of magnitude of the distance covered during a time t being $\sqrt{2Dt}$. The limitations of the nonreal initial conditions [$C(x = 0, t = 0) = \infty$] implies that Eq. (3) cannot be compared with experiments for very short times.

To approach a situation more related to the lung, at some stage of the modeling a wall representing the end of the alveolar sacs will be placed in a duct. Let us assume a rigid wall perpendicular to the duct axis, located at $x = -1$. At that point, the reflection of the molecules from the walls results in a concentration gradient of zero [i.e., $\partial C(x = x_1, t)/\partial x = 0$]. In other words, it comes from Fick's law of diffusion [Eq. (2)] that there is no flow across a rigid wall. Now, for the same initial condition, the solution of the diffusion equation is

$$C(x,t) = \frac{M}{\sqrt{\pi}} \int_{x/2\sqrt{Dt}}^{\infty} e^{-\eta^2} \, d\eta \tag{4}$$

η being the integration variable. However, the manipulation of this type of solution becomes much more difficult. We are nevertheless still very far from a geometry approaching lung anatomy.

Whatever the technique used, a second factor should be considered if we wish to describe more realistically gas mixing in the lung (i.e., the convective movement which is simultaneous with diffusion). If all the molecules displace themselves with the same velocity u in the tube already considered, it can be shown from matter balance and Fick's law that the adequate equation is

$$\frac{\partial F}{\partial t} = D \frac{\partial^2 F}{\partial x^2} - u \frac{\partial F}{\partial x} \tag{5}$$

The solutions of Eq. (5) with the initial and boundary conditions already considered in Figure 3 are presented by the dashed lines in the same figure. The same spread occurs concurrently with a displacement of the mean value with velocity u. The spread doubles each time the mean distance covered by convection quadruples.

The advent of modern digital computers was the key for the solution of this type of equations in situations where the analytical solutions are unobtainable. This is usually the case in physiological systems, due to their natural complexity. Nevertheless, we will see in the next section that the classical analytical manipulations are still obligatory in some circumstances.

B. Numerical Solutions

The numerical techniques to solve differential equations are old, but their application increased dramatically with the development of digital computers. The basic idea is to divide the duct into a certain number of nodes a distance of Δx apart (distance between the vertical lines in Fig. 4). The concentration is computed in those nodes which represent slices Δx thick. The choice of Δx depends on the precision wanted for the concentration curves. The implicit assumption is that within each slice there is perfect gas homogeneization. Equation (5) is replaced by a system of differential equations, the solution of each one giving the concentration in one node. In the previous example, the concentration in node n is given by

$$\frac{dF_n}{dt} = D \frac{(F_{n+1} - F_n) - (F_n - F_{n-1})}{\Delta x^2} - u_n \frac{F_{n+1} - F_{n-1}}{2\Delta x} \tag{6}$$

We now use normal d for the derivation (instead of ∂) because, at node n, F_n depends only on time, the spatial derivative being computed numerically: the right-hand side of Eq. (6). There are different ways of computing numerical derivatives, the one used in Eq. (6) being the commonest. These differential equations are solved by standard numerical techniques. The corresponding computer programs are found in any computer program library.

The solution of the same problem already discussed is represented in Figure 4 for t = 4 sec together with the analytical solution (solid line) and

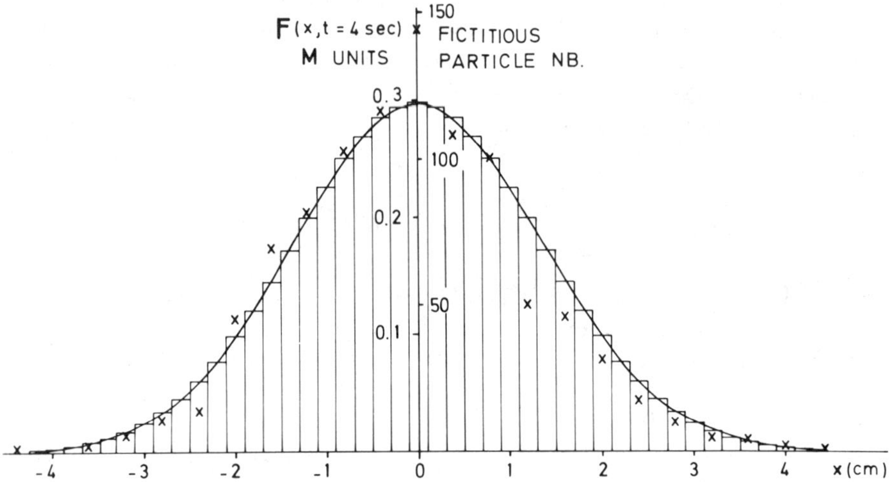

Figure 4 Comparison of the analytical, numerical, and stochastic solution of the diffusion equation for a δ function as initial condition. See the text for details.

with $\Delta x = 0.2$ cm. The precision of the solution is limited only by computer time availability. The enormous advantage of using a digital computer is that it solves the diffusion equation with the same ease whatever the initial and the boundary conditions are. If node i represents the origin of coordinates, the initial condition equivalent to $\delta(x)$ corresponds to $F_i = 1$ and $F_n = 0$ ($n \neq i$). The nonphysical concentration for very short times related to the δ function (which is infinity for t = 0) disappears and the volume of O_2 is simply given by S Δx. We have used 51 nodes with an integration step time equal to 5 msec. It is obvious from Figure 4 that the exact solution is accurately approached.

C. Stochastic Solutions

Another method to solve Eq. (1), first used by Dirac to study neutron diffusion, is based on a very simple principle. The x axis is also divided in a finite number of nodes. In the case previously considered, where all the particles are at the same node for t = 0, anyone can simulate the diffusion process with a simple tossing of a coin and much patience. Consider one fictitious particle in node i (Fig. 4) and move it to the right every time the coin falls heads and to the left every time it falls tails. This is the random walk, which can be proved to be equivalent to diffusion. The x in Figure 4 show the result corresponding to tossing 45 times a coin and repeat the operation 1000 times, each one for one fictitious particle initially situated in the central node. Even throwing 45,000 times only roughly approaches the analytical or the numerical solution. This shows that this is a very time consuming method. Although using a coin is a boring method, the use of the random generator number of any small personal computer can give the same result, and its use is an instructive way for grasping what diffusion is. For example, the slowness of diffusion becomes apparent when we see that one particle often crosses the origin of coordinates several times before reaching the "final" position. In the air, the real O_2 and N_2 molecules travel at a speed of about 0.5 km/sec and we saw that the real displacement is less than 1 cm in 1 sec (Chap. 1).

One of the crucial points in the understanding of the mechanisms of binary mixing can also be easily grasped by the stochastic method. When one particle representing O_2 moves to the right, automatically a N_2 particle moves to the left. When the convective velocity is zero, the net flow of matter (O_2 + N_2) is zero although each type of molecule has an opposite diffusion flow if the concentration gradient is not zero. This means that when considering inspired gases to have concentration 1 and residual gases concentration zero, if after mixing the inspired gas concentration is F(x,t), we automatically know that residual gas concentration is 1 - F(x,t). This is no longer valid when ternary diffusion is considered (Chap. 1), which makes intuitive predictions much more difficult.

The stochastic method most closely simulates the random motion of molecules. Another principle that can be grasped by this type of exercise is the realization that Fick's law of diffusion is merely a consequence of random motion. It is possible to demonstrate that the fictitious particles moving according to the tossing of a coin satisfy Fick's law of diffusion and consequently the diffusion equation. Except for pedagogical reasons or for producing personal computer games, does the stochastic method present an interest? Indeed, even with fast digital computers this method is very slow. However, there is a mathematical technique derived from the probability theory which permits a very fast solution (Cox and Miller, 1965). This gives a practical interest to this method.

The first attempt to use a stochastic method for a lung model was by Stibitz (1969) and the stochastic method was also used in the formulation of the current transport equation of gas mixing in the lung (Paiva and Paiva-Veretennicoff, 1972). During the past 10 years of development of model analyses of gas transport in the lung, the three techniques previously described have been used in a complementary way. A fruitful utilization of these techniques is the possibility of solving the same problem by independent methods. When the result is the same we almost have the assurance that there are no errors. We shall see in the next section that each one of these three techniques presents some unique characteristics which were applied to our modeling approach.

III. Trumpet Model

The anatomical data published by Weibel, particularly Table XI.2 (symmetrical model) of his famous book (Weibel, 1963), have been extensively utilized for model analyses. This table was probably one of the most useful contributions ever given to lung modeling workers. That was the obvious purpose of Weibel reflected in the poem that opens his book, both poem and book being dedicated to D. Gómez. The graphical representation of the same table for the 13 last lung generations gives a cumulative cross-sectional area of the airways which presents a trumpet shape (Fig. 5) when plotted against a linear distance. Usually, the origin of the coordinates (x_0) from which the distance is taken is chosen as the end of the alveolar sacs (twenty-third generation). The entry of the model (x_1) corresponds to the entry of genera-

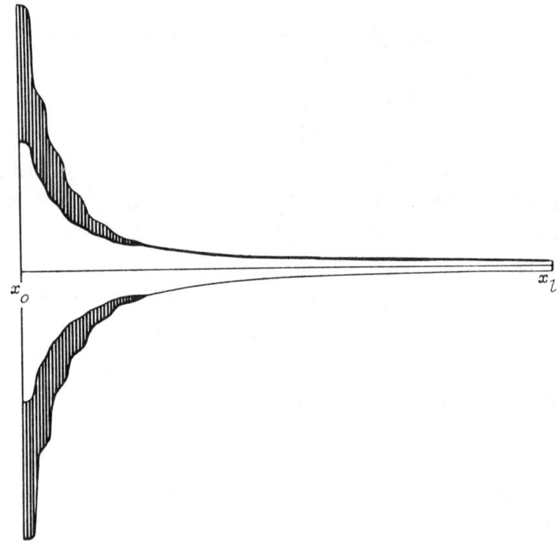

Figure 5 Graphical representation of the cumulative cross-sectional area of the last 13 lung generations of Weibel model. The origin of the coordinates (x_0) is the end of the alveolar sacs and x_1 corresponds to the entry of generation 11. The shaded zone of this trumpet-shaped model corresponds to the volume occupied by the alveoli. (From Paiva, 1972.)

tion 11. The distance between x_0 and x_1 is equal to 2.2 cm. In this case the lung is considered to be equivalent to 2048 (2^{11}) of those geometrical figures, the dashed zone of which corresponds to the volume occupied by the alveoli. The trumpet shape is a consequence of replacing each pair of branches of generation 12 by only one where the cross section is doubled, each four branches of generation 13 by only one where the cross section is quadrupled, and so on until generation 23. This is a consequence of one of the basic assumptions (instantaneous radial diffusion) subtending the present model. Those assumptions are the following:

1. The first 10 generations only introduce a delay equal to the ratio between the volume of those generations and the flow; that is, the flow is of piston type (with no radial velocity gradients).
2. The diffusion coefficient is constant and represents the molecular diffusion coefficient of a binary gas mixture.
3. Radial diffusion is instantaneous so that there are no radial concentration gradients.
4. The molecules inside the alveoli do not diffuse axially (i.e., there is no diffusion across the alveolar walls).
5. The geometry is rigid. It is as if the volume changes took place only at the end of the alveolar sacs.
6. The gases are incompressible and the temperature is constant.

Before discussing each assumption and its domain of validity, it is more convenient to accept them a priori and to understand the transport equation which they necessarily imply. We therefore give only an intuitive feeling which guided the establishment of these assumptions and will discuss them in more detail later.

During the inspiration, the difference between the real motion of the gases passing the first 10 generations and the simulated one, according to assumption 1, lies in the shape of the front between the inspired and the resident gases: It is spread for the real gases because some axial mixing occurs and it is perfectly sharp in the model where no mixing is considered. In the lung, once the front between inspired and residual gases has crossed the first 10 generations, the concentration (in these generations) is equal to the inspired gas concentration. The same is true for the model. Assumption 1 can therefore affect only the first part of the inspiration. During a normal breath, the tidal volume is much larger than the dead space and we can accept that this assumption is reasonable.

The basis for the consideration of assumption 2 is related to the way we imagine gas mixing in the last lung generations. Most of the lung volume is located within the alveoli and the convective velocity is very small therein. We have therefore considered only the molecular diffusion as the mechanism of mixing. Furthermore, the dependence of the molecular diffusion coefficient on the gas concentrations or on the presence of other gases is well known. We consider only simulations where the gases concentrations are such that the molecular diffusion coefficient can be taken constant.

The logic of assumption 3 comes from the rapidity of the radial concentration equilibration by molecular diffusion which is given by $d^2/2D$, d being the duct diameter and D the diffusion coefficient. This are only few milliseconds in the zone of the respiratory bronchioles.

Assumption 4 is the basis for the consideration of the delay in axial spread due to the alveolar septa. We can look at Figure 6 and imagine the motion of a molecule inside an alveolar duct. It is clear that the assumption of instantaneous radial mixing inside this structure overestimates mixing. On the other hand, assuming that the molecules inside the alveoli do not diffuse axially underestimates mixing because the real molecules can indeed displace inside each alveolus. Due to the geometry of the alveoli, which have a depth close to their width, both effects should approximately compensate each other.

The relative variation of volume of the different lung structures is not yet clearly established but they probably change more or less isotropically. The consideration of a rigid geometry (assumption 5) consists in assuming that all the volume changes takes place at the origin of the model (x_0 in Fig. 5) that is, at the end of the alveolar sacs. The reasoning for this assumption is that the larger part of volume change takes place in the alveolar zone of the lung where gas equilibration by diffusion is very rapid. This should make the different ways of making the model to expand equivalent.

Finally, the assumption 6 is a consequence of the small variation of pressure and temperature within the lung for a large range of breathing conditions.

A. Transport Equation

The previous six assumptions lead to one—and only one—transport equation, which is only slightly more complex than Eq. (5) describing the transport and mixing in a duct of constant cross section. Indeed, the application of the principle of matter balance and Fick's law of diffusion in a geometry of variable cross section with a zone corresponding to the alveoli leads to the equation (Paiva, 1972)

$$\frac{\partial F}{\partial t} = D\,\frac{s}{S}\,\frac{\partial^2 F}{\partial x^2} + \frac{D}{S}\,\frac{ds}{dx}\,\frac{\partial F}{\partial x} - u\,\frac{\partial F}{\partial x} + Q \qquad (7)$$

where Q is the source term, negative for O_2 and positive for CO_2. We only consider in this chapter the case where Q = 0. F is the fractional gas concentration, which is a function of time (t) and distance (x) from the alveolar end of the model. s(x) and S(x) are the cross-sectional area of the conducting airways alone, and the total cross section of airways plus alveoli, respectively, at given values of x (Fig. 5). D is the binary diffusion coefficient between inspired and residual gas, and u the convection velocity. Equation (7) was published simultaneously and independently by Scherer et al. (1972) and used extensively since.*

There are only two differences between Eq. (7) with Q = 0 and Eq. (5) describing the transport in a cylinder of constant cross section: On the one hand, D is multiplied by the factor s/S and on the other hand a new term is introduced. The factor s/S, which is the ratio between the duct cross section without and with alveoli, is only different from unity in the alveolar zone. It represents the delay in the axial spread of the molecules due to the reflections from the alveolar septa. We have used for the last lung generations the model proposed by Weibel (1963) where the alveolar ducts are represented by two axisymmetrical cylinders and the alveoli by 1/8 of an annular ring (Fig. 6). In this model s/S = 1/4. The new term is $(D/S)(ds/dx)(\partial F/\partial x)$ and it reflects the spatial structure of the bronchial tree. Indeed, the characterization of the geometrical boundaries of the model requires, a priori, the three spatial coordinates. If we could represent such a complex structure by such a simple term, using only one spatial coordinate (x), it is because of the use of the assumption of instantaneous radial diffusion and the use of a symmetrical model of the airways. The other spatial coordinates are implicitly included in S and s. The price to pay for this simplification is that, as we only have one spatial variable, we cannot distinguish between different pathways: All the pathways are necessarily equivalent. It is of interest to note that (D/S)(ds/dx) has the dimensions of a velocity. However, such a velocity is not a direct description of a real convective movement of particles but a merely mathematical consequence of the nonphysical assumption of instantaneous radial diffusion in a variable cross-sectional structure.

---

*Jacobs was probably the first to give an explicit equation for the diffusion in a system of nonuniform varying cross section (Jacobs, 1935). He obtained an equation that is identical to Eq. (7) when S = s and u = 0. However, Jacobs only studied solutions with steady-state conditions ($\partial F/\partial t = 0$) and for uniform varying cross sections (ds/dx = constant). Furthermore, he did not consider the assumption of instantaneous radial diffusion, the system studied by him thus being valid only for very small values of ds/dx.

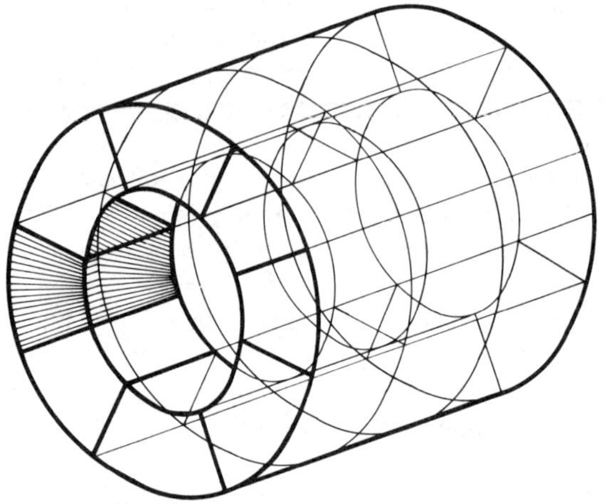

Figure 6 Model of an alveolar duct. Each alveolus is represented by 1/8 of an annular ring. (From Paiva, 1974.)

Having an equation [Eq. (7)] that is supposed to describe the gas concentration inside the human lung (insofar as the Weibel model is an adequate representation), the first thing to do is to solve it with initial and boundary conditions representing situations of physiological interest. We will first consider a 2-sec inspiration of O_2 followed by a 2-sec expiration with a constant flow of 250 ml/sec. For simplicity, the inspired and the residual gas concentrations are assumed to be equal to 1 and 0, respectively. We also neglect the gas exchange. As during quiet breathing only 4 ml/sec of O_2 crosses the alveolar capillary membrane, the concentration profiles are only slightly modified. Furthermore, during the expiration, we will consider only N_2 concentration curves. As the respiratory quotient (flow of CO_2 from the blood/flow of O_2 into the blood) is close to 1, the errors introduced during quiet breathing are small. The initial condition is then chosen $F(x, t = 0) = 0$. The boundary conditions during inspiration are $\partial F/\partial x = 0$ at $x = 0$ (reflexive condition) and $F(x_1,t) = 1$ for $t_1 \leqslant t \leqslant 2$ sec, t_1 being the time needed for the inspired gas to cross the first 10 generations. The simple boundary condition $F = 1$ at the entry of the model is convenient because the diffusion flow therein is negligible compared with the convective flow. During the expiration, the velocity is reversed and the concentration at the entry of the model is given by the solutions of Eq. (7).

Figure 7 shows solutions of Eq. (7) for the conditions described. Curves 1 to 10 (panel A) are the solutions (F(x,t) for $t = 0.4n$ sec ($n = 1, \ldots, 10$) (i.e., every 0.4 sec). The concentration is plotted as a function of the distance to the origin of coordinates (lower abscissa) or the Weibel generation (upper abscissa). Curves 1 to 5 correspond to the inspiration and

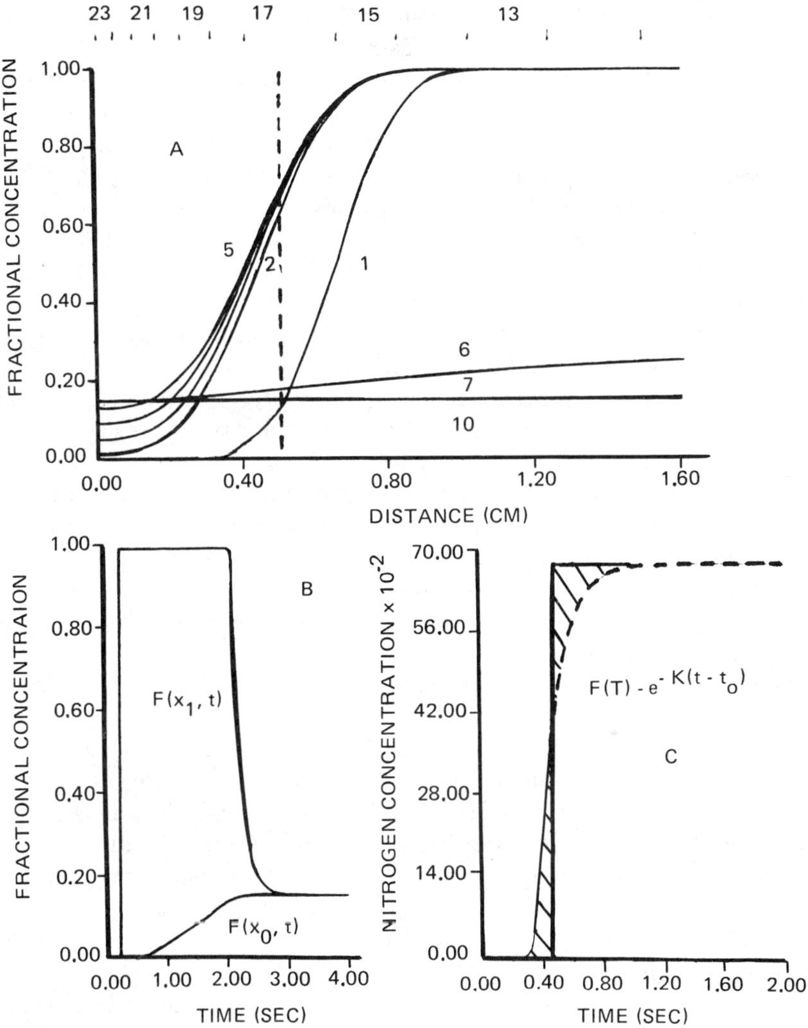

Figure 7 Solutions of Eq. (7) for a constant flow ($\dot{V}$ = 250 ml/sec). Period of the respiratory movement equal to 4 sec. (A) Solutions (F(x,t) for t = 0.4 n sec (n = 1, . . . , 10). (B) Solutions at $x = x_0$ and $x = x_1$ for $0 \leqslant t$ (sec) $\leqslant 4$. (C) Simulation of the expired N_2 concentration measured at the entry of the trachea. The two shaded zones have equal areas and indicate the traditional manner of computing Fowler dead space, which is equal to 115 ml when computed from the beginning of the trachea. The dashed curve is an exponential, fitted on the second part of phase II, from which it is indistinguishable. See the text for further details. (From Paiva, 1973.)

6 to 10 to the expiration, curves 5 and 10 being the end of inspiration and expiration, respectively. The vertical dashed line is such that (for a model extended until the beginning of the trachea) the volume proximal to it is equal to 115 ml. Instead of representing the concentration as a function of x we can use t as the abscissa axis. Panel B represents the concentration at the entry of the model–$F(x_1,t)$–and at the alveolar end–$F(x_0,t)$. Finally, panel C gives the simulated expiratory N_2 concentration curve. The two shaded zones have equal areas and indicate the traditional manner of computing Fowler dead space, which is equal to 115 ml. The interest of comparing these two manners of computing the volume of 115 ml is discussed below. The dashed curve is an exponential, fitted on the concentration curve, from which it is indistinguishable.

Curves 2 to 5 in panel A are almost stationary. This striking behavior means that insofar as this model represents the real system, the gas concentration in the lung does not change during most of the inspiration when the flow is constant. Between the mouth and generation 15 the concentration is 1 and then falls. Only the last 8 mm of the bronchial tree would present a concentration different from the inspired one. The concentration profile represented by curves 2 to 5 is usually called the (quasi) stationary front or more appropriately the diffusion front (between inspired and residual gases). In the last lung generations, where the convective velocity is very small, the concentration increases steadily due to the arrival of O_2 molecules by diffusion.

Perhaps the simplest way to grasp the physical meaning of the diffusion front is to think about the behavior of a N_2 molecule [the N_2 concentration profile is equal to $1 - F(x,t)$]. On the one hand, these molecules are pushed by bulk flow toward the last generations, this physical force (a pressure gradient) decreasing toward the last generations and being zero at the end of the alveolar sacs. On the other hand, the molecular agitation that makes the molecules diffuse in all directions tends to oppose this bulk movement. Although diffusion and convection take place simultaneously, we can artificially separate them by thought as far as this separation takes place during very short time intervals, short enough not to change significantly the concentration profiles. If we consider, for example, curve 5 of Figure 7 and stop the convection, the diffusion flow at any point is given by the Fick's law of diffusion [Eq. (2)] and equal to $DS(dF/dx)$ for N_2. If we stop diffusion and make the gas flow by convection only, it is given by $F\dot{V}$ or FuS. The diffusion front therefore represents the balance between the N_2 bulk flow towards the periphery and the diffusion flow in the opposite direction, that is, $D(dF/dx) = Fu$ (Engel et al., 1973).

It is of equal interest to understand why during the expiration the concentration becomes very rapidly constant everywhere in the model (curves

6 to 10). Now diffusion and convection both contribute to equalize the concentrations. Even without diffusion, the convective movement would decrease the concentration gradient of curve 5 but a small gradient would remain in the last generations. However, the distances therein are sufficiently small to enable an equilibration by diffusion.

The time-dependent representation of concentrations (Fig. 7B) offers a different view of the same phenomenon. The curve $F(x_1,t)$ is zero during the time needed to cover the first 10 generations. It becomes equal to 1 instantaneously (piston-type flow) and remains equal to 1 during the beginning of the expiration. This first part of the expiration corresponds roughly to the part of curve 5 in Figure 7A, where $F = 1$. There is then a rapid decrease in concentration, corresponding to the transition between curves 5 to 7 of Figure 7A, and finally the concentration remains constant until the end of the expiration. Curve $F(x_0,t)$ shows the same initial delay (first 10 generations passage) but more than twice the same delay before the concentration begins to increase. Now the molecules covered the 13 last generations first by convection, then by convection and diffusion, and finally only by diffusion. During the whole inspiration the O_2 concentration rises continuously (corresponding to curves 2 to 5) and also rises slightly at the beginning of the expiration. This means that although the convective flow is toward the mouth, the diffusive flow in the opposite direction was not zero at the beginning of the expiration, the O_2 molecules diffusing according to its (large) concentration gradient. However, because of the convective velocity, this gradients decreases rapidly and the concentration at $x = x_0$ ceases to increase. It remains constant until the end of the expiration. Finally, both curves $F(x_1,t)$ and $F(x_0,t)$ joined together, which is another way of expressing the constant concentration everywhere within the model.

Figure 7C is also of interest. It represents the simulation of the single-breath test (for a 0.5-liter inspiration). The slope is flat and the computed Fowler dead space equal to 115 ml. For the considered flow and tidal volume, the model indeed behaves as if there were only two compartments: one with a volume equal to 115 ml and no mixing at all and another compartment where the mixing is perfect. However, as the dead space depends on several variables (flow, tidal volume, model volume, diffusion coefficient), this analogy is of little help. It is nevertheless of interest to see to which volume in the trumpet model the dead space corresponds. This is represented by the vertical dashed line of Figure 7A. If there were no diffusion during the expiration, the curve of Figure 7C could be obtained directly from curve 5 of Figure 7A if this last curve was expressed as a function of lung volume instead of distance. The simulation of an expiration without molecular diffusion results in rather different curves and in a Fowler dead space increased by 30%. This demonstrates the crucial role played by diffusion during the beginning of the expiration.

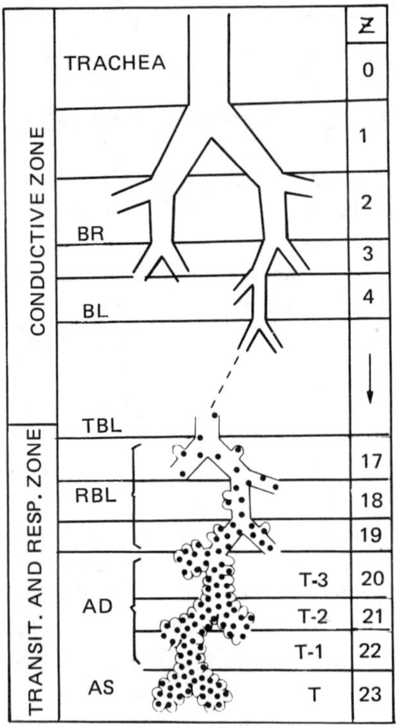

Figure 8 Symmetrical Weibel model with a graphical visualization of curve 5 of Figure 7. The black dots represent N_2 molecules and its density is in proportion to the N_2 concentration. (Adapted from Weibel, 1963.)

The Bohr dead space (V_D) is traditionally computed using the equation

$$\frac{V_D}{V_T} = \frac{F_E - F_A}{F_I - F_A} \tag{8}$$

where V_T is the tidal volume and F_I and F_E the mean concentration of inspired and expired inert gas, respectively. F_A is the mean alveolar concentration. It is easy to demonstrate that the symmetrical trumpet model generates identical Bohr and Fowler dead spaces. The reason is that the expired alveolar plateau and the mean alveolar concentrations are identical in this model.

We have represented in Figure 8 the symmetrical Weibel model with a graphical visualization of curve 5 of Figure 7. The density of the black dots is in proportion to the N_2 concentration (curve 10 would correspond to an uniform density). This figure represents schematically the N_2 molecules, which on the one hand are pushed by convection toward the last lung generations, and on the other hand tend to move proximally by diffusion (according to Fick's law). Only few N_2 molecules reach generation 16 because the larger convective velocity therein. The half-density zone is situated between generations 17 and 18. How can this be more accurately expressed in mathematical terms? The time independence of a concentration profile is mathematically expressed by $\partial C/\partial t = 0$. The transport equation (7) becomes space dependent only, and after dividing it by D and using $u = \dot{V}/S$, we have

$$s \frac{d^2 F}{dx^2} + \left(\frac{ds}{dx} - \frac{\dot{V}}{D}\right)\frac{dF}{dx} = 0 \tag{9}$$

If F is time independent, so must be the boundary conditions. For $x = x_1$ the boundary chosen ($F = 1$) is already time independent. For $x = 0$, the large volume of the lung with respect to the tidal volume makes $F = 0$ a reasonable approximation. The error due to this boundary condition can be seen from the values of curves 2 to 5 in Figure 7. Particularly for small tidal volumes, this error is small. The model geometry being rigid, S and s are also time independent, and therefore Eq. (9) depends only on the ratio $\dot{V}/D$, which is constant. The model then predicts that a sixfold increase in the flow is equivalent to a sixfold increase in the diffusion coefficient, which corresponds to changing SF_6 into He as tracer gases.

The solution of Eq. (9) with the boundary conditions $F = 0$ and $F = 1$ for $x = 0$ and $x = x_1$, respectively, is a well-known differential equation boundary value problem (Lieberstein, 1972) and the solutions are given in Figure 9. For a flow $\dot{V} = 500$ ml/sec, curves 1, 2, and 3 correspond to $D = 0.1$, 0.225, and 0.6 cm^2/sec, representing the gas pairs, SF_6-air, N_2-O_2, and He-air, respectively. Curves 4 and 5 correspond to $D = 0.6$ cm^2/sec, but the flow is equal to 125 ml/sec and zero, respectively. For a given flow, the smaller the diffusion coefficient, the more peripheral the diffusion front. When seen as an equilibrium between convection flow and backward diffusion flow, this means that when D decreases, the diffusion flow at the same point decreases and the equilibrium with the convective flow is reached more peripherally, where the velocities are lower. We have used for the computation of the curves of Figure 9 a geometry derived from Hansen and Ampaya (1975) in order to compare with other published results using that geometry (see below). This corresponds to a lung volume of 3.7 liters, whereas the previous values were obtained from a lung volume of 2.625 liters.

The diffusion front is spread over several lung generations. The value corresponding to the larger concentration gradient of the diffusion front may be used to localize it (Paiva et al., 1976). In a function presenting an inflection point, the maximum of its derivative is located at the point where its second derivative is zero ($d^2F/dx^2 = 0$). From Eq. (9) it results that such a condition is fulfilled for

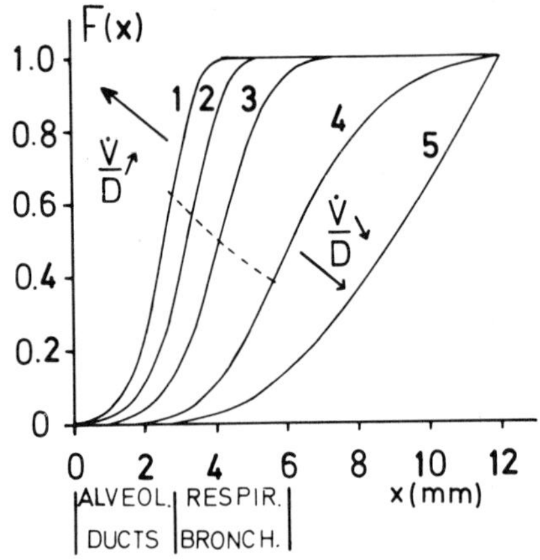

Figure 9 Solutions of Eq. (9) with the boundary conditions F = 0 and F = 1 for x = 0 and x = x_1, respectively. Curves 1, 2, and 3 correspond to D = 0.1, 0.225, and 0.6 cm^2/sec, respectively, and $\dot{V}$ = 500 ml/sec. Curves 4 and 5 correspond to $\dot{V}$ = 125 and $\dot{V}$ = 0 ml/sec, respectively, both solutions with D = 0.6 cm^2/sec.

$$\frac{ds}{dx} = \frac{\dot{V}}{D} \tag{10}$$

This is a surprisingly simple relation between the structure (ds/dx) and function (the position of the diffusion front) of the lung. For each curve, the inflection point is its intercept with the dashed line of Figure 9. When a reflexive condition ($\partial F/\partial x = 0$) is assumed at x = 0 (Fig. 7A), although the concentration increases during inspiration, the inflection point remains at the same position. Unfortunately, the zone of the lung where the diffusion front is situated (respiratory bronchioles) is at the present time beyond the possibilities of direct concentration measurements. If we compute the model volume proximal to the inflection point we find 210.8, 162.1, 144.3, and 126.6 ml for curves 1 to 4, respectively. The equivalent Fowler dead space is equal to 194.4, 158.6, 137.9, and 130.1 ml, respectively. This is a surprising good agreement and establishes a link between the Fowler dead space measured at the mouth and the lung anatomy. The use of Weibel's anatomical data instead of Hansen-Ampaya's data does not modify the previous considerations, the absolute values of the dead space being slightly larger. The importance of this result should not be overestimated, as the inflection point is situated in a zone of the front which is almost linear. A small error in its determination results, therefore, in a very different value for the volume of the model proximal to the inflection point.

If $\dot{V}/D$ increases toward ∞, the curves approach the constant $F(x) = 1$, $x > 0$. If $\dot{V}/D$ decreases toward zero, the curves approach curve 5. This last curve does not present an inflection point and therefore Eq. (10) does not apply. Curve 5 is only of academic interest because it does not correspond to any physiological situation. If the model cross section were constant, this curve would have been a straight line from the point ($x = 0, F = 0$) to ($x = 12$ mm, $F = 1$), the difference between both curves being due to the trumpet-shaped geometry of the model.

How would it be possible to test the prediction of the diffusion front dependence on the $\dot{V}/D$ ratio only? Because the diffusion front can only be measured in its very proximal part, it comes from the previous considerations that the Fowler dead space probably is the more adequate parameter. To support this view, we have computed the Fowler dead space for different $\dot{V}$ and D. If we consider the reference value of 158 ml for $\dot{V} = 0.5$ liter/sec, $V_T = 1$ liter and $D = 0.225$ cm^2/sec, doubling or halving both flow and D changes the dead space by less than 1 ml. We shall see in the next section how the measured dead space depends on flow.

Another parameter suggested by the trumpet model is the exponential behavior of the second part of phase II of the single-breath expiration curves (the dashed line of Fig. 7C). For the previous simulation conditions, the following exponential fits the second half of phase II:

$$F(T) - F(t) = e^{-k\dot{V}(t-t_0)} \tag{11}$$

with $k = 30$ liter^{-1}. F(T) is the end expiratory concentration and $\dot{V}$ the flow. A useful property of any exponential function–exp(-kx)–is expressed by the fact that ln 2 divided by k gives the distance x on the abscissa, which halves the difference between the exponential and its asymptote. Thus the exponent 30 liter^{-1} indicates that the difference between phase II and the simulated alveolar plateau is halved every ln 2/0.03 = 23 ml.

The phase II of real single-breath washouts is indeed very close to a single exponential and the computation of k from any single-breath expiratory curve in normal subjects shows that this value is about 10 liter^{-1} (i.e., one-third of the simulated one). Such a large difference is not surprising, as the trumpet model does not take into account several factors that tend to decrease k. Here we only briefly analyze two of them: the adequacy of the anatomical data and the role of the transit-time distribution in the proximal generations of the bronchial tree. Concerning the first factor, it is of interest to study the sensitivity of the computed k on the geometry of the model.

We have chosen to simulate the He and SF_6 single-breath expirations and have represented in Figure 10 the sensitivity of k_{He} and k_{SF_6} on the geometry of the model. We have considered the trumpet divided in slices 0.02 cm thick and have changed (radially) the volume of those slices by a

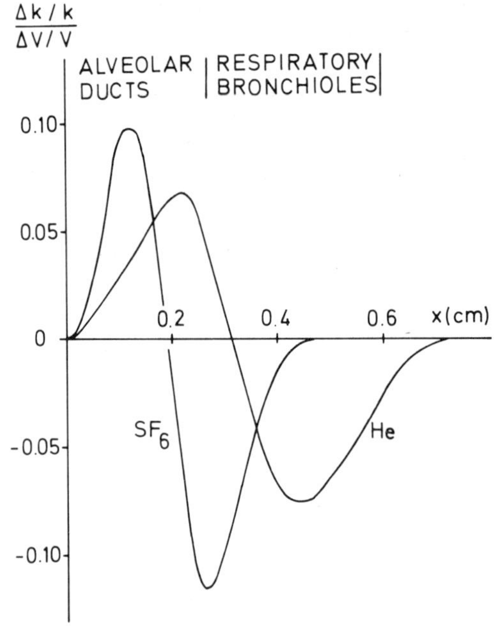

Figure 10 Sensitivity of the exponent (k) fitted on the simulated He and SF_6 phase II of single-breath washouts. The trumpet was divided in slices 0.02 cm thick. The abscissa is the distance of the slices center to the alveolar end of the model. The volume of each slice was changed (radially) by a small amount ΔV. The ordinate is the relative variation of k divided by the relative variation of V, which is the mathematical definition of the sensitivity of k with respect to the slice volume V.

small amount ΔV. The slices' cross sections s and S are increased by small amounts Δs and ΔS such that s/S remains constant. We computed the relative variation of k divided by the relative variation of V, which is the mathematical definition of the sensitivity of k with respect to the slice volume V. The minima of both curves correspond to the position of the diffusion front of these gases. Therefore, increasing the geometry of the model in the zone where the diffusion front is situated decreases the value of k (approaching the observed values); that is, it delays the establishment of the alveolar plateau. The left parts of these sensitivity curves (positive values) correspond to the distal part of the diffusion fronts, where there is an opposite effect: an increase in the cross section accelerates the concentration homogenization. In this zone, where diffusion transport dominates, the diffusion front flattens by an increase of the cross section s which increases diffusion mixing, and the concentration equilibration during the beginning of the expiration is more rapid. Increasing the model volume proximal to x = 0.7 cm has no effect at all on k. This corresponds to the consideration of a dead space which only delays phase II but does not change its shape.

An interesting aspect of the curves in Figure 10 is that their general shape remains unchanged when the flow is varied. Increasing the flow displaces both curves to the left, and decreasing it displaces them to the right. A consequence of this is that even if we could find a geometry such that the experimental data were approached for a given flow, the discrepancy would have been even larger for other flows. Indeed, the experimental k values are relatively insensitive to the flow variations (Lacquet, unpublished observations).

The combined effect of decreasing the cross section in the last generations and increasing it proximally is exactly what happens when the trumpet-shaped model is replaced by a cone. The comparison between the He and SF_6 expiratory curves generated by these two types of geometrical boundaries was previously reported in detail (Paiva, 1980), showing that gas mixing is not very sensitive to the geometry of the last lung generations. This demonstrates the impossibility of fitting the geometry of a series space model based on single-breath expiratory curves. This is a useful result, as several authors have attempted to determine the shape of the trumpet model simulating the same expired concentration curve as the one measured experimentally. This attractive idea was introduced by Baker et al. (1975) but ignores all the other factors that play an important role in the genesis of the single-breath expirates and which are considered as geometrical factors.

Another factor influencing the phase II is the transit-time distribution of the proximal generations of the bronchial tree. Horsfield and Cumming (1968b) published the distribution function of transit times between the carina and the lobular branches defined as the first branch of diameter 0.07 cm or less. The incorporation of their transit time distribution in the simulations decreases k only by about 1%. However, extending the same distribution until the entry of the acini decreases k by about 15% and when the distribution is extended until the diffusion front location, a rather adequate description of the experiments can be obtained. We hope that these preliminary results stimulate anatomists to describe with greater detail the morphometry of the last generations of the conducting zone of the lung.

We have also simulated a breath with D = 0 during the expiration. The exponent of Eq. (11) becomes equal to 8 liter^{-1}. This (compared with 30 liter^{-1}) gives a quantitative evaluation of the role of the diffusion whose influence on k takes place mainly at the beginning of the expiration.

B. Comparisons with Experiments

A direct comparison between simulations and experiments concerns the slope of the alveolar plateau simulated by the model, which is flat contrary to experimental evidence. Based on the model analysis it was concluded that the gas transport and mixing in the series spaces of the lung is not the cause of the sloping alveolar plateau (Paiva, 1973). However, even if we accept our model verdict, we have only eliminated one possible cause, but we have not proposed an alternative explanation for the sloping alveolar plateau.

Although a direct measurement of gas concentration in the zone of the diffusion front is not yet possible, Fukuchi et al. (1976) were able to measure, by intrapulmonary gas sampling, its proximal part and could verify that the model predictions are qualitatively correct: The front moves peripherally when increasing the flow or decreasing the lung volume.

To test the validity of the model, more quantitative comparisons between simulations and experiments were needed. Of particular interest were the studies where the influence of several variables on a given physiological parameter were compared with the corresponding model predictions. This was the case of the multibreath H_2-SF_6 washout performed by Lacquet (Lacquet et al., 1975; Paiva et al., 1976), where the dead space was calculated as a function of breathing frequency and tidal volume both for H_2 and SF_6. The results shown in Figure 11 correspond to 87 simultaneous washouts of H_2 and SF_6, both 3% in air, obtained in two normal male subjects, aged 27 and 37, respectively: frequency, tidal volume, and flow in each experiment were analogous to the simulated conditions. Continuous analysis of mixed expired air was done with a mass spectrometer, and the dead-space volumes were obtained by parameter fitting of a lumped-parameter model similar to the one developed by Wise and Defares (1959) or by Weber and Bouhuys (1959).

In the left panel the tidal volume was kept constant and equal to 600 ml and the respiratory frequency was variable. In the right panel the respiratory frequency was constant but the tidal volume varied. Solid and dashed lines are the corresponding simulations using Weibel and Hansen-Ampaya data, respectively. The qualitative agreement between simulations and experiments can be considered rather satisfactory taking into account that there was no attempt to fit the model parameters on those points (V_D). Only published anatomical data and classical physical laws were used. The larger values of the dead space compared with previous simulations can be largely accounted for by the incorporation of mouth and instrumental volumes into the measured values. The main conclusion from the previous comparison is that the model predicts a separation between H_2 and SF_6 which is about twice the experimental one. Then, although both gases equilibrate completely in the

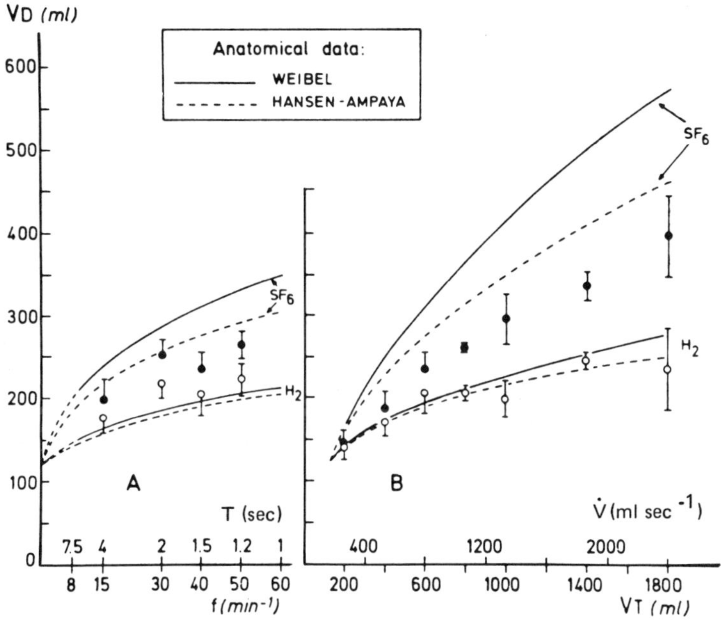

Figure 11 Dead space is represented on the ordinate, frequency (A) and tidal volume (B) on the abscissa. Circles (open circles: H_2; closed circles: SF_6) and vertical lines are the mean value and standard deviation of dead spaces computed from experimental multibreath washout curves. Solid and dashed lines represent the simulated dead space using the Weibel and the Hansen-Ampaya geometry, respectively. See the text for further details. (From Paiva et al., 1976.)

model during one respiratory cycle, the model nevertheless underestimates the gas mixing in the lung. The authors concluded that molecular diffusion is the main but not the only physical phenomenon that intervenes in gas mixing. From Figure 11A it is apparent that the simulated dead space increase for a 7.6-fold increase of $\dot{V}$ (f = 8 and 60 min^{-1}) is indeed almost the same that for a 7.6-fold increase of D (D_{SF_6} = 0.1 and D_{H_2} = 0.76 cm^2/sec), as discussed before. The experimental results are not incompatible with this observation but the variability is large.

The overestimation by the model of the H_2-SF_6 separation was confirmed by the analysis of He-SF_6 single-breath experiments (Engel et al., 1979). Figure 12 shows the model simulation of a 1-liter inspiration of a He-SF_6 mixture in O_2 followed by a 1-liter expiration both at a constant flow of 1 liter/sec. Only the end-inspiratory and end-expiratory concentra-

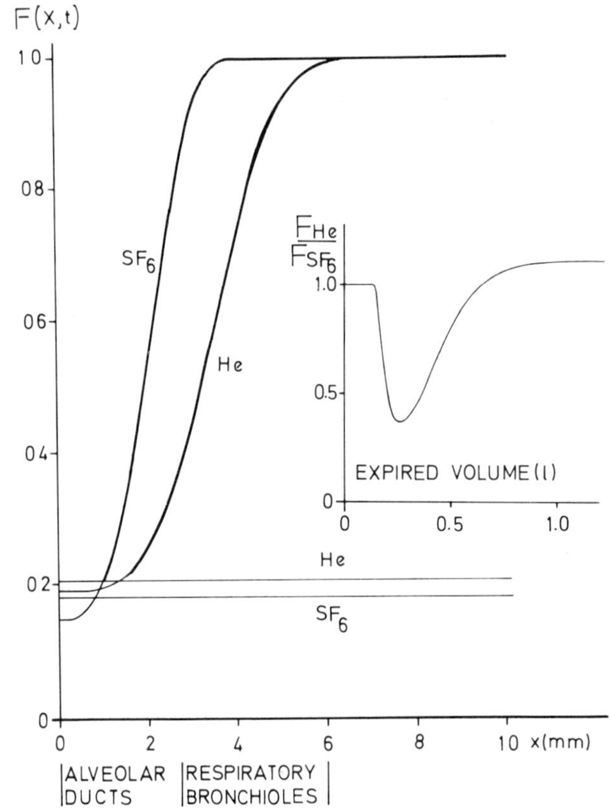

Figure 12 Simulation of a 1-liter inspiration of a He-SF_6 tracer mixture in O_2, followed by a 1-liter expiration both at a constant flow of 1 liter/sec. The ordinate is the He and SF_6 concentration relative to the inspired concentration and the abscissa is the distance to the alveolar end of the model. Only the end inspiratory and end expiratory concentration profiles are shown. The He/SF_6 ratio at the exit of the model plotted against expired volume is represented in the inset. (From Paiva and Engel, 1979.)

tion profiles are shown. They illustrate the different position of the diffusion fronts and the end-expiratory concentration differences. At the end of the expiration the He/SF_6 concentration ratio is about twice the experimental value in humans and in dogs and one order of magnitude larger than in pigs (Engel et al., 1979; Kelly et al., 1982a). This confirms that the model overestimates the separation between gases. The simulation of the expired He/SF_6 concentration ratio is in the inset. Its comparison with experiments

(Engel et al., 1979) also shows a larger He-SF_6 separation. For example, the minimum value of FHe/FSF_6 is much smaller in experiments, which indicates a much sharper phase II in the simulations or a larger exponent of the exponential phase II as discussed above.

C. Analysis of the Model Assumptions

When they model a simple physical process, the aim of physicists is an exact description. This cannot be the case when they study a biological system where they make a compromise between a correct description of reality and the necessary simplification leading to handy mathematical techniques. A sound analysis of the model assumptions is therefore a fundamental step. It not only gives a justification of the validity of the model but can also be the starting point for further improvements (i.e., for a better description of the experimental observations). We present now an analysis of the assumptions underlying the trumpet model.

1. The first 10 generations only introduce a delay equal to the ratio between the volume of these generations and the flow (piston-type flow).

The validity of this assumption has been extensively studied and the gas transport in the conducting airways is the subject of Chapter 3. The major step in this analysis came from the work of Scherer et al. (1975), who measured the axial spread of gases in a cast based on human anatomical data. They have shown that the axial dispersion is proportional to the mean gas velocity and that in the trachea it is about three orders of magnitude larger than molecular diffusion. This result was confirmed by other studies both in casts (Ultman and Blatman, 1977) and in humans (Ultman et al., 1978). How can our assumption of zero (!) axial diffusion and instantaneous radial diffusion (piston-type flow) in the first 10 generations be adequate? The main reason is that during a normal breath, this axial dispersion affects only the concentration profile of the front between inspired and resident gases. Once the front crosses the first 10 generations, the concentration becomes uniform therein. However, a quantitative analysis was possible with Scherer's formulas; when incorporating them in the appropriate transport equation (Engel et al., 1979) the influence of gas spread in the first generations on the solutions of the transport equation appeared to be very small indeed.

One of the interesting implications of the diffusion front is that it gives strong support to the nonconsideration of axial mixing in the first generations, at least during inspiration. Indeed, whatever the importance of axial mixing in the first generations, once the diffusion front is established, this can only influence concentration in the zone where the concentration is smaller than 1. But in this zone the velocities are very small and the molecular diffusion probably approaches total axial mixing. It is evident that this explanation does not apply for high-frequency breathing or for small-tidal-volume experiments where the front has no time to be established.

2. The diffusion coefficient is constant and represents the molecular diffusion of a binary gas mixture.

This assumption presents two aspects. The first is the consideration of the molecular diffusion (D) as the only mixing process in the lung; the second consists of assuming that D can be taken as a constant, given by the diffusion coefficient of a binary mixture. The last aspect was extensively studied by Chang et al. (Chang et al., 1975; Chang and Farhi, 1980) and it is also discussed in Chapter 1. It can be shown from their work that in the situations considered in the present chapter this is indeed a very good assumption. Also of utmost usefulness were the experiments by Göttingen's group giving reliable values for the diffusion coefficients of respiratory gases (Worth and Piiper, 1978; Worth et al., 1978). In the case of the pairs of gases discussed above, the experiments gave D values very close to those already commonly used.

The consideration of D as the only mixing process in the lung is clearly an oversimplification. It offers the advantage of giving a lower limit for axial mixing. If other mixing mechanisms apply at the level of the diffusion front (if this is the case it will probably be in its proximal part, where the Reynolds number is larger), the front will be more spread. At the present time, we have no basis to establish a quantitative approach to such mechanisms.

3. Radial diffusion is instantaneous, so that there are no radial concentration gradients.

One of the powerful aspects of modeling is the common possibility of establishing lower or upper limits for a variable. This is the case for the axial dispersion of a gas in the bronchial tree during normal breathing, where the upper limit is given by the Taylor-Aris equation (Taylor, 1953; Aris, 1956);

$$D + \frac{r^2 \bar{u}^2}{48D} \qquad (12)$$

where D is the molecular diffusion coefficient, r the duct radius, and $\bar{u}$ the mean convective velocity. Equation (12) results from the analysis of transport by diffusion and convection in a cylinder of circular cross section, where the gases diffuse radially and axially and the flow is laminar. It was first applied to the lung by Wilson and Lin (1970). Equation (12) can be incorporated into a transport equation [Eq. (7) for a variable D)] and it was shown that using only D instead of Eq. (12) gives almost indistinguishable results (Lacquet et al., 1975). For example, the simulated dead spaces represented in Figure 11 decrease approximately 1 ml for SF_6 and much less for H_2. The use of D instead of both terms of Eq. (12) corresponds indeed to the assumption of instantaneous radial diffusion.

4. The molecules inside the alveoli do not diffuse axially.

The analysis of diffusion in a model representing an alveolar duct was carried out simultaneously by several authors (Chang et al., 1973; Davidson and Fitzgerald, 1974; Paiva, 1974). One of those analyses was specifically done with the aim of testing the validity of describing the transport in an alveolar duct by coupling two assumptions: instantaneous radial diffusion and no axial diffusion inside an alveolus. The diffusion in the structure represented in Figure 6 was simulated by a stochastic method and the results compared with the solution of Eq. (7) under the same conditions. The agreement was very good (Paiva, 1974).

5. The geometry is rigid.

The choice of models other than isotropically expansile is related to technical difficulties in the numerical computations. Different type of expansile models have been used in identical simulations, allowing a direct comparison between them. Of particular interest is the comparison with the results of Scherer's model (Scherer et al., 1972) and the present one. They are equivalent with the exception of the assumption under discussion. In Scherer's model, the alveoli expand uniformly (not the airways). In the present model, the volume changes take place at the end of the alveolar sacs (at $x = 0$). The results of both models are almost indistinguishable for simulations of normal breathing. We shall see in the next section that for vital capacity simulations an expansile model is more appropriate. In a radially expansile model, Eq. (7) remains unchanged but the velocity at any point takes now into account the variation of volume proximal to that point. Also, for a vital capacity maneuver, comparison of a radial expansile with a radial-axially expansile (isotropic) model results in a very similar concentration curves (Engel and Paiva, 1981).

6. The gases are incompressible and the temperature is constant.

This assumption of the model is the easiest to justify, since it is known that during quiet breathing the variation of pressure (Mead, 1961) and temperature (McFadden, 1983) in the last 13 lung generations are negligible. It is evident that the driving force for gas movement within the lung is a pressure gradient. However, as far as gas mixing is concerned, it is easier to assume that the pressure is constant within the lung and to impose a given flow.

D. Critique of the Trumpet Model

If the foregoing assumptions on which the trumpet model is based are indeed realistic, what causes the differences between simulations and experiments? Why is the simulated slope flat? Why does the model overestimate the He-SF_6 (or H_2-SF_6) separation?

One of the factors not taken into consideration is the asymmetry of the proximal generations of the bronchial tree. This factor was considered in detail by Horsfield and Cumming, who analyzed the consequences of airway morphology on the single-breath test and have shown that it does not influence the alveolar plateau (Horsfield and Cumming, 1968b). Neither can a difference in the transit times from our 2^{11} (2048) trumpet models representing the lung influence the He-SF_6 separation.

We have already pointed out one of the conclusions drawn from the trumpet model: Mechanisms other than molecular diffusion probably intervene in gas mixing (i.e., assumption 2 using molecular diffusion as the only mixing process should perhaps be modified). One of the possible mechanisms is cardiogenic mixing (Engel et al., 1973). We shall see in the next section that it is not likely to explain the discrepancies observed. We have also used the empirical formulas of Scherer obtained for the first generations (Scherer et al., 1975) and assumed they are valid for all the lung (Paiva et al., 1976). This can partially explain the experimental observation concerning H_2 and SF_6 dead spaces shown in Figure 11, but the simulated alveolar plateau is reached even faster than when using molecular diffusion only. Furthermore, we have no physical basis for extrapolating Scherer formulas and this subject is still open. It is studied at present by several groups because of its implications on the explanations of the mechanisms of mixing during high-frequency ventilation (Chap. 4).

Another weakness of the model is related to the use of the symmetrical geometry of the last generations of the bronchial tree. This point was stressed by Mon and Ultman (1976), who simulated convection and diffusion in the asymmetrical airway system proposed by Parker, Horsfield, and Cumming (1971) for the last lung generations. Their model produced a sloping alveolar plateau for the single-breath test and they concluded: "The origin of the plateau slope could be the longitudinal stratification of tracer concentration along the airway paths or could alternatively be an effect of geometric asymmetries; the plateau could not be due to the presence of the alveoli since radial concentration differences in alveolated airways have been shown to be negligible. Since the analyses of Scherer et al. and Paiva in symmetric geometries did not produce a physiologically significant plateau, it remains that it must be produced by the geometric asymmetries."

The work of Mon and Ultman remained without continuation mainly because the stochastic technique used is very time consuming to handle. Presumably because of that, the authors did not show that the same technique, applied to a symmetric model, produces indeed a flat plateau. They nevertheless opened a new line of research which found a conceptual basis with the introduction of the interdependence concept that we discuss in the next section.

A different approach to gas mixing in the lung has been attempted, mainly by the Göttingen group, and a review of that work was done by Piiper (1979). Briefly, it consists of characterizing the lung by a few compartments defined by their volume and the conductances between them. For example, the complexity of the gas mixing described in this section is bypassed by assuming that the diffusive mixing between inspired and resident gas occurs at a single plane whose diffusive resistance or conductance was computed. We also saw that there is an intrinsic difference in gas transport between inspiration and expiration due to the velocity reversal. In those models the computed conductance is a consequence of the overall mixing during all the breath and its physical and physiological meaning is therefore not clear. It is nevertheless possible that such models are useful for fitting experimental data if they can be described by a reduced number of parameters. They represent an operational or phenomenological approach to the description of gas mixing in the lung and will not be discussed further.

IV. Two-Trumpet or One-Branch-Point Model

A. Interdependence Concept

The mammalian lung presents a unique characteristic which to our knowledge is not found in any other natural or artificial structure: a to-and-fro convective movement in a multibranch cul-de-sac system. A direct consequence of this type of structure is a decreasing convective velocity toward the periphery. Somewhere within the lung, molecular diffusion and convective flow are of the same order of magnitude.

The relative contribution of convective and diffusive transport is usually expressed by the Péclet number (Pe), given by Pe = ud/D, where u is the mean convective veolcity, d the duct diameter, and D the molecular diffusion coefficient. The Péclet number provides a measure of the relative magnitude of mass transfer by convection to mass transfer by diffusion. The zone of the lung where this occurs was called by Gómez the critical zone (Gómez, 1965). It is noteworthy that according to the anatomical model of Weibel the inflection point of the diffusion front concentration profile [Eq. (9)] is found at the boundary between generations 17 and 18 for a flow of 250 ml/sec (Fig. 7), which corresponds to Pe = 0.2 (i.e., the mass transfer by diffusion appears to be therein five times the mass transfer by convection). The reason for this is that Pe is independent of any type of structure or boundary conditions, whereas the diffusion front results from the diffusion and convection in a trumpet-shaped structure. Furthermore, the diffusion front of Figure 7 is a consequence of the particular boundary conditions chosen to simulate a respiratory movement.

The concept of interdependence of transport can be grasped from an analysis of the diffusion front. It is clear from Figure 7 that during most of the inspiration, the transport is purely convective in all the generations proximal to generation 15. The concentration is equal to 1 and consequently $\partial C/\partial x = 0$, which implies a zero diffusion flow (Fick's law). The consequence of a purely convective flow at a given branch point is that the amount of inspired gas goes into each parallel unit in proportion to the flow: The units are independent from the transport point of view. In an isotropically expanding lung, the flow at each branch point is proportional to the volume of each of the two groups of units subtented by that branch point.

At the other extreme of the bronchial tree, corresponding to generation 23, the convective velocity approaches zero and the parallel units with a very peripheral branch point equilibrate very fast by diffusion mixing. Their concentrations will be equal and the units can therefore be considered as one single unit with a volume equal to the sum of the volumes of each one. It was the quantitative formulation of the transport in the intermediate zone that led to the new concept of interdependence or convection-diffusion interaction (Paiva and Engel, 1979).

We have represented in Figure 13 three branches in the zone where the transport by convection and by diffusion is of the same order of magnitude. We show a two-dimensional random walk simulation of a fictitious particle represented at equal time intervals both for $u = 0$ (open circles) and for $u \neq 0$ (closed circles). If there were no convection, the particle trajectory would have been one of the infinite possibilities whose axial dispersion is statistically described by the gaussian function (Fig. 4). If we add a convective displacement such that the velocity profile is flat (piston-type flow), the trajectory is given by the continuous line. It is clear from the comparison of both trajectories without and with convection that the particle went to the right branch because, for the velocity considered, the particle approached, by random walk, the right branch and was swept into that branch by the bulk flow. Unequal velocities in the daughter branches as well as different cross sections of the branches would have altered the trajectory of the particle. For example, a small cross section in one of the branches would have reduced the probability of the particle entering that branch. It therefore seems clear that the velocities in each branch and the cross sections play a crucial

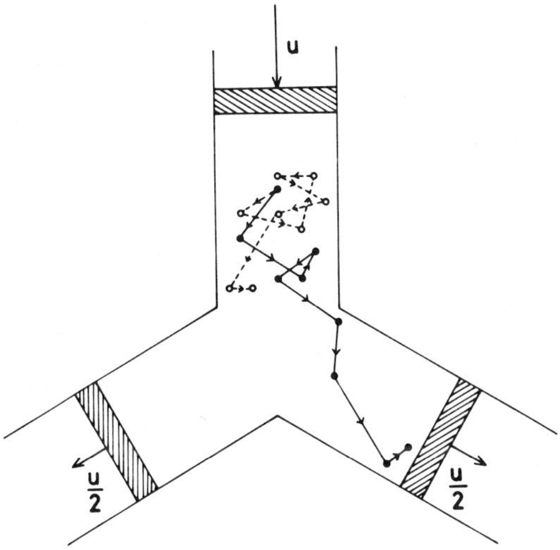

Figure 13 Two-dimensional random walk simulation of a fictitious particle represented at equal time intervals both for u = 0 (open circles) and for u ≠ 0 (closed circles). In the last case, the convective velocity in the daughter branches is identical and the three branches represent the zone of the lung where the transport by convection and by diffusion is of the same order of magnitude.

role on the transport of one inspired particle in one or the other branch and consequently on the concentration profiles in each branch. However, these considerations, based on Figure 13, would have been of little use if not based on a mathematical formalization of the problem.

Mon and Ultman (1976) used the random walk approach (visualized in Fig. 13) to describe convection and diffusion in the Parker model of the acinus (Parker et al., 1971). However, that approach presents a drawback: It is very difficult to describe the results as a function of the parameters of the model, such a velocities, diffusivities, or cross sections. This probably explains why the pioneering work of Mon and Ultman was not pursued. We have used a different approach (Paiva and Engel, 1979). We have already discussed the fact that the diffusion equation is nothing more than Fick's law of diffusion and a matter balance in an element of volume. We have extended this formalism for a branching tube (Fig. 14). Probably because nobody has ever been faced with the problem of describing simultaneous diffusion and convection in a branching tube, such a formalism is not, to our knowledge, to be found in any textbook of mathematics or physics. We shall describe here only briefly how we dealt with it.

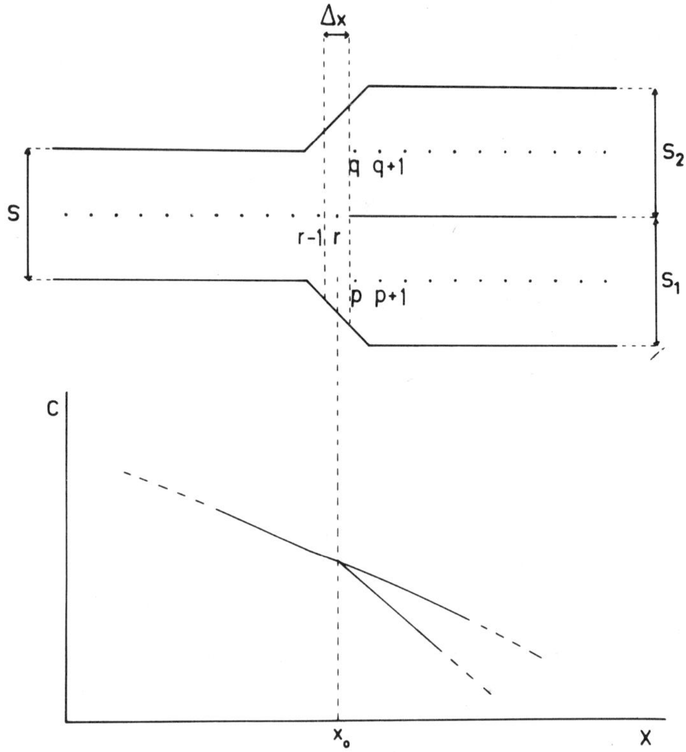

Figure 14 Representation of a branching tube for the one-dimensional analysis of transport by the solution of Eqs. (13) and (14). Nodes r, p, and q enable the writing of a continuity condition at the branch point. The lower diagram represents schematically the concentration curve with a bifurcation at $x = x_0$. (From Paiva, 1983.)

We have represented in Figure 14 three ducts where the concentration is computed in the nodes (closed circles). The link between the three ducts is established by the equations that express the matter balance at the branching point (node r), taking into account both convection and diffusion flow. It can be shown that such conditions are given by

$$\frac{dF_r}{dt} = D\left(\frac{F_{r+1} - 2F_r + F_{r-1}}{\Delta x^2} \; \frac{1}{S_r} \; \frac{S_p + S_q - S_r}{\Delta x} \; \frac{F_{r+1} - F_r}{\Delta x} \right.$$

$$\left. - \frac{1}{S_r} \; \frac{F_p u_p S_p + F_q u_q S_q - F_r u_r S_r}{\Delta x}\right) \qquad (13)$$

with

$$F_{r+1} = \frac{F_p S_p + F_q S_q}{S_q + S_q} \qquad (14)$$

The present analysis differs from the classical diffusion equation for two nontrivial reasons. On the one hand, in the classical numerical description of a spatial variable it is always possible to reduce the errors due to the space discretization by reducing Δx. In the present case a discontinuity always exists at the level of the bifurcation between node r and nodes p or q, even for a very small Δx. On the other hand, the concentration profiles bifurcate at the node r or $x = x_0$ (lower panel of Fig. 14); that is, there are two (right) derivatives of the concentration for $x = x_0$. Each derivative multiplied by the cross section and D gives the diffusion flow into each one of the two daughter branches. The interdependence of transport is a consequence of the matter balance at the branch point. If there is a large concentration gradient at the entry of one unit, the diffusion flow will be high therein and fewer molecules remain available to go to the other branch whatever the convective flow may be. The convective flow also obeys the matter balance, the sum of the convective flow in the two daughter branches being equal to the convective flow in the parent branch. We do not consider here gas transfer to or from the blood, which would introduce sink and source terms.

Even if all the previous considerations are accepted, it is not evident, a priori, that gas transport in a three-dimensional structure can be simulated using a one-dimensional diffusion equation. Indeed, in the zone of branching, the transport takes place by convection and diffusion in three-dimensional space. How can we be sure that such a complex phenomenon can be realistically described by the conditions at a single point? To answer this question the diffusion convection equation in a two-dimensional network was solved and the solutions were compared to those obtained from Eqs. (13) and (14) (Paiva, 1983). For a very large range of velocities, the two approaches gave very similar results. Furthermore, other velocity profiles of convective flow were simulated and showed no differences in the results. This analysis validated the use of the one-dimensional approach to the study of gas transport and mixing in a branching structure. It is nevertheless likely that for larger Péclet numbers, such as those found in more proximal conducting airways, the approach is not valid, for both normal and high-frequency breathing (Chap. 4).

The concept of interdependence can perhaps better be grasped from the similation shown in Figure 15, representing a 1-liter inspiration of O_2 with He and SF_6 as tracers. We assumed a trumpet-shaped geometry, but where peripheral to a branch point situated at the level of the respiratory

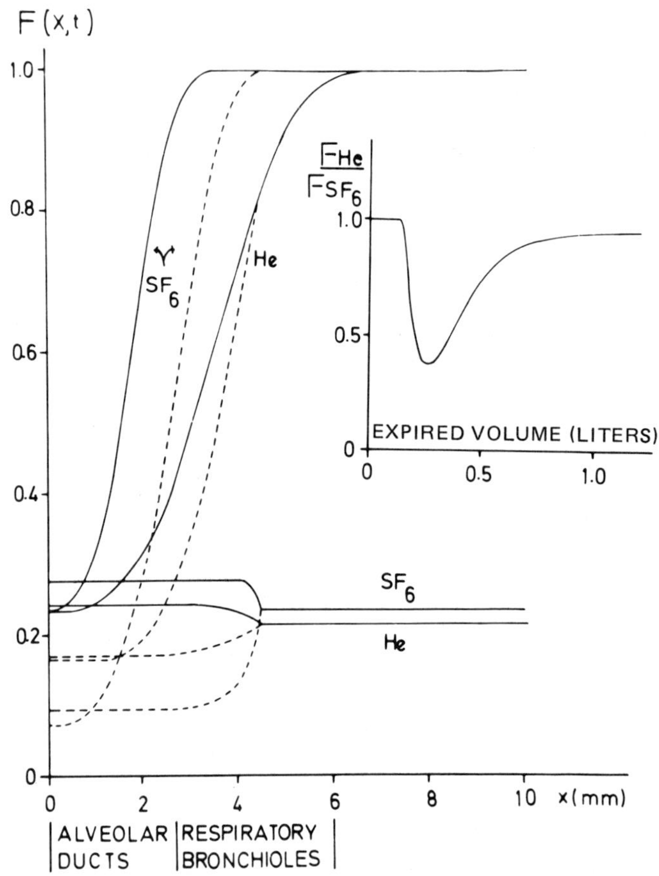

Figure 15 Simulation of a 1-liter inspiration of a He-SF_6 tracer mixture in O_2, followed by a 1-liter expiration both at a constant flow of 1 liter/sec. The ordinate is the He and SF_6 concentration relative to the inspired concentration and the abscissa is the distance to the alveolar end of the model. We assumed a trumpet geometry, but peripheral to a branch point situated at the level of the respiratory bronchioles (at x = 4.3 mm from the alveolar end) the flow in half of the lung is three times the flow in the other half (0.75 and 0.25 liter/sec, respectively). Solid and dashed lines represent gas concentrations in the better- and lesser-ventilated unit, respectively. Only end-inspiratory and end-expiratior curves are represented. The He/SF_6 ratio at the exit of the model plotted against expired volume is represented in the inset. (From Paiva and Engel, 1979.)

bronchioles (at x = 4.3 mm from the alveolar end) the flow in half of the lung is three times the flow in the other half; that is, for the total flow at the mouth of 1 liter/sec, the flow is 0.75 liter/sec and 0.25 liter/sec in each half of the lung, respectively. The ordinate is the He and SF_6 concentration relative to the inspired concentration and the abscissa is the distance to the alveolar end. Solid and dashed lines represent gas concentrations in the better and lesser ventilated unit, respectively. Only end inspiratory and end expiratory curves are represented.

For the flow and branch point positions of Figure 15, the SF_6 front is distal to the branch point, whereas the He front falls on it. Thus SF_6 enters each unit independently, in proportion to the volume flows (in the ratio of 3:1), while He transport is more uniformly distributed. Hence the high-flow unit is SF_6 enriched. On expiration, greater weighting of the better ventilated unit results in a mean expired He/SF_6 that is less than that from an equivalent uniformly ventilated lung. This is represented in the inset (He/SF_6 expired concentration ratio), which clearly shows that the expired concentration curves are a bad representation of alveolar concentration. Indeed, during the expiration and within the alveolar zone, the mean He concentration largely exceeds the mean SF_6 concentration, the reverse being true for the expired gases. The reason for this is that the interdependence mechanism "traps" the He molecules in the less expansile unit.

Do the previously described paradoxical results have a practical interest? A He/SF_6 concentration profile of the type shown in Figure 15 was indeed observed in pig lungs after breath holding, which has been interpreted as being due to the fast He diffusion in the less ventilated unit (Kelly et al., 1982a), a mechanism similar to the one described above. Some paradoxical results where O_2 exchange was improved by breathing dense gases (Martin et al., 1972; Saltzman et al., 1971) could also be explained by the interdependence concept. At the present time, however, it is not possible to know if such explanations indeed correspond to what goes on within the lung. It is possible that other phenomena account for such paradoxical results. It is also possible that if the explanation holds, the parallel units within the lung between which the interdependence applies are larger than those proposed by the present simulations, which consider molecular diffusion as the only mechanism of axial spread. Indeed, if the spread is larger than the one predicted by molecular diffusion, the diffusion front will be more proximal and branch points subtending larger units are now located on it. Those branch points were situated proximal to the diffusion front when the spread was given by molecular diffusion only.

Two interesting observations arose from the simulations of the two-trumpet model. First, the alveolar gas concentration within terminal units at end inspiration is not necessarily proportional to their relative volume expansions even in the absence of phase differences and asynchrony. Volume flow per unit volume (or specific compliance) in two units may be identical, yet alveolar concentration of inspired gas may differ greatly. Furthermore, the pattern of gas concentration throughout the respiratory cycle in the two units may be quite dissimilar. Second, diffusion-dependent separation of inert gases could be interpreted in terms of a parallel model, whereas all the previous interpretations were based on transport in the series spaces only.

Finally, the previous explanations perhaps also apply to some paradoxical results reported by Hogg et al. (1972). Those authors observed that after insufflation of beads into the bronchi of excised lobes, the inspiration of a He-SF_6 mixture resulted, after expiration, in the alveolar gas being SF_6 enriched, which was attributed to a deeper penetration of the heavier gas due to Taylor diffusion. It is clear from Figure 15 that during the inspiration, with the exception of the terminal part of the less ventilated unit, all the lung is SF_6 enriched ($F_{SF_6} > F_{He}$). It is possible that some collateral channels connect SF_6-enriched zones with the obstructed zones which are ventilated only via collateral channels and which were found to be SF_6 enriched.

B. Slope of the Alveolar Plateau

The formalization of the transport in a branching structure [Eqs. (13) and (14)] made feasible the quantitative analysis of the intra-acinar asymmetry and its possible influence on the genesis of the sloping alveolar plateau. Hansen and Ampaya (1975) described the acinus as an asymmetrical structure, the entry of which (terminal bronchiole) corresponds to generation 15 and extends to generation 26 (Chap. 1). Most of the alveolar sacs are situated at orders 23 and 24. The use of Eqs. (13) and (14) made possible consideration of the acinus as a structure ending at two different generation orders. We consider simulations in an acinar model where half of the lung branches end at generation 23 (as in the one-trumpet model) and half at a more proximal generation. Different analyses were proposed by Luijendijk et al. (1980) and Nixon and Pack (1982). We show in Figure 16 the simulation of a 1-liter O_2 inspiration at a constant flow of 1 liter/sec in a model where the branch point is at the end of the respiratory bronchioles (entry of the alveolar ducts), which corresponds to the entry of generation 19 in the Weibel model. The ordinate is the O_2 concentration and the abscissa (x) is the distance from the terminal end of the longer unit. The dashed and the solid lines are the O_2 concentrations in the shorter and longer units, respectively. The numbers 5 to 10 represent concentrations at 0.2-sec intervals. Curves 5 and 5′ correspond to the end of the inspiration (beginning of the expiration). The inset represents O_2 concentration at model exit (generation 13/14) plotted against expired volume.

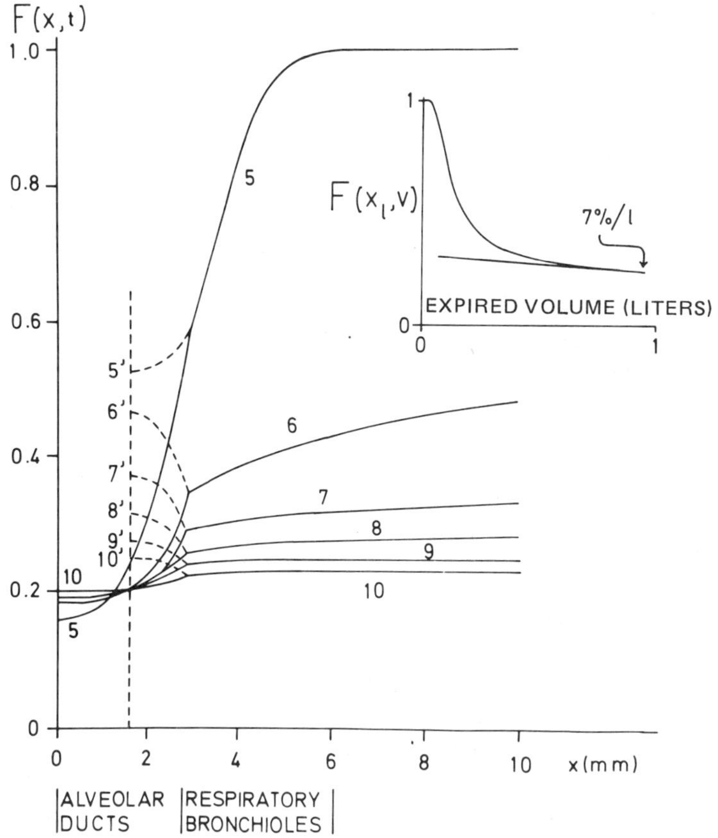

Figure 16 Pattern of O_2 concentration (F) during expiration after a 1-liter inspiration of O_2 at 1 liter/sec into an asymmetrical two-trumpet model. Dashed lines: shorter unit (volume V_2); solid lines: longer unit (volume V_1), and common pathway ($V_2/V_1 = 0.12$). Branch point is at x = 2.7 mm. Numbers 5 to 10 represent concentration at 0.2-sec intervals as a function of distance (x) from the terminal and of the longer unit. Inset: O_2 concentration at exit of model plotted against volume expired. Note that in the shorter unit alveolar concentrations are relatively greater and fall during expiration when the gradients are reversed. This results in a changing concentration in the common airway and a sloping alveolar plateau. (From Paiva and Engel, 1981.)

The alveolar O_2 concentration in the shorter unit is higher than in the longer unit, the magnitude of this difference depending on the degree of asymmetry (Paiva and Engel, 1981). During expiration, the alveolar concentration in the longer unit is essentially unchanged, with rapid equilibration in most of the unit volume. A small axial gradient persists near the branch point due to back diffusion of O_2 against the convective flow. In contrast, the alveolar F_{O_2} in the shorter unit falls during expiration, the rate of fall depending both on degree of asymmetry and the magnitude of the volumes subtended by the branch point. Furthermore, equilibration of gas concentration does not occur and a reversed concentration gradient is apparent even near the terminal boundary (despite a gradient of zero at the boundary).

The foregoing results are a consequence of the interdependence of gas transport among parallel pathways. During inspiration convective flow into the smaller unit is less than that into the larger unit (in proportion to the relative volumes). At the branch point this corresponds to a difference of velocity in the same proportion. The lower convective velocity into the smaller unit, together with its shorter diffusive pathlength, contribute to a more proximally situated diffusion front during inspiration. On the other hand, the diffusion flow in each unit is in proportion to the concentration gradient and the cross section (Fick's law), both cross sections being the same in the simulation. As a consequence, the diffusive flow in the smaller unit per unit of volume of this unit is larger than the diffusive flow per unit of volume in the larger unit. Thus the smaller unit is "better ventilated" despite equivalent inspiratory flow per unit volume in the two units.

During expiration there is also an interdependence of gas transport between the two paths at the branch point. The relatively poorly ventilated larger unit has a higher N_2 concentration (F_{N_2}), or lower F_{O_2}, at the onset of expiration. The relatively large convective velocity ensures rapid equilibration of gas concentration within the unit. At the branch point, gas with a high F_{O_2} is convected at a relatively low velocity (because of its small volume) from the shorter unit. The gradient of F_{O_2} at the branch point favors diffusive flux of O_2 out of (N_2 into) the smaller unit and because of its short diffusion path length and low velocity, the flux is sufficient to progressively lower F_{O_2} even in the terminal divisions. The presence of an O_2/N_2 concentration gradient at the branch point causes some diffusion of O_2 back into the larger unit, explaining the curvilinearity of the concentration curve near the branch point during expiration (Fig. 16). However, this back diffusion of O_2 is opposed by a relatively large convective flow, resulting in a quasi-stationary concentration gradient and no significant change in the alveolar F_{O_2} within the unit.

Since during expiration the gas concentration at the branch point and downstream is determined by the concentrations leaving the two units, the decreasing alveolar F_{O_2} in the shorter unit necessarily causes a progressive decrease in the expired O_2 concentration as expiration proceeds, resulting in a sloping alveolar plateau. The magnitude and pattern of this fall depend on the degree of asymmetry (Paiva and Engel, 1981). There need not be any sequential filling or emptying in the convective sense (i.e., all volume changes are synchronous and in constant proportion to each other). Seen in terms of N_2, some of the N_2 expired from the larger unit to the branch point initially diffuses back into the shorter unit (countercurrent) as a consequence of the small convective flow in this unit due to its small volume.

A consequence of the mechanism generating the slope of the alveolar plateau within an asymmetrical acinus is that the simulated alveolar plateau is not a straight line but presents a curvilinear shape. Indeed, during expiration, the concentration differences between the parallel units generating the slope decrease (if not, the slope would have been nil), and consequently the slope of the alveolar plateau also decreases.

An intuitive feeling of the different factors discussed above can be grasped from Figure 17. We have represented N_2 molecules by closed circles, the density of which are roughly proportional to 1 - F(x,t) (Fig. 16). We have considered gas transport during inspiration (Fig. 17A) and during expiration (Fig. 17B). The thin arrows indicate displacement by diffusion and the heavy arrows the displacement by convection. We have indicated the diffusion arrows according to the concentration gradient of N_2 (Fig. 16), but it is clear that they have only a statistical meaning, showing that the majority of the molecules move according to the indicated direction. On

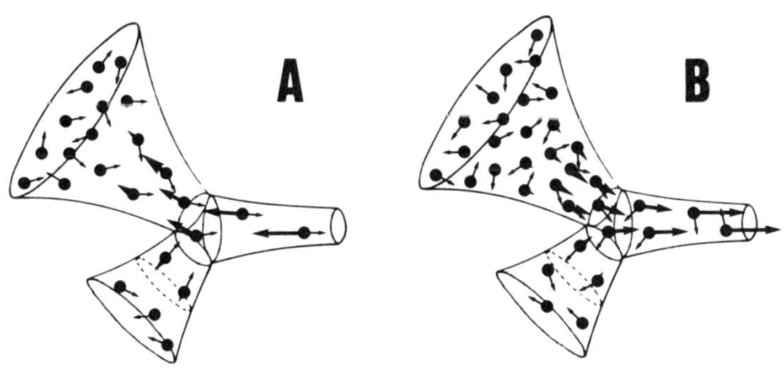

Figure 17 Schematical representation of the interdependence of transport by diffusion and convection in an asymmetrical two-trumpet model. The N_2 molecules are represented by closed circles during an O_2 inspiration (A) and during the subsequent expiration (B). The thin arrows indicate displacement by diffusion and the heavy arrows the displacement by convection. See the text for further details.

the other hand, the convection arrow is a deterministic arrow and the molecules indeed always move by convection according to the indicated direction.

During inspiration (Fig. 17A) we described above a larger diffusion O_2 flow in the small unit relatively to its volume, giving a larger O_2 concentration therein. This is seen as the small unit having a smaller N_2 concentration. In terms of N_2 molecular displacement, this means that N_2 molecules in the small unit approach the branch point by diffusion and are swept away by the bulk flow (which is larger at the entry of the larger unit). At the alveolar end of both units, the diffusion movement has no preferential direction (zero concentration gradient). The same explanation of the diffusion front given for the (one) trumpet model also holds here in both trumpets (one diffusion front in each trumpet). The proximal part of the front is close to the entry of the model and we have represented therein a smaller number of N_2 molecules. The large arrow of convection in the peripheral direction is balanced by a small arrow of diffusion in the opposite direction. Indeed, the convection flow is equal to $F_{N_2}\dot{V}$ and F_{N_2} is very small. The uniform dimension of the diffusion arrows indicates that the intrinsic diffusive movement is the same everywhere.

During expiration (Fig. 17B), the only significant concentration gradient appears in the zone of the branch point. The N_2 molecules diffuse countercurrent into the smaller unit. Those molecules are therefore prevented from being expired and the N_2 concentration at the output of the model is smaller than it would be if this countercurrent diffusion into the small unit did not occur. During expiration, this effect decreases as the N_2 concentration between the two parallel units equilibrates and more N_2 is available to go out of the model, producing a sloping alveolar plateau. The magnitude of the slope is therefore a consequence of a large number of parameters: structure of the branch point region (in the zone of the diffusion front), whose location is itself a consequence of flow; the diffusion coefficient; and the volume of the units subtended by the branch point, which determines the convective flows at the branch point. We shall see in the next section that a more accurate description of the interdependence of transport needs the consideration of multibranch-point models (MBPMs).

An equivalent description of the interdependence of transport by convection and diffusion in an asymmetrical structure can be given by a model with two identical parallel units, except at the branch point, where one of them is narrowed (De Vries et al., 1981; Kelly et al., 1982b; Engel, 1983). If the branch point is in the zone of the diffusion front, the smaller diffusion flow into the narrowed unit, during inspiration, creates a concentration inhomogeneity despite identical volume change in both units. During expiration, countercurrent diffusion of N_2 from the narrowed unit into the nonnarrowed unit can also produce a sloping alveolar plateau by the same mechanism as discussed for the two-trumpet asymmetrical model.

C. First In-Last Out Pattern of Breathing

An interesting (and surprising) application of the interdependence concept was the demonstration that the "first in-last out" pattern of breathing can be generated in an asymmetrical acinus. We show in Figures 18 and 19 the simulation of the transport and mixing of a He bolus injected at 20 and 80% of a vital capacity (VC) inspiration, followed by a VC expiration. The branch point was assumed to be situated 3.7 mm from the terminal end of the longest unit, which corresponds to a volume ratio of the two subtended units equal to 0.23. The position of the branch point was selected to coincide with the inflection point of the diffusion front established in a symmetrical trumpet in which volumes, flows, and diffusivity correspond to those of the experiments. The simulations shown correspond to the inhalation of a 1.54-ml bolus of He at 20 (Figs. 18 and 19B) and 80% (Fig. 19C) VC during a constant-flow VC inspiration and expiration at 100 ml/sec. The diffusion coefficient chosen was 0.6 cm^2/sec, corresponding to that of He/N_2. The simulated volume flow into each trumpet was always in proportion to its volume and synchronous. There was no sequential convective filling or emptying at any time.

Because of the VC changes in volume we modified our previous rigid, nonexpansile model so that volume change (ΔV) was associated with gradual increase in the cross-sectional area (ΔS). Thus $\Delta S \propto \Delta V$. This is the radially expansile model (Engel and Paiva, 1981).

Figure 18 shows the He concentration profiles during the inspiration for a bolus inspired at 20% VC and for the time values indicated by vertical bars in Figure 18A. The interface between the inspired bolus and residual gas advances to the branch point (BP), from where transport by diffusion to the two units is very close whereas the total volume of gas entering the shorter unit is less, in proportion to its volume. This results in relatively greater initial F_{He} in the shorter unit (curves 2 and 3 in Fig. 18). Later, in inspiration, the non-He-containing air inhaled subsequent to the He bolus is also preferentially transported (by diffusion) into the shorter unit, diluting the initially higher F_{He}. At the same time He molecules diffuse back to the branch point, from where they are convected into the larger unit. Curves 1 to 4 in Figure 18 show the progressive decrease in the concentration difference between the short and long units. At some point in time between curves 4 and 5 the concentrations are identical, and at end inspiration (curve 5) F_{He} is higher in the longer unit. Thus a volume of air in excess of 30% VC needs to be inhaled following a He bolus to cancel out the initially greater F_{He} in the shorter unit.

When the He bolus is inhaled at 80% VC the initial F_{He} is again greater in the short unit. The remaining 20% VC of air is insufficient to reverse the relative F_{He} in the two units so that at end inspiration the shorter unit still

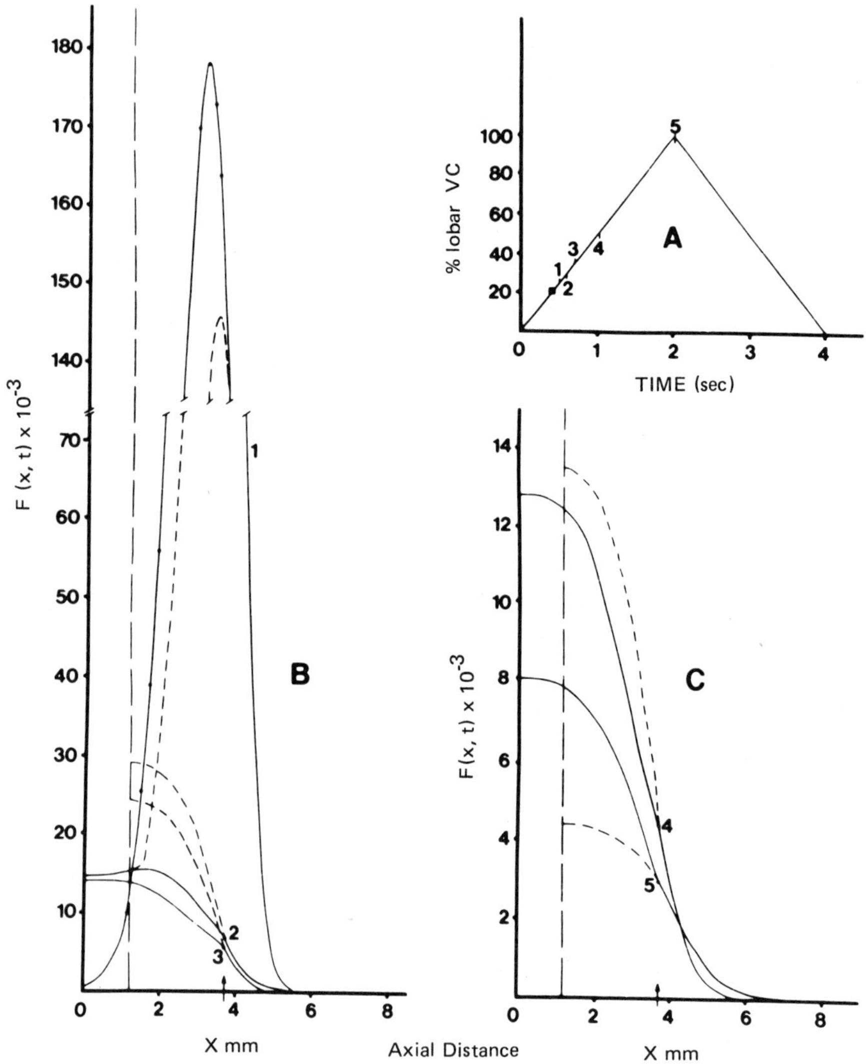

Figure 18 Concentration profiles within an asymmetrical two-trumpet model during inspiration of a 1.54-ml He bolus at 20% of lobar VC. (A) Lobar volume change as a function of time. Closed square: point of inhalation of the bolus. Numbers 1 to 5 are points corresponding to concentration profiles shown in (B) and (C). In (B) and (C), solid lines: concentrations in longer trumpet and common stem; dashed lines: concentration in shorter trumpet; arrow: position of branch point at x = 3.7 mm; solid ordinate (x = 0): terminal end of the longer trumpet; dashed ordinate: terminal end of the shorter trumpet. (From Engel and Paiva, 1981.)

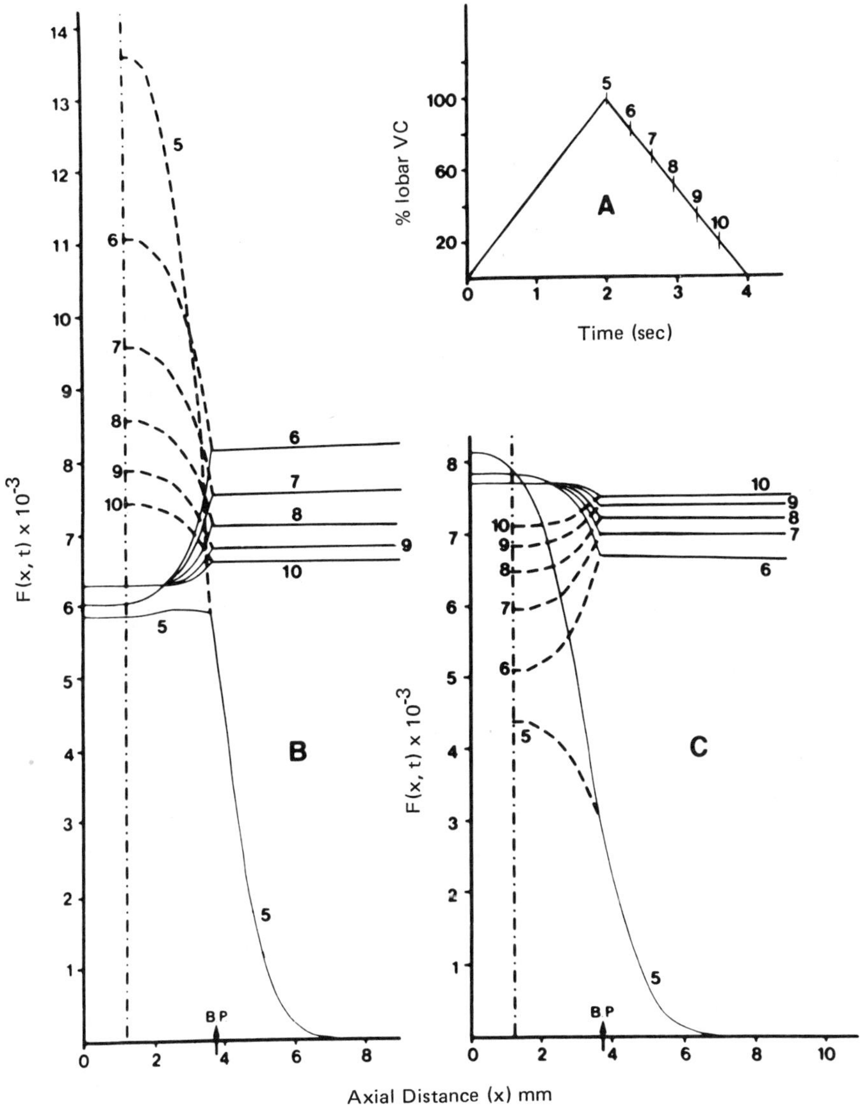

Figure 19 He concentration profiles within an asymmetrical model during expiration after inhalation of 1.54-ml He bolus at 80% lobar VC (B) and 20% VC (C). (A) Volume change as a function of time. Points 5 to 10 represent volume and time for corresponding concentration profiles. Axes and arrow as in Figure 18. Note increasing F after 20% VC bolus, decreasing F after 80% VC bolus. (From Engel and Paiva, 1981.)

has a higher F_{He} (curve 5 in Fig. 19B). When the He bolus is inhaled at an intermediate lung volume the F_{He} in the two units at end inspiration differs to a lesser extent.

During expiration the large concentration gradient between the BP and the end of the shorter unit results in a marked diffusive transport. Although some back diffusion takes place into the larger unit, the mean concentration at the BP and downstream progressively falls (curves 6 to 10 in Fig. 19B). Thus the expired F_{He} measured at the exit of the model also decreases. This changing concentration, when plotted against expired volume, constitutes a downward-sloping alveolar plateau.

After the 20% VC bolus inhalation F_{He} at the BP increases during expiration (curves 6-10 in Fig. 19C). This is associated with marked back diffusion of He into the shorter unit, whose F_{He} consequently increases throughout expiration. In contrast, the decrease in F_{He} within the longer unit is small and transient. Hence the expired F_{He} measured at the exit of the model gives rise to an upward-sloping alveolar plateau. The direction of the slope simulated for boluses inhaled at different points in the VC shows a gradual change from a positive slope after a 20% VC bolus to a negative one after an 80% VC bolus, as observed experimentally (Fukuchi et al., 1980).

The main findings of previous analyses are the observations that diffusive interaction between asymmetrical intra-acinar units, ventilated in parallel, can simulate the first in-last out pattern of sequential filling and emptying observed experimentally. Classically, the changing expired concentration during single-breath washouts was thought to represent temporal or volume-dependent convective sequencing of units, those better ventilated emptying early and those less well ventilated emptying late. The present analysis offers a different concept of gas transport contributing to the apparent first in-last out sequence. The analysis suggests that shorter units within the acinus are preferentially ventilated (by diffusion) at all lung volumes. This is not due to incomplete axial equilibration of gas concentration in the terminal airway as initially proposed by Krogh and Lindhard (1917). On the contrary, axial concentration gradients are less prominent in the longer pathways, and in the shorter pathway they are actually reversed!

The same model has also been used to simulate breath holding and the result is a complete gas equilibration after 5 sec. We shall see in the next section that the use of a model with a large number of branch points predicts a much slower equilibration.

To what extent the previous mechanism can explain the first in-last out pattern of breathing is still unknown. It points, however, to an unsuspected possibility which could be displayed only by a model approach of gas transport in the lung. Although the mechanism of interdependence of transport can be understood without mathematics, its formulation without formalization would probably have been too complex to get a good grip on. On the other hand, as the mechanism described previously is a consequence of different factors than those responsible for the classical explanation (different time constants or different regional compliances), it gives a new insight into the subject.

D. Simulation of Cardiogenic Mixing

Sampling from conducting airways of dog lungs postmortem, Fukuchi et al. (1976) observed that during inspiration of 100% O_2 at physiological flow rates the F_{N_2} fell to zero. However, when flow was below 50 ml/sec, F_{N_2} did not reach zero but stabilized at a progressively higher value the smaller the flow. The authors interpreted these results to reflect mouthward displacement of a stationary diffusion front so that at the low inspiratory flows, the tail of the diffusion front encroached on the sampling site. This effect, simulated in an asymmetrical model, is shown in Figure 20.

The volume of the two trumpet units together (inset) is 23.4 ml and the whole lung is represented by 64 such pairs of units (i.e., a volume of 1500 ml, corresponding roughly to the lung volume of dogs used in physiological experiments). The volume ratio of the two trumpets is 3, which is close to the volume ratio of alveoli subtended by those bronchi in a dog's lung (Horsfield and Cumming, 1976). The distance between the alveolar end of the longest unit and the entry of the model is equal to 3 cm. Lung asymmetry is represented by the second trumpet joining up at a branch point 2 cm from the alveolar end of the longest trumpet and 0.95 cm from the alveolar end of the shorter one.

Figure 20 demonstrates the influence of flow rate on the position of the diffusion front in each trumpet following the inspiration of 100 ml of O_2 at a constant flow. At a flow of 40 ml/sec (curve 3), gas concentration at the branch point (location 3) is equivalent to inspired gas ($F = 1$) and the two diffusion fronts are independent. At lower flows (curves 1 and 2) diffusion into the smaller trumpet becomes significant, resulting in a decreased F at the branch point. This influences the concentration of gas transported into the larger trumpet by convection.

Within each trumpet unit a constant-flow inspiration results in a diffusion front. Along each bronchial pathway, during inspiration, the inspired gas concentration (F_{O_2}) progressively falls (F_{N_2} rises). However, due to the asymmetry of the bronchial tree, the linear velocities, as well as diffusion distances, in each of the daughter branches differ, resulting in substantially different values of F_{N_2} at points in the airway equidistant from the branch point. When inspiratory velocities are sufficiently low, diffusion within the smaller unit results in N_2 appearing at the branch point. For the large trumpet unit the presence of alveolar gas at the branch point is "inappropriate," as the transport into this unit is entirely convective at this point. Conse-

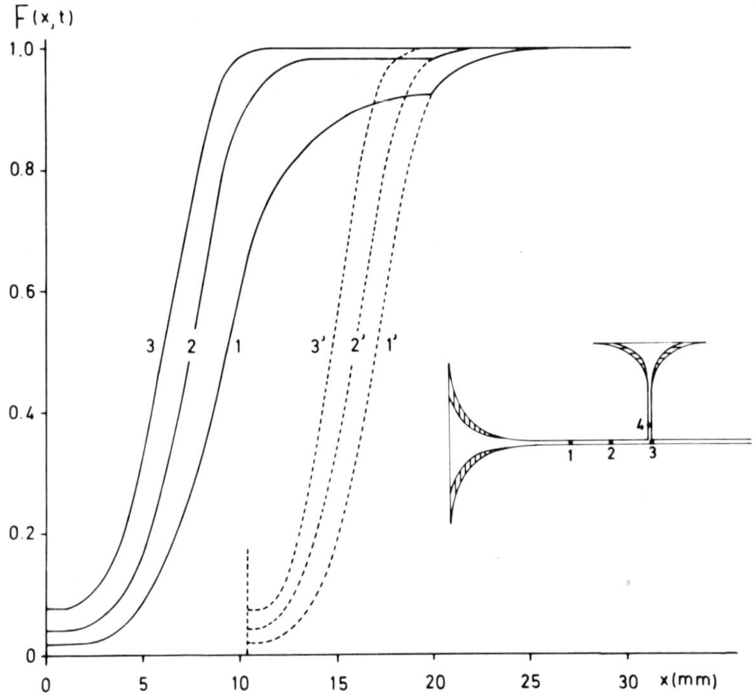

Figure 20 Oxygen concentration (F) plotted against distance from the alveolar end of the longest unit in the two-trumpet model (inset) at end inspiration. Curves 1, 2, and 3 indicate position of diffusion front in larger unit; curves 1′, 2′, and 3′ that in smaller unit, at constant inspiratory flows of 10, 20, and 40 ml/sec, respectively. Vertical dashed line represents the alveolar end of the smaller unit. Note progressive decrease in inspired gas concentration at the branch point (x = 20 mm) at lower flows. (From Paiva and Engel, 1982.)

quently, the effect of diffusion from the smaller unit is to lower the gas concentration (FO_2) inspired into the larger unit. This illustrates a diffusive interaction between the two units due to the low inspiratory flow rates used.

When inspiratory flow is not constant but is interrupted by cardiogenic flow pulses, the pattern of gas concentrations may be deduced from Figure 20. At a point in the airway corresponding to location 2 a decrease in flow to both units or a mouthward-directed cardiogenic pulse will result in a large rise in FN_2 (drop in FO_2) due not only to a mouthward displacement of the diffusion front but also to transient interaction between the two units at the branch point located upstream. The intermittent interaction between the two trumpet units at the branch point is irreversible. It results in pulses of N_2 diffusing out of the smaller unit and being convected into the larger unit, effectively reducing its FO_2.

From comparison between the rate of rise of FN_2 on the oscillations recorded during inspiration of O_2, Engel et al. (1973) concluded that the cardiogenic pulses almost invariably reversed the direction of flow in the airway sampled. This conclusion was based on the assumption of a symmetrical lung and may not be correct. The asymmetrical model analysis shows how FN_2 oscillations could be recorded in an airway without flow reversal. In fact, large FN_2 fluctuations could take place in a given airway without any flow oscillation if the latter were confined to a smaller unit upstream.

The mean FN_2 simulated at end inspiration in locations 1, 2, and 3 was substantially greater in the presence of flow oscillations than without oscillations. In fact, at the same inspiratory flow the airway FN_2 differed approximately 3 to 15-fold. This is consistent with experimental findings. Fukuchi et al. (1976) quantified the relationship between airway FN_2 and inspiratory flow both in vivo and postmortem. Assuming a symmetrical lung, they calculated from the ratio of flows necessary to achieve a given airway FN_2 that the effective diffusion coefficient (D′), incorporating effects of cardiogenic mixing, was 5-10 times greater than molecular diffusivity (D). The simulation of the same curves with the two-trumpet model approximates very closely those described by Fukuchi et al. (1976). Using these authors' calculations, a value for D′/D of 5.0 is obtained (Paiva and Engel, 1982). Therefore, the results of these simulations indicate that flow oscillations within an asymmetrical bronchial tree may produce patterns of gas concentration similar to those observed experimentally and attributed to cardiogenic gas mixing. Furthermore, the apparent enhancement of gas mixing can be simulated using the well-defined physical processes of convection and molecular diffusion, assuming blunt velocity profiles.

When molecular diffusion is the only mechanism of gas mixing, oscillatory flows (with blunt velocity profiles) in a symmetrical lung do not significantly enhance the mixing process. For this reason Engel et al. (1973) proposed that some form of enhanced diffusion based on Taylor-type phenomena (Taylor, 1953) may explain cardiogenic gas mixing. Recently, Slutsky (1981) described a quantitative, theoretical model of enhanced gas mixing secondary to cardiogenic oscillations based on the concept of augmented diffusion applicable to high-frequency ventilation (Slutsky et al., 1980). Indeed, there may be a similarity between the augmented diffusion which must take place in the bronchial tree to maintain gas exhange during high-frequency ventilation (Bohn et al., 1980) and the enhancement of gas mixing due to cardiac action. However, the latter takes place at a substantially lower frequency and is associated with asynchronous flows throughout the lung. Whether mixing mechanisms based on nonblunt velocity profiles contribute to cardiogenic mixing is still not known. However, asymmetry of the bronchial tree is well documented (Horsfield and Cumming, 1976) and the physical processes of convection and molecular diffusion are well defined. Our results do not preclude the possibility that cardiogenic gas mixing may be contributed to by mechanisms related to nonblunt velocity profiles as modeled by Slutsky (1981) and described in Chapter 4.

What are the implications of the foregoing simulations of cardiogenic gas mixing? Clearly, at any given point in the airway gas mixing is enhanced in the presence of flow oscillations. This enhancement may be represented quantitatively by an effective diffusion coefficient (D′). However, any conclusions based on a geometrically symmetrical model may not be valid. Therefore, measurement of a given value for D′ in one airway does not allow generalization to other parts of the lung. Actually, this is true not only because of the asymmetry in bronchial anatomy, but also because the magnitude of the cardiogenic impulse may vary in different parts of the lung. Therefore, the experimental results of enhanced mixing in conducting airways do not allow generalization to other parts of the lung. Indeed, it is still not clear whether cardiac motion plays a significant role in gas mixing within the gas-exchanging zone of the lung. Recent work by Jones et al. (1982) seems to indicate that such a role is negligible.

V. Multibranch-Point Models

The two-trumpet model described in the preceding section suggested that some experimental observations could be explained with the interdependence concept: the paradoxical results with gases of different diffusivities, the intraregional first in-last out pattern of breathing, the apparent increased diffusivity due to cardiogenic mixing, and the intraregional component of the sloping alveolar plateau, which would be due partially to intra-acinar asymmetry. Those possible explanations are only suggestions for further research and can be confirmed only by experimental observations.

The main weakness of the two-trumpet model is the arbitrariness of the branch point location subtending two asymmetrical units. It assumes a symmetrical dichotomy proximal and distal to the branch point. To overcome this difficulty, a fixed position of the branch point in the diffusion front can be chosen: the inflection point of the concentration curve (Lacquet and Van Muylem, 1982). This choice nevertheless suffers from the drawback of the dependence of the diffusion front spread on several parameters: flow, lung volume, and diffusion coefficient. The number of interdependent branch points is therefore not constant. Furthermore, the use of one branch point necessarily considers the lung as if the alveolar end was located at the level of only two different generation orders (generation 23 and a proximal one in the model described in the preceding section). Finally, if the transport in each branch point was independent of the transport in the others, the one-branch-point model could be used successively with different locations of the branch point and the solution of each simulation could be added using a superposition technique. However, this is not, a priori, the case for the branch points located in the zone of the diffusion front. The one-branch-point model is unable to deal with the influence that serially distributed branch points have on each other.

The simple generalization of the one-branch-point model is the consideration of a large number of branch points. Once the conditions at one branch point are established, the extension to a large number of branch points is a trivial, time-consuming computer programming problem. Four papers dealing with multibranch-point models (MBPMs) were recently published (Davidson and Engel, 1982; Bowes et al., 1982; Paiva, 1982; Paiva and Engel, 1984). We summarize briefly here their main results.

Davidson and Engel (1982) utilized the acinar model of Parker et al. (1971) to simulate gas transport and mixing in that model, consisting of five identical subunits, each one with five branch points. Those authors confirmed the unequal distribution of inspired gas between parallel pathways. After the simulation of a 1-liter inspiration followed by a 1-liter expiration at a constant flow of 1 liter/sec, the alveolar N_2 slope measured at the entry of the model during the last 0.25 liter of the expirate was equal to 3.3% per liter. This compares well with the results obtained by Mon and Ultman (1976) using the same model. These authors found a slope of 3.5% per liter measured between 0.75 and 1.25 liters of the expirate for a flow of 0.5 liter/sec and an inspired volume of 0.75 liter. Davidson and Engel (1982) also demonstrated that the interdependence of transport by diffusion and convection at the branch points subtending asymmetrical units can account for a persistent axial gradient observed within the model.

Bowes et al. (1982) considered an arbitrary structure of the acinus with perfect symmetry between the terminal bronchioles and the last respiratory bronchioles and a very asymmetrical pattern of branching distally (at the level of the alveolar ducts). After a 1-liter O_2 inspiration (with a flow equal to 0.5 liter/sec), those authors measured the slope of the alveolar plateau between 0.75 and 1.25 liters of expired volume. They found 3.4% per liter, which lies within the range of values for normal subjects as in the previous model analysis. These authors also computed the efficiency of gas mixing, which was defined as the volume of N_2 expired divided by the volume expected if mixing were complete. They found a 97% efficiency from their model and concluded that the acinar asymmetry is insufficient to account for the failure of complete gas mixing found in normal subjects, where the efficiency is close to 85%.

The third of these MBPMs (Paiva, 1982) used an acinar model derived from the anatomical data of Hansen and Ampaya (1975) and addressed more specifically the question of evaluating the persistent intra-acinar concentration inhomogeneity after breath holding. After 10 sec of breath holding, significant concentration inhomogeneities would persist within the acinus, contrary to the two-trumpet model predictions, which suggests a complete homogenization. The reason for this difference is that each unit of the two-trumpet model indeed represents a very large number of branch points subtending units with different concentrations. The path of each molecule in that complex network needed to reach an homogeneous concentration is much larger than in the two-trumpet model, where there are no branch points within each unit.

The conclusions of the previous MBPM are probably qualitatively correct, as they are based on well-established physical laws describing molecular transport in an asymmetrical structure. However, even if the concepts described were beyond dispute, the quantitative values vary as a function of the anatomical structure chosen. We therefore decided (Paiva and Engel, 1984) to perform some single-breath simulations using the Hansen and Ampaya anatomical data, which provide a more realistic description of the human acinar anatomy.

The MBPM used by us consists of the structure represented partially in Figure 21. The entry of the model (top) corresponds to a terminal bronchiole and we represented one of the eight groups of units subtended by the fourth generation of the acinus. This model was built in such a way that the total cross section of all the units of the same generation is identical to the values given by Hansen and Ampaya (1975). Almost an infinite number of different models fulfill this condition. We chose one at random.

A comparison of the models of Parker et al. (1971) and Bowes et al. (1982) with ours (Paiva and Engel, 1984) can be done by computing, for each generation, the volume ratio of the two groups of units subtended by this generation for each model (Table 1). The analysis of Table 1 clearly shows the very different type of asymmetry in the three models. Furthermore, the total cross section of the model of Parker et al. (1971) is one order of magnitude smaller than that of Bowes et al. (1982) and our model. It is therefore not surprising that simulations using those models predict different slopes for the alveolar plateau.

We have represented in Figure 21 the expired concentration computed at the entry of the model but where a delay corresponding to the transport in the generations proximal to the terminal bronchioles was introduced (using

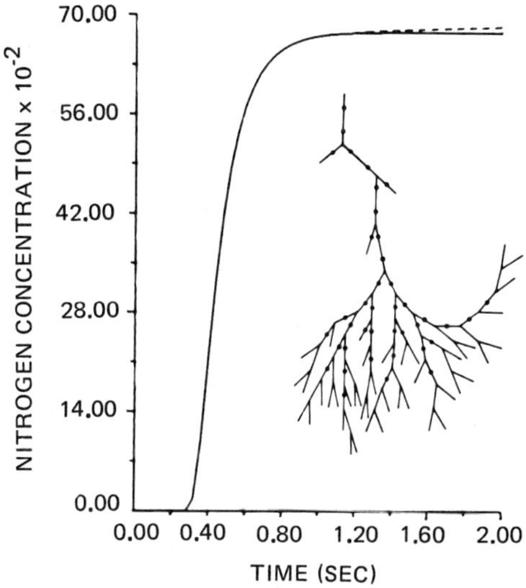

Figure 21 Simulation of the expired N_2 concentration, as a function of time, measured at the entry of the trachea using the MBPM (dashed line). The conditions of the simulation are the same as those used in Figure 7 and the continuous curve is the one already represented in that figure. The only difference between the simulation using the trumpet model and the MBPM is found in the alveolar plateau, which presents now a nonnegligible slope. The structure of the MBPM is partially represented; the entry of the model (top) corresponds to a terminal bronchiole and one of the eight groups of units subtended by the fourth generation of the acinus is also represented.

Weibel data). The conditions of the simulation were the same as in Figure 7. The continuous line is the simulation using the one-trumpet model and the dashed line using the MBPM, the only difference being the appearance of a sloping alveolar plateau. The influence of the acinar asymmetry on phase II is negligible.

We computed (Fig. 22) the slope of the alveolar plateau for a constant flow of 0.5 liter/sec and a variable tidal volume, the slope being computed for the last 0.25 liter of the expired volume. A very strong dependence of the slope on the tidal volume is apparent. The main reason for this behavior is the gas equilibration between the parallel units of the model during the expiration. Indeed, for larger tidal volumes, the parallel units have more time to equilibrate. Both this strong dependence on tidal volume and the slope values themselves are different from experimental observations. The shape of phase III also differs; it is almost linear in experiments but presents

Table 1 Comparison of the Degree of Asymmetry of the Acinar Models of Parker, Horsfield, and Cumming (PHC); Bowes et al. (B); and Ours (PE): For the First Five Generations, the Volume Ratio of the Two Groups of Units Subtended by Them Was Computed[a]

Generation number													
1		2			3			4			5		
B	PE	PHC	B	PE	PHC	B	PE	PHC	B	PE	PHC	B	PE
												0.042	0.799
									0.581	0.696		0.042	0.947
						1	0.870	0.167			0.286	0.042	0.642
			1	0.831	0.118				0.581	0.473		0.042	1.000
												0.042	0.485
						1	0.756		0.581	0.864	0.118	0.042	0.296
												0.042	0.897
								0.423	0.581	0.747		0.042	0.348
1	0.935	0.276										0.826	0.490
									0.581	0.859	0.815	0.826	0.466
						1	0.938					0.826	0.695
									0.581	0.763		0.826	0.634
			1	0.995	0.286							0.826	0.630
						1	0.771	0.118	0.581	0.590	0.167	0.826	0.812
												0.826	0.696
									0.581	0.603		0.826	0.402

[a]The PHC model does not consider the first generation of the acinus; the volume ratio therefore begins on generation 2 for that model.

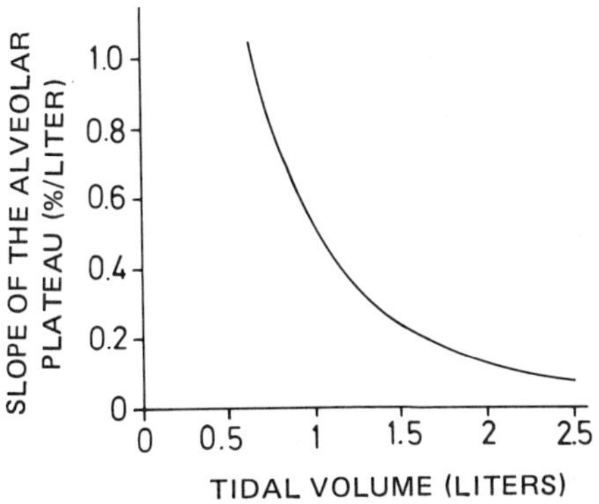

Figure 22 Slope of the alveolar plateau as a function of tidal volume. The slope was computed for the last 0.25 liter of the expired volume from the expired N_2 concentration curves simulated using the MBPM.

an exponential shape in the simulations. The mixing efficiency computed with this model is equal to 98.7% compared with 100% in the one-trumpet model, where the alveolar concentration is homogeneous and equal to the end-expired concentration. Now, the end-expired and alveolar concentrations are different and we cannot therefore infer the gas concentration inside the lung from the expired concentration curves.

One of the interesting results using the one-branch-point model is the conclusion that an (isotropically) expanding asymmetrical structure automatically generates an inhomogeneous concentration of the inspired gases. A representation of the degree of that intrinsic acinal inhomogeneity is given in Figure 23. $\Delta V_{O_2}/V_0$ was computed using the formula $\Delta V_{O_2}/V_0 = \bar{F}_{O_2}/(1 - \bar{F}_{O_2})$, where $\bar{F}_{O_2}$ is the mean O_2 concentration averaged throughout a 1-liter expiration after a 1-liter O_2 inspiration with a constant flow of 0.5 liter/sec. We have used a logarithmic scale because if we assume the acinus to be homogenously perfused, that distribution closely approaches the $\dot{V}/\dot{Q}$ distribution, which is conventionally represented on a log scale. Despite the homogeneous volume change, a twofold range of inspired gas per unit volume is found (range between 0.7 and 0.5 on the log scale), although the slope of the alveolar plateau is only 0.53% per liter. In agreement with the other MBPMs, this indicates that the slope of the alveolar plateau underestimates the concentration inhomogeneity. When Figure 23 is compared with the $\dot{V}/\dot{Q}$ distribution of a normal subject derived from the inert gas technique, it appears to be much narrower. Part of the difference is probably due to the method of computation of the $\dot{V}/\dot{Q}$ distribution, which overestimates the spread, particularly of the very narrow distributions. The remaining difference, if any, would indicate that the acinar inhomogeneity contributes little to the $\dot{V}/\dot{Q}$ distribution.

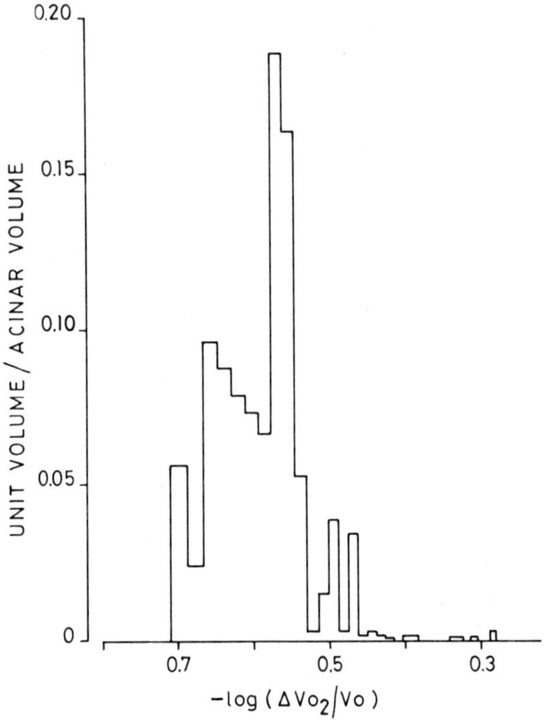

Figure 23 Intrinsic acinar inhomogeneity of the inspired O_2. $\Delta VO_2/V_0$ was computed using the formula $\Delta VO_2/V_0 = \bar{F}O_2/(1 - \bar{F}O_2)$, where $\bar{F}O_2$ is the mean O_2 concentration averaged throughout 1-liter expiration after a 1-liter O_2 inspiration with a constant flow of 0.5 liter/sec.

The previous considerations suggest that either the anatomical data used are not representative of a normal lung, or that the intra-acinar gas inhomogeneities, although substantial, constitute a small fraction of the overall impairment in gas mixing.

We finally show the simulation of an experiment consisting of a single breath with a He-SF_6 tracer mixture. The MBPM is particularly useful in this type of simulation where the diffusion fronts presenting different spreads for He and SF_6 are located at different places within the acinus. We have represented in Figure 24 a simulation corresponding to a 1-liter inspiration, a 1-liter expiration, and a flow equal to 0.5 liter/sec. The abscissa is the expired volume and the ordinate the He and SF_6 concentrations divided by their inspired concentrations. We have also represented the He/SF_6 concen-

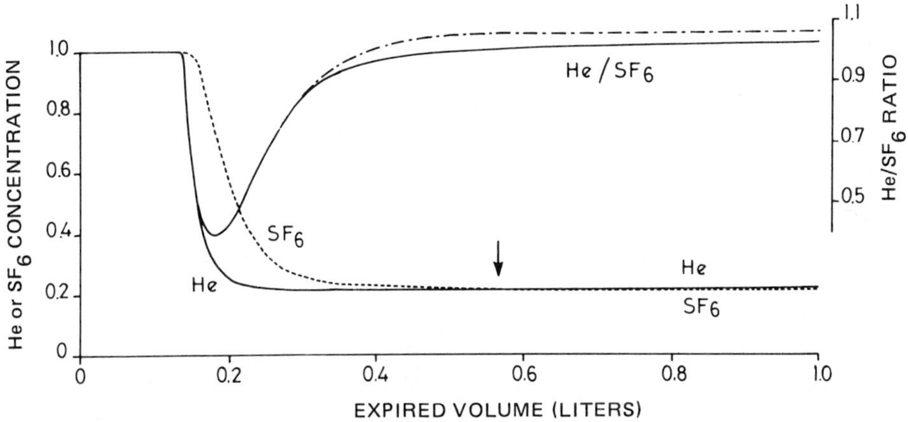

Figure 24 Simulation of an experiment consisting of a 1-liter O_2 inspiration with a He-SF_6 tracer mixture, followed by a 1-liter expiration ($\dot{V}$ = 0.5 liter/sec). The abscissa is the expired volume and the ordinate the He and SF_6 concentrations divided by their inspired concentrations. The He/SF_6 concentration ratio is represented both for the simulation using the MBPM (solid line) and the equivalent trumpet model (dotted-dashed line).

tration ratio using both the MBPM (solid line) and the equivalent trumpet model (dotted-dashed line), where the He/SF_6 slope ratio corresponding to phase III is constant. This last point was discussed in detail in Section III. The main difference between the simulation and the experiments on humans consists in simulated phases II which are much sharper than in experiments, and in phases III, the slopes being much smaller than the observed ones. The main reason for the difference in phase II is nonconsideration by the model of the different transit times due to the asymmetry of the first lung generations of the bronchial tree, as well as to the different flows from different lung regions. The reason for the discrepancy between simulated and observed slopes can be the inadequacy of the anatomical data, the existence of interacinar inhomogeneities, or the nonisotropical acinar movement. The differentiation between possibilities is the subject of work in progress.

VI. Conclusions

During the last 10 years the modeling approach to intrapulmonary gas mixing has contributed greatly to its understanding. We have tried in this chapter to give the mathematical basis necessary to understand the new concepts, such as the diffusion front and the interdependence of transport by convection and diffusion. We have subsequently shown the possible interest of those concepts in the interpretation of experimental data. Finally, we have focused on the latest developments of modeling gas mixing in the lung periphery, called the multibranch-point models. One of the interesting results of these simulations is the demonstration that within a zone as small as an acinus (0.16 ml), the range of inspired gas per unit volume is almost twofold (i.e., similar to that observed between the top and bottom of the lung in upright subjects).

The simulations using three different acinar structures have shown the dramatic need for more anatomical data. Such data, not only from humans (normal and pathological) but also from animals, would be invaluable for progress in this field. The development of computer-assisted morphometric techniques will probably soon make the anatomical data available. Some improvements on the MBPM analysis can also be attempted, such as the consideration of inert gas transport across the alveolar walls between neighboring alveoli or via collateral channels.

The direct link between the acinar structure and the inert gas expiratory concentration curves opens a new way for research: the possibility of obtaining indirect information about the acinar structure from a new analysis of single and multiple inert gas washouts. Another promising direction for future work is that of the incorporation of gas exchange into the modeling analysis. Although preliminary attempts have been made, a systematic approach to the problem is still missing. Unfortunately, knowledge of the intra-acinar perfusion distribution is very limited. Finally, all the previous considerations on intrapulmonary gas mixing assume a given mass transport law independent of the intrinsic elastic properties of the lung. Again, the physiological basis for that analysis, such as the elastic properties of sublobar lung units, is still very scarce. Probably modeling and experimental work should be carried on in parallel. We hope that this chapter will stimulate physiologists and modeling workers to continue their pursuit of a better understanding of this fascinating aspect of physiology.

Acknowledgments

A large part of this chapter's content is the direct consequence of a longstanding friendly collaboration with Ludwig Engel. I am particularly grateful for his many suggestions, which improved the manuscript considerably. I am indebted to H. K. Chang and A. De Troyer for their critical reading of the manuscript, to A. Van Muylem for the computations leading to Fig. 10, and to Mrs. D. Leemans for the preparation of the manuscript.

References

Anthonisen, N. R., Robertson, P. C., and Roos, W. R. D. (1970). Gravity-dependent sequential emptying of lung regions. *J. Appl. Physiol.,* **28**: 589-595.

Aris, R. (1956). On the dispersion of a solute in a fluid flowing through a tube. *Proc. R. Soc. Lond.,* **235A**:67-77.

Baker, L., Ultman, J., and Rhoades, R. (1975). Characterization of lung geometry from the single-breath nitrogen washout test. *Comput. Biomed. Res.,* **8**:254-266.

Bohn, D. J., Miyasaka, K., Marchak, B. E., Thompson, W. K., Froese, A. B., and Bryan, A. C. (1980). Ventilation by high frequency oscillation. *J. Appl. Physiol. Respir. Environ. Exercise Physiol.,* **48**:710-716.

Bowes, C., Cumming, G., Horsfield, K., Loughhead, J., and Preston, S. (1982). Gas mixing in a model of the pulmonary acinus with asymmetrical alveolar ducts. *J. Appl. Physiol. Respir. Environ. Exercise Physiol.,* **52**:624-633.

Buist, A. S., and Ross, B. B. (1973). Quantitative analysis of the alveolar plateau in the diagnosis of early airway obstruction. *Am. Rev. Respir. Dis.,* **108**:1078-1087.

Chang, H. K., and Farhi, L. (1980). Ternary diffusion and effective diffusion coefficients in alveolar spaces. *Respir. Physiol.,* **40**:269-279.

Chang, H. K., Cheng, R. T., and Farhi, L. (1973). A model study of gas diffusion in alveolar sacs. *Respir. Physiol.,* **18**:386-397.

Chang, H. K., Tai, R. C., and Farhi, L. (1975). Some implications of ternary diffusion in the lung. **23**:109-120.

Cox, D. R., and Miller, H. D. (1965). *The Theory of Stochastic Processes.* London, Methuen.

Davidson, M. R., and Engel, L. A. (1982). Gas transport in an asymmetrical acinus. *Bull. Eur. Physiopathol. Respir.,* **18**:203-214.

Davidson, M. R., and Fitzgerald, J. M. (1974). Transport of O_2 along a model pathway through the respiratory region of the lung. *Bull. Math. Biol.,* **36**:275-303.

De Vries, W. R., Luijendijk, S. C. M., and Zwart, A. (1981). Helium and sulfur hexafluoride washout in asymmetric lung models. *J. Appl. Physiol. Respir. Environ. Exercise Physiol.,* **51**:1122-1130.

Engel, L. A. (1983). Gas mixing within the acinus of the lung. *J. Appl. Physiol. Respir. Environ. Exercise Physiol.,* **54**:609-618.

Engel, L. A., and Paiva, M. (1981). Analyses of sequential filling and emptying of the lung. *Respir. Physiol.,* **45**:309-321.

Engel, L. A., Wood, L. D. H., Utz, G., and Macklem, P. T. (1973). Gas mixing during inspiration. *J. Appl. Physiol.,* **35**:18-24.

Engel, L. A., Utz, G., Wood, L. D. H., and Macklem, P. T. (1974). Ventilation distribution in anatomical lung units. *J. Appl. Physiol.,* **37**:194-200.

Engel, L. A., Paiva, M., Siegler, D. I. M., and Fukuchi, Y. (1979). Dual tracer single breath studies of gas transport in the lung. *Respir. Physiol.,* **36**:103-119.

Fick, A. (1855). Ueber Diffusion. *Ann. Phys. Leipzig,* **170**:59-86.

Fowler, W. S. (1949). Lung function studies: III. Uneven pulmonary ventilation in normal subjects and in patients with pulmonary disease. *J. Appl. Physiol.,* **2**:283-299.

Fukuchi, Y., Roussos, C. S., Macklem, P. T., and Engel, L. A. (1976). Convection, diffusion and cardiogenic mixing: an experimental approach. *Respir. Physiol.,* **26**:77-90.

Fukuchi, Y., Cosio, M., Murphy, B., and Engel, L. A. (1980). Intraregional basis for sequential filling and emptying of the lung. *Respir. Physiol.,* **41**:253-266.

Gómez, D. M. (1965). A physico-mathematical study of lung function in normal subjects and in patients with obstructive pulmonary diseases. *Med. Thorac.,* **22**:275-294.

Hansen, J. E., and Ampaya, E. P. (1975). Human air space shapes, sizes, areas and volumes. *J. Appl. Physiol.,* **38**:990-995.

Hogg, W., Brunton, J., Kryger, M., Brown, R., and Macklem, P. (1972). Gas diffusion across collateral channels. *J. Appl. Physiol.,* **33**:568-575.

Horsfield, K., and Cumming, G. (1968a). Morphology of the bronchial tree in man. *J. Appl. Physiol.,* **24**:373-383.

Horsfield, K., and Cumming, G. (1968b). Functional consequences of airway morphology. *J. Appl. Physiol.,* **24**:384-390.

Horsfield, K., and Cumming, G. (1976). Morphology of the bronchial tree in the dog. *Respir. Physiol.,* **26**:173-182.

Jacobs, M. H. (1935). Diffusion processes. *Ergeb. Biol.,* **12**:1-137.

Jones, H. A., Chakrabarti, M. K., Davies, E. E., Hughes, J. M. B., and Sykes, M. K. (1982). The contribution of heart beat to gas mixing in the lungs of dogs. *Respir. Physiol.,* **50**:177-185.

Kelly, S., Cohen, C., Powell, E., Paiva, M., and Engel, L. A. (1982a). Gas mixing in the lungs of dogs and pigs. *Respir. Physiol.,* **47**:341-349.

Kelly, S., Paiva, M., and Engel, L. A. (1982b). Bronchoconstriction and gas mixing in canine and pig lungs. *Bull. Eur. Physiopathol. Respir.,* **18**:229-237.

Krogh, A., and Lindhard, J. (1917). The volume of the dead space in breathing and the mixing of gases in the lungs of man. *J. Physiol. Lond.,* **51**:59-90.

Lacquet, L. M., and Van Muylem, A. (1982). He and SF_6 single-breath expiration curves. Comparison with the Paiva-Engel model. *Bul. Eur. Physiopathol. Respir.*, **18**:239-246.

Lacquet, L. M., Van der Linden, L. P., and Paiva, M. (1975). Transport of H_2 and SF_6 in the lungs. *Respir. Physiol.*, **25**:157-173.

Lieberstein, H. M. (1972). *Theory of Partial Differential Equations.* New York, Academic Press.

Luijendijk, S. C. M., Zwart, A., De Vries, W. R., and Salet, W. M. (1980). The sloping alveolar plateau at synchronous ventilation. *Pflugers Arch.*, **384**:267-277.

Martin, R. R., Zutter, M., and Anthonisen, N. R. (1972). Pulmonary gas exchange in dogs breathing SF_6 at 4 Ata. *J. Appl. Physiol.*, **33**:86-92.

McFadden, E. R., Jr. (1983). Respiratory heat and water exchange: physiological and clinical implications. *J. Appl. Physiol. Respir. Environ. Exercise Physiol.*, **54**:331-336.

Mead, J. (1961). Mechanical properties of lungs. *Physiol. Rev.*, **41**:281-330.

Michels, D. B., and West, J. B. (1978). Distribution of pulmonary ventilation and perfusion during short periods of weightlessness. *J. Appl. Physiol. Respir. Environ. Exercise Physiol.*, **45**:987-998.

Milic-Emili, J., Henderson, J. A. M., Dolovich, B. M., Trop, D., and Kaneko, K. (1966). Regional distribution of inspired gas in the lung. *J. Appl. Physiol.*, **21**:749-759.

Mon, E., and Ultman, J. S. (1976). Monte Carlo simulation of simultaneous gas flow and diffusion in an asymmetric distal pulmonary airway model. *Bull. Math. Biol.*, **38**:161-192.

Nixon, W., and Pack, A. I. (1982). Effect of gaseous interaction between lung units on the expired concentration of nitrogen. *J. Appl. Physiol. Respir. Environ. Exercise Physiol.*, **53**:496-504.

Otis, A. B., McKerrow, C. B., Bartlett, R. A., Mead, J., McIlroy, M. B., Selverstone, N. J., and Radford, E. P., Jr. (1956). Mechanical factors in distribution of pulmonary ventilation. *J. Appl. Physiol.*, **8**:427-443.

Paiva, M. (1972). Computations of the boundary conditions for diffusion in the human lung. *Comput. Biomed. Res.*, **5**:585-595.

Paiva, M. (1973). Gas transport in the human lung. *J. Appl. Physiol.*, **35**: 401-410.

Paiva, M. (1974). Gaseous diffusion in an alveolar duct simulated by a digital computer. *Comput. Biomed. Res.*, **7**:533-543.

Paiva, M. (1980). Boundary conditions and geometry in pulmonary gas transport models. *Comput. Biomed. Res.*, **13**:271-282.

Paiva, M. (1982). Model analysis of inert gas mixing in the lung. *Bull. Eur. Physiopathol. Respir.*, **18**:189-201.

Paiva, M. (1983). Diffusion and convection in a branching tube. *Comput. Biomed. Res.*, **16**:190-198.

Paiva, M., and Engel, L. A. (1979). Pulmonary interdependence of gas transport. *J. Appl. Physiol.,* **47**:296-305.

Paiva, M., and Engel, L. A. (1981). The anatomical basis for the sloping N_2 plateau. *Respir. Physiol.,* **44**:325-337.

Paiva, M., and Engel, L. A. (1982). Influence of bronchial asymmetry on cardiogenic gas mixing in the lung. *Respir. Physiol.,* **49**:325-338.

Paiva, M., and Engel, L. A. (1984). Model analysis of gas distribution within human lung acinus. *J. Appl. Physiol. Respir. Environ. Exercise Physiol.,* **56**:418-425.

Paiva, M., and Paiva-Veretennicoff, I. (1972). Stochastic simulation of the gas diffusion in the air phase of the human lung. *Bull. Math. Biophys.,* **34**:457-466.

Paiva, M., Lacquet, L. M., and Van der Linden, L. P. (1976). Gas transport in a model derived from Hansen-Ampaya anatomical data of the human lung. *J. Appl. Physiol.,* **41**:115-119.

Parker, H., Horsfield, K., and Cumming, G. (1971). Morphology of distal airways in the human lung. *J. Appl. Physiol.,* **31**:386-391.

Piiper, J. (1979). Series ventilation, diffusion in airways, and stratified inhomogeneity. *Fed. Proc.,* **38**:17-21.

Rauwerda, P. E. (1946). Unequal ventilation of different parts of the lung. Ph.D. thesis, University of Groningen, Groningen, The Netherlands.

Saltzman, H. A., Salzano, J. V., Blenkarn, G. O., and Kylstra, J. A. (1971). Effects of pressure on ventilation and gas exchange in man. *J. Appl. Physiol.,* **30**:443-449.

Scheid, P., and Piiper, J. (1980). Intrapulmonary gas mixing and stratification. In *Pulmonary Gas Exchange,* Vol. 1: *Ventilation, Blood Flow, and Diffusion.* Edited by J. B. West. New York, Academic Press, pp. 87-130.

Scherer, P. W., Shendalman, L. H., and Greene, N. M. (1972). Simultaneous diffusion and convection in single breath lung washout. *Bull. Math. Biophys.,* **34**:393-412.

Scherer, P. W., Shendalman, L. H., Greene, N. M., and Bouhuys, A. (1975). Measurement of axial diffusivities in a model of the bronchial airways. *J. Appl. Physiol.,* **38**:719-723.

Sikand, R., Cerretelli, P., and Farhi, L. E. (1966). Effects of $\dot{V}A$ and $\dot{V}A/Q$ distribution and of time on the alveolar plateau. *J. Appl. Physiol.,* **21**:1331-1337.

Slutsky, A. S. (1981). Gas mixing by cardiogenic oscillations: a theoretical, quantitative analysis. *J. Appl. Physiol.,* **51**:1287-1293.

Slutsky, A. S., Drazen, J. M., Ingram, R. H., Kamm, R. D., Shapiro, A. H., Fredberg, J. J., Loring, S. H., and Lehr, J. (1980). Effective pulmonary ventilation with small volume oscillations at high frequency. *Science,* **209**:609-611.

Stibitz, G. R. (1969). Calculating diffusion in biological systems by random walks with special reference to gaseous diffusion in the lungs. *Respir. Physiol.,* **7**:230-262.

Taylor, G. (1953). Dispersion of soluble matter in solvent flowing slowly through a tube. *Proc. R. Soc. Lond.,* **219A**:186-203.

Ultman, J. S., and Blatman, H. S. (1977). Longitudinal mixing in pulmonary airways. Analysis of inert gas dispersion in symmetric tube network models. *Respir. Physiol.,* **30**:349-367.

Ultman, J. S., Doll, B. E., Spiegel, R., and Thomas, M. W. (1978). Longitudinal mixing in pulmonary airways—normal subjects respiring at a constant flow. *J. Appl. Physiol. Respir. Environ. Exercise Physiol.,* **44**: 297-303.

Weber, J., and Bouhuys, A. (1959). Theoretical considerations on lung clearance. *Acta Physiol. Pharmacol. Neerl.,* **8**:121-136.

Weibel, E. R. (1963). *Morphometry of the Human Lung.* Heidelberg, Springer-Verlag.

Wilson, T. A., and Lin, K. (1970). Convection and diffusion in the airways and the design of the bronchial tree. In *Airway Dynamics Physiology and Pharmacology.* Edited by A. Bouhuys. Springfield, Ill., Charles C Thomas, pp. 5-19.

Wise, M. E., and Defares, J. G. (1959). A model for unequal ventilation of a common dead space and two separate dead spaces. *Bull. Math. Biophys.,* **21**:343-362.

Worth, H., and Piiper, J. (1978). Diffusion of helium, carbon monoxide and sulfur hexafluoride in gas mixtures similar to alveolar gas. *Respir. Physiol.,* **32**:155-166.

Worth, H., Nüsse, W., and Piiper, J. (1978). Determination of binary diffusion coefficients of various gas species used in respiratory physiology. *Respir. Physiol.,* **32**:15-26.

7

Intraregional Gas Mixing and Distribution

LUDWIG A. ENGEL

Westmead Hospital
Sydney, New South Wales, Australia

I. Introduction

The terms "intraregional" and "interregional" were introduced as a consequence of topographical studies of ventilation and perfusion distribution in the lung using radioactive gases. A region thus corresponded to a single detector field when up to 12 external scintillation detectors were used to map intrapulmonary distribution of radioactive markers. Since in different studies varying numbers of detectors were used or, alternatively, a gamma camera image was arbitrarily subdivided into a number of regions, no strict definition of the size of a region exists. However, assuming 12 detectors (6 on each lung) and a total lung capacity (TLC) of 6 liters, each region corresponds to 500 ml of lung at TLC. Therefore, at functional residual capacity (FRC), the average regional volume would approximate 250 ml. On the other hand, the volume of an acinus, calculated from morphometric or radiological studies, corresponds roughly to the volume of a sphere 7 mm

---

This work was supported by National Institutes of Health Grant Number HL26330.

in diameter (i.e., 0.12 ml). Thus each lung region may contain over 2000 acini! It is important, therefore, when speaking of structure or function, to recognize that the terms "intraregional" and "intra-acinar" may refer to lung units of substantially different size. In this book topographical or interregional ventilation distribution has been dealt with in Chapter 5 and the theoretical aspects of gas mixing within the acinus were described in Chapter 6. In this chapter we focus on experimental data that bear on intraregional gas mixing and ventilation distribution.

II. Historical Aspects

Mixing of inspired gas with that present in the lung began to be studied early in the nineteenth century. Humphry Davy was the first to use an inert gas (hydrogen) as a tracer to calculate his own lung volume. In 1860, Gréhant also used hydrogen to measure his resting end expiratory lung volume. He coined the term "coefficient of ventilation" referring to the ratio of fresh inspired gas to the FRC. The similarity between this coefficient and the ventilation per unit volume ($\Delta V/V_0$) makes that the starting point for the extensive studies of intrapulmonary distribution of inhaled gases carried out in recent years.

The concept of pulmonary dead space was first clearly formulated by Zuntz (1882). Loewy (1894) made plaster of paris casts of the airways of collapsed lungs and measured the anatomical dead space to be 144 ml (excluding the intralobular bronchi). In 1890, Christian Bohr introduced his equation for calculating the respiratory dead space in terms of alveolar and expired gas concentrations, and Haldane and Priestly used it to calculate dead space for carbon dioxide and oxygen. Siebeck (1911) was the first to use the Bohr equation and an inert gas (hydrogen) to measure dead space.

Krogh and Lindhard (1917) first proposed that inspired gas was not homogeneously distributed in the lung. In a classic paper they suggested that the more deeply situated spaces (alveoli) received less inspired gas than the more superficial ones (alveolar ducts). To distinguish between effects of gas exchange and alveolar gar distribution, Roelsen (1938) used an apparatus for multiple sampling of alveolar gas during the course of a single expiration to study the intrapulmonary distribution of hydrogen. He postulated that as expiration proceeds, a larger proportion of the expirate is contributed by parts of the lungs that received less of the inspired gas.

The period of study of ventilation distribution using discontinuous fractional gas analyses was brought to a conclusion by Rauwerda (1946). His work was influential for many years in discrediting the concept of inhomogeneity of gas tensions within the primary lobule. The development of rapid analyzers for respiratory and other gases from 1940 on gave rise to a multitude of physiological and clinical studies of ventilation distribution which will be discussed below.

III. Mechanisms of Gas Mixing

A. Convection or Bulk Flow

This refers to the transport of gas as a consequence of a pressure gradient and results in a change in the total amount of gas present in the lung or any part of it. Convection is the predominant mechanism of gas transport in the conducting airways during normal breathing and conventional ventilation of the lung. This subject has been discussed in detail in Chapter 3.

B. Molecular Diffusion

This is the principal mechanism of gas concentration equilization in the lung periphery and has been discussed in detail in Chapters 1 and 6.

C. Cardiogenic Mixing

The fact that heart contractions shake the lung about must have been obvious to biologists for centuries. Actual studies of this effect on gas flow date back to over 100 years ago. Flow pulses synchronous with the heart beat and differing in phase were demonstrated within airways of human subjects by West and Hugh-Jones (1961). The exact means by which the heart produces these pulses is not clear. However, the effect is likely to be due to the heart itself rather than pulsation of intrapulmonary vessels. Total obstruction of a lobar branch of the pulmonary artery does not alter the pattern of gas concentrations in an airway within that lobe (Engel et al., 1973a). Furthermore, mechanical oscillation of the heart in situ by means of a thread reproduces the gas oscillations as well as the mixing effects postmortem. In contrast, a small volume of saline in the pericardial space abolishes the oscillations without a measurable change in cardiac output (Fukuchi et al., 1977). It is likely that the asymmetric motion of the heart during each cycle creates a pressure wave which is transmitted throughout the parenchyma. If the time constant of a unit exposed to the pressure stimulus is short enough, transient volume changes will occur, resulting in flow oscillations within the airway. These transient volume changes may be reflected in the radiologically apparent movements of bronchovascular bundles (Palmieri, 1949) and of the lung parenchyma (Wei et al., 1984).

The mechanism by which flow pulses within the airways equalize gas concentration differences is also not clear. Taylor-type dispersion was among the first mechanisms suggested (Engel et al., 1973a). Slutsky (1981) proposed a quantitative theoretical model based on theories of gas transport used to explain gas exchange during high-frequency ventilation. However, other mechanisms may also play a part. Pendelluft in the presence of gas concentration inequality should enhance diffusive mixing among parallel units. Even if flow were synchronous, the movement of gas from units with different concentrations into a common airway and back again would result in mixing between the units. In the presence of airway asymmetry, flow oscillations during inspiration may result in small volumes of alveolar gas being transported from more proximally situated units to the lung periphery (Paiva and Engel, 1982). Depending on the initial gas distribution, this effect could either create or minimize concentration differences. Although cardiogenic gas mixing is important in conducting airways and reduces the size of the dead space (see below), measurable effects on alveolar gas mixing have not been demonstrated (Horsfield et al., 1982).

D. Taylor-Type Dispersion

Interaction between axial convection and lateral diffusion, and gas mixing within conducting airways, is dealt with in Chapters 3 and 4. Despite its importance in high-frequency ventilation (Chap. 4) it is likely that Taylor dispersion plays a small role in alveolar gas mixing during normal breathing or conventional ventilation. The reason is that the mechanism is significant only where gas transport by convection predominates over that due to axial diffusion (i.e., in the conducting airways). However, there the concentration differences are present only during the first part of each inspiration (i.e., during the washin of the dead space). In view of the relatively small volume of the dead space in relation to the tidal and alveolar volume, a major effect on alveolar gas concentrations would not be expected. Equally predictable is the increasing importance of such mechanisms when tidal volume becomes smaller.

IV. Potential Mechanisms of Gas Mixing Inhomogeneity

Perfect mixing between the inspired air and that present in the lung requires that the volume of fresh gas inspired into each lung unit (ΔV) bear a constant relationship to the volume of the unit (V_0). Furthermore, the volume changes should be synchronous and in phase with the overall volume change recorded at the mouth. This would result in every part of the lung having an identical specific ventilation ($\Delta V/V_0$), which would be the same as that of the whole lung.

In practice the two principal mechanisms of gas transport (convection and diffusion) do not achieve such success. The length of the conducting airways in relation to their total cross-sectional area constitutes a large diffusion resistance which prevents gas equilibration within the time of the respiratory cycle. This results in the series or Fowler dead-space concept, a volume that needs to be subtracted from the inspired volume when considering alveolar ventilation and gas exchange. In addition, the structural inhomogeneity of the alveolated part of the lung makes it unlikely that expansion is truly homogeneous even in the excised lung. In vivo, effects of lung weight and interaction between the lung and chest wall contribute further to nonhomogeneous gas distribution. Since convection and molecular diffusion constitute the principal mechanisms for gas mixing and distribution in the lung, impairment of this process may be conveniently discussed under these two headings.

A. Convection Dependent Inhomogeneity

Convection within the lung is determined by respiratory mechanics. Ignoring the effect of inertia, the volume of gas going to any lung unit (ΔV) and the flow rate ($\dot{V}$) may be related to the pressure applied (ΔP) by the equation $\Delta P = \Delta V/C + \dot{V}R$, where C is the compliance of the unit and R the resistance of its airway. This equation can be used as a framework for discussing the convective mechanisms underlying inhomogeneity of gas distribution in the lung.

Differences in Static Mechanical Properties

When volume changes are relatively slow, then, for a given pressure applied to two units (A and B),

$$\frac{\Delta V_A}{\Delta V_B} = \frac{C_A}{C_B}$$

Hence if the compliances of the two units differ, the proportions of inspired gas will be unequally distributed. If the ratios of compliance to unit volume [i.e., specific compliance (C/V_0)] are not the same, differences in alveolar gas concentration will exist between the two units.

Sequential Filling and Emptying

Because of the nonlinear pressure-volume (P-V) relationships an unequal specific compliance between two units implies a different shape for the two P-V curves. Two such curves are illustrated in Figure 1. When the volumes are normalized at total lung capacity, compartment B, which in this example is the smaller one, has the more curvilinear pressure-volume relationship. Con-

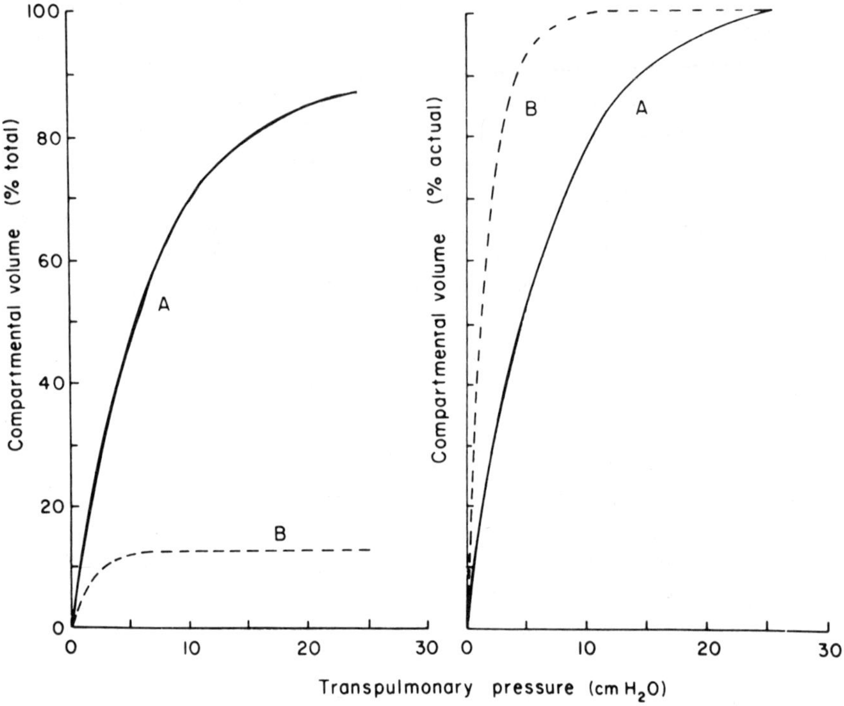

Figure 1 Pressure-volume curves of two compartments (A and B). Left: Volume expressed as percent of sum of the two compartments. Right: Volume as percent of maximum of each compartment. See the text for details. (From Fukuchi et al. 1980.)

sequently, as transpulmonary pressure is decreased during expiration, the contribution from unit B to the expirate will progressively increase relative to that from unit A. Similarly, during inspiration a reversed sequence of volume changes will take place. This sequential filling and emptying results from the unequal curvilinear pressure-volume relationships and reflects a first in-last out pattern. However, there appears to be no a priori reason for the unit with the lower specific compliance to have a more curvilinear P-V curve. The fact that experimental data in normal lungs never indicate late emptying of the better ventilated units suggests a fundamental functional characteristic of which we are totally ignorant.

Differences in Applied Pressure Swings

When volume changes are slow but the applied pressure (ΔP) to the two units differs,

$$\frac{\Delta V_A}{\Delta V_B} = \frac{\Delta P_A C_A}{\Delta P_B C_B}$$

Thus, even if the mechanical properties of the units were identical, inspired gas distribution could differ. This mechanism has been shown to influence gas distribution among topographically distributed lung zones (Chap. 5), but it is possible (although unproven) that unequal stress distribution within the lung parenchyma also influences gas distribution among acini or groups of acini.

Differences in Dynamic Mechanical Properties

As stated above, when volume changes are slow, $\Delta V_A/\Delta V_B = C_A/C_B$. When volume changes are relatively rapid (i.e., $\dot{V}$ is large, $\Delta V_A/\Delta V_B = R_B/R_A$, where R_A and R_B refer to the "personal" resistances of each unit and exclude any common resistance. Hence $\Delta V_A/\Delta V_B$ is time independent when $R_A C_A = R_B C_B$. The RC product is the mechanical time constant of the lung unit and may serve as the basis for an operational definition of "static" and "dynamic" distribution of gas flow. For practical purposes, when time is greater than 3RC, $\Delta V_A/\Delta V_B$ will be time independent even when $R_A C_A \neq R_B C_B$. This defines "static" gas distribution. When time is less than 3RC, $\Delta V_A/\Delta V_B$ will change with time (or flow or breathing frequency), resulting in asynchronous filling and emptying of the units (Otis et al., 1956). Furthermore, the sequence of filling and emptying will differ from that due to unequal static mechanical properties in that it will resemble a first in-first out pattern. Thus the time or frequency dependence of gas distribution will have both a temporal and a spatial component (unequal $\Delta V/V_0$).

Asymmetry of Conducting Airways

Because of the marked asymmetry of conducting airways in both human and canine lungs (Chap. 2), the dead-space volume is likely to be distributed preferentially to units situated in the lung periphery. Indeed, calculations made on the human lung indicate that the inspired volume required to bring fresh inspirate into lobules subtended by different airways ranges from 102 to 271 ml (Horsfield and Cumming, 1968). Thus, following a 500-ml breath of O_2, differences in alveolar N_2 concentration of about 5% could be attributed to unequal distribution of dead space alone.

Collateral Ventilation

This may be thought of as an imperfect compensation for unequal mechanical impedance to gas transport among units ventilated in parallel. Although ventilation by collateral channels is easily demonstrable, the anatomy of these pathways is not yet clear. Theoretically, if the route taken passes through the alveolated portion of the lung, the inspirate would be diluted by alveolar gas so that the collaterally ventilated units would be relatively poorly ventilated even if the inspired volume were normal. Alternatively, if collateral ventilation takes place by channels akin to small airways, the increased resistance of these may be such as to diminish the convective volume flow as discussed above (see "Differences in Dynamic Mechanical Properties"). In addition, a relatively smaller cross section of such collateral channels may constitute an increased diffusive resistance, limiting the transport of fresh gas by diffusion (see below). It is likely that collateral ventilation plays a major role only in diseased lungs.

Airway Closure

Although massive closure of airways takes place at low lung volumes (Engel et al., 1975), some airways may close even above FRC, the number increasing as lung volume and transmural pressure decrease (Forkert et al., 1979). The proportion of closed airways is not uniform in different lung regions and the P-V relationship of lung zones with different proportions of closed airways should differ. Gas trapping within a zone with a greater number of closed airways would result in a higher resting volume (V_0) and a relatively low specific ventilation. Furthermore, the sequence of airway opening and closure would be reflected in a first in-last out pattern of gas distribution. Although superficially analogous to the behavior of units with unequal static mechanical properties, this mechanism depends on a nonuniformity of critical closing pressures within airways rather than on elastic properties of the lung parenchyma. Also, it may be relatively time dependent, as collateral ventilation of obstructed units may compensate for ventilatory changes due to gas trapping (Ruff et al., 1981). It is likely that gas inhomogeneity due to airway closure is prominent in diseased lungs where airway inflammation and luminal secretions markedly enlarge the range of critical opening and closing pressures found in normal lungs.

B. Inhomogeneity Dependent on Convection-Diffusion Interaction

Intra-acinar Branching Asymmetry

Because the relative role of convective to diffusive gas transport (Peclet number) falls progressively with decrease in airway size, distribution of inspired gas among small intra-acinar units depends to a large degree on molecular diffusion. Thus although here too mechanical factors control convection, the overwhelming influence of diffusion determines alveolar gas concentrations. The normal asymmetrical structure of an acinus may result in at least a two-fold range of alveolar gas concentrations as a consequence of the interaction between convection and diffusion within the confines of acinar geometry. During the respiratory cycle this dynamic interaction results in a diffusive pendelluft, producing patterns that may be analogous to both the first in-first out and first in-last out convective sequences (Chap. 6).

Unequal Narrowing of Airways in the Lung Periphery

Because of the very large total cross-sectional area of small airways, the time constant of small lung units is very short. Thus even in the presence of marked inhomogeneity of airway diameter, the distribution of volume expansion may remain unaltered. However, because diffusive transport is proportional to the cross section available for diffusion, the diffusive flux of inspired fresh gas will be in proportion to the relative cross-sectional areas. Indeed, a diffusive interaction, similar to that due to branching asymmetry, will result in inequality of alveolar gas concentrations and an apparent sequence of filling and emptying (Chap. 6).

V. Single-Breath Inert Gas Washouts

Ever since the pioneering work of Krogh and Lindhard (1917) it has been accepted that to trace the movement of O_2 and CO_2, it is useful to follow the movement of inert gas diluents either present in the inspired breath or preexisting in the lung spaces. Concentration differences within alveolar gas and between alveolar and dead-space gas are caused by both dilution and gas exchange. An obvious advantage of the physiological gases is that measurements can be made during steady-state conditions because an inspired-to-alveolar gas concentration difference is maintained by gas exchange. In contrast, measurements of dead space and of gas mixing using inert gases apply to unsteady states only. Nevertheless, the smaller fluctuations of inert gas concentration within a breath, as well as the ability to indicate how the O_2-carrying inspired gas moves, make the inert gas tests both more convenient and more important.

A. Fowler Dead Space and Phase II

After a single breath of fresh gas, the initial part of the expiration consists of pure inspirate (phase I) followed by a relatively sharp transition to alveolar

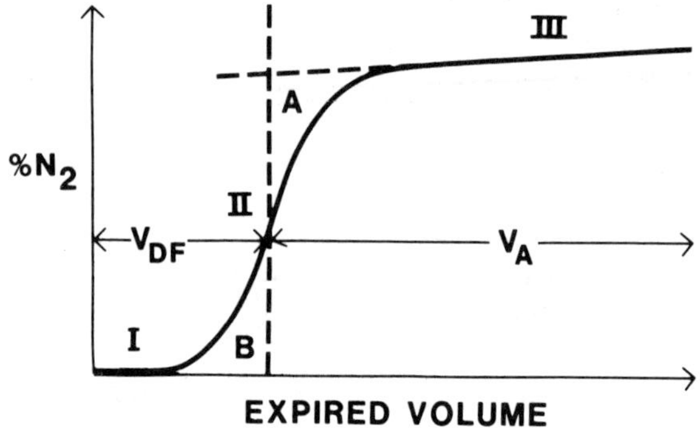

Figure 2 Plot of nitrogen concentration (% N_2) against expired volume after a breath of O_2, showing phases I, II, and III of washout curve. Vertical dashed line divides phase II into equal areas A and B and expired volume into the Fowler dead Space (VDF) and an alveolar volume (VA).

gas which then occupies the rest of expiration. Fowler (1948) utilized the single-breath N_2 washout after an inspiration of O_2 to solve graphically Bohr's equation for the calculation of dead-space volume (Fig. 2). According to Fowler the dead space corresponded to "the volume of the conducting airways down to the location at which a large change in gas composition occurs." On expiration, this large concentration change corresponds to phase II of the N_2 washout. As originally envisaged, the sigmoid curve is a consequence of axial mixing between the inspired gas within the conducting airways and the alveolar gas in the lung periphery. In its simplest form the Fowler dead-space model assumes synchronous emptying from all parallel pathways which are symmetrical, so that the arrival of the "large change in gas composition" at the mouth sweeps out the volume exactly equivalent to that of the conducting airways.

More recent analyses of simultaneous convection and diffusion within the airways have confirmed the general validity of the model described above. To a first approximation in normal lungs, phase II probably does reflect the diffusion front between inspired and alveolar gas within the lung periphery. However, the position of this front at end inspiration depends on the dynamic equilibrium between convection of the inspirate toward the periphery and the mixing of alveolar gas with that in the conducting airways (Chap. 6). Since the inspiratory flow sweeps the diffusion front peripherally, one would expect a positive relationship between dead space and inspiratory flow. However, any breathhold at end inspiration would rapidly conceal such a relationship, due to the mouthward displacement of the diffusion front caused by

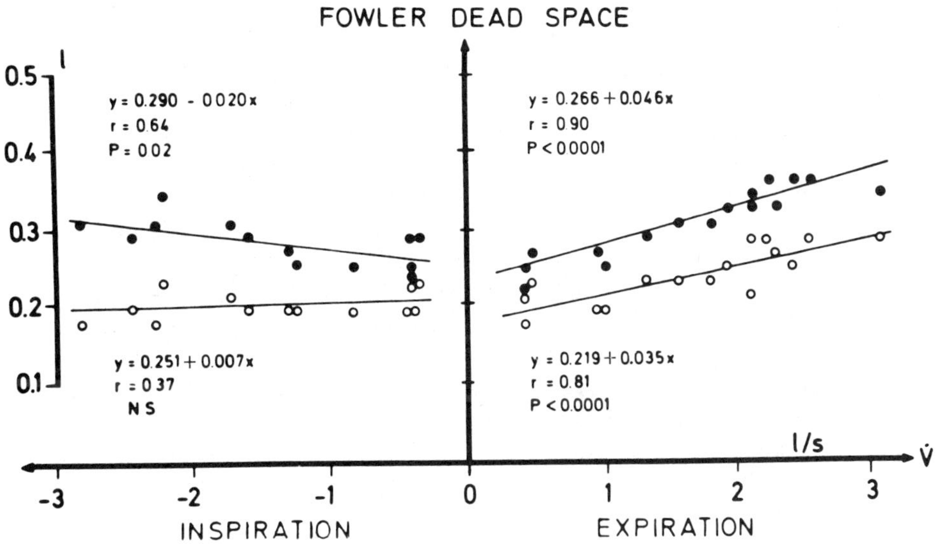

Figure 3 Relationship between Fowler dead space and inspiratory flow rate at an expiratory flow of 1 liter/sec (left); relationship between Fowler dead space and expiratory flow rate at an inspiratory flow of 1 liter/sec (right). Closed circles: SF_6; open circles: helium. Note the steeper positive slope for expiratory flow. (From Lacquet and Van Muylem, 1982.)

the flux of alveolar gas across the relatively large cross-sectional area of the airways. Similarly, a slow expiratory flow rate would allow substantial gas mixing to occur during the first part of expiration, reducing the size of the dead space measured at the mouth. Indeed, when expiratory flow is kept constant at 1 liter/sec, a small positive relationship between dead space and inspiratory flow (Fig. 3) is measurable at the mouth (Lacquet and Van Muylem, 1982). Comparison of dead space measured in the trachea and small airways of anaesthetized dogs showed that increases in inspiratory flow increased dead space at both sites but the relative changes in the lung periphery were much greater (Engel et al., 1973b). This was consistent with a peripheral displacement of the diffusion front, so that the additional dead-space volume was entirely located distal to the small airways.

Similarly, when inspiratory flow is maintained at 1 liter/sec, a positive relationship exists between expiratory flow and the Fowler dead space (Lacquet and Van Muylem, 1982). The slope of this relationship is steeper than that for inspiratory flow (Fig. 3), but the slope probably depends in part on the selected magnitude of the inspiratory flow. Predictably, when breathing frequency is increased at a constant tidal volume, dead space increases (Roos et al., 1954). When flow rates are increased even further by concomitant increases in tidal volume, the large increases in physiological dead space in normal subjects (Lifshay et al., 1971) are probably also due in part to the peripheral displacement of the diffusion front. In contrast to these findings, Bashoff et al. (1967) observed consistent reduction of dead space during forced expirations. The most likely explanation for this paradoxical finding is that during the very high flow rates used (4.6-7.2 liters/sec), a large change in the interregional pattern of emptying took place, so that phase II appeared earlier. Indeed, studies with radioactive gases demonstrate a much greater emptying of upper lung regions early during a rapid expiration (Millette et al., 1969).

During breath holding at end inspiration, the volume of the dead space decreases rapidly at first and then more slowly (Fowler, 1948). This is a direct consequence of gas mixing and the decrease in cross-sectional area of the airways between the lung periphery and the trachea. These dead-space changes can readily be visualized by model simulation of simultaneous convection and diffusion (Chap. 6).

The mechanism responsible for reduction of dead space during breath holding is of interest. Horsfield and Cumming (1968) inferred from Fowler's data (1948) that alveolar N_2 must advance up to the main bronchi during 30 sec of breath holding and concluded that the linear distance (8 cm) is too great to explain in terms of simple gaseous diffusion. Indeed, direct measurement of gases sampled from small airways shows conclusively that cardiogenic mixing contributes significantly to the reduction of dead space during breath holding (Fig. 4). Measurements made after stopping the heart show a systematically greater dead space and correspondingly lower N_2 concentrations within small airways during end inspiratory breath holds (Engel et al., 1973a). The more rapid gas mixing seen in vivo may be reproduced postmortem by artificial mechanical oscillation of the heart simulating the mechanism of cardiac churning. The studies utilizing intrapulmonary gas sampling clearly demonstrate that the reduction of Fowler dead space during breath-holding is a relatively crude measure of the rate of gas mixing within the airways. Despite a three- to eightfold decrease in the time for N_2 to reach 50% of the alveolar value within small airways, only one-fourth of the reduction in dead space recorded in the trachea could be attributed to the cardiogenic component of gas mixing.

Although in the presence of a constant inspiratory flow an increase in lung volume displaces the diffusion front mouthward (Engel et al., 1973b), the measured dead space increases by 2 to 3 ml per 100-ml increase in end-inspiratory lung volume (Fowler, 1948; Birath, 1959). This is almost certainly due to the dilatation of the major airways at higher lung volumes.

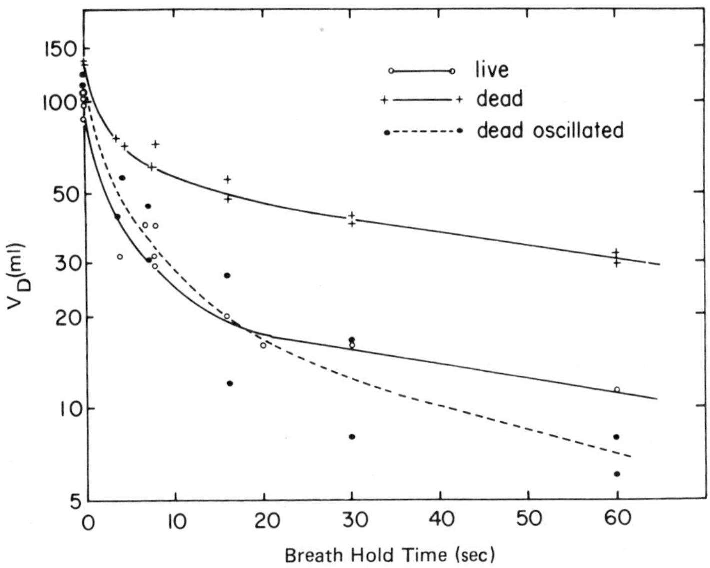

Figure 4 Fowler dead space (VD) as a function of breath hold time in one dog in vivo, postmortem, and during manual oscillation of the heart after death. Rate of decrease in VD in vivo may be equaled postmortem by manual oscillation of the heart. (From Engel et al., 1973a.)

Theoretically, gas diffusivity should also influence the position of the diffusion front (Chap. 6). Indeed, experimental studies have invariably shown a larger dead space for a dense gas (e.g., SF_6) than for a light gas (e.g., H_2 or He) (Fig. 3) (Power 1969; Lacquet et al., 1975).

In a symmetrical, homogeneously ventilated lung the shape of phase II would merely reflect diffusive mixing between the dead space and alveolar gas. In an asymmetrical, homogeneously ventilated lung phase II would incorporate the transit-time distribution due to bronchial asymmetry (Horsfield and Cumming, 1968). However, in the presence of unequally ventilated parallel units, phase II must also reflect the differences in flows from the different units (Paiva, 1973). Figure 5 illustrates such an experimental result. The normalized slope of phase II, measured between 25 and 75% of the value at which phase II becomes phase III, has been plotted as a function of breath number during a multiple-breath N_2 washout with tidal volumes of 1 liter. The gradual flattening of the slope illustrates the contribution of parallel unequally ventilated units to this part of the washout curve.

In disease states not only is the inequality of compartmental gas con-

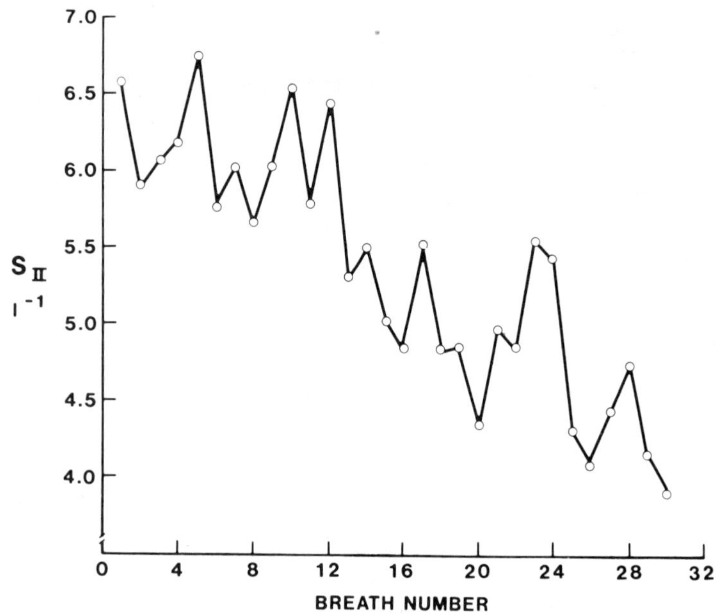

Figure 5 Normalized slope of the midportion of phase II of a N_2 washout (S_{II}) for consecutive 1-liter breaths of a multiple-breath N_2 washout. Progressive flattening is consistent with unequal ventilation of parallel units. (After Crawford et al., 1985.)

centrations greater, but the emptying may become markedly sequential. Both these factors would be expected to spread out phase II over a larger expired volume range. Indeed, measurements of phase II in patients with chronic airflow obstruction show a consistently greater volume of the expirate occupied by phase II (Worth and Smidt, 1982). For the same reason, the transition between phase II and phase III becomes less distinguishable. Under these circumstances calculation of dead space using the Fowler technique becomes not only technically difficult but physiologically questionable.

B. Alveolar Gas Inhomogeneity

After a single inspiration of O_2 the N_2 concentration in the expired gas (FE_{N_2}) increases rapidly as dead space gas is cleared, reaching a plateau (phase III) which in normal subjects slopes gently upward (Fig. 2). The gas expired after the first 750 ml has been generally accepted to represent gas coming from the alveolated portion of the lung. The fact that the alveolar plateau is not horizontal but slopes upward indicates that alveolar gas is not uniformly distributed. The magnitude of the slope has been widely used as a measure of the nonuniformity of gas distribution in the lung. However, a sloping plateau requires not only that concentration differences be present, but also that the units empty to some degree sequentially. Therefore, changes in the slope cannot discriminate between different degrees of sequential emptying and different degrees of alveolar gas concentration inequality. Furthermore, since over any volume range most units contribute to the expirate, the change in FE_{N_2} during an expiration must underestimate the differences that exist among the units.

Following the initial description (Fowler, 1949) the measurement of the slope of the alveolar plateau was standardized by Comroe and Fowler (1951). In this test the subject inspired a vital capacity (VC) breath of O_2 from RV and expired fully to RV. The rise in FE_{N_2} between an expired volume of 750 and 1250 ml (ΔN_2) was taken as an expression of alveolar gas inhomogeneity. Although no attempt was made to control flow rates, differences between age groups were observed (Greifenstein et al., 1952) and ΔN_2 was obviously greater in a variety of pulmonary diseases. The test also differentiated between a group of subjects who smoked cigarettes and those who either did not smoke or smoked a pipe or cigars only (Olsen and Gilson, 1960). After modification of the test by Kjellmer et al. (1959) wherein the subject inhaled 1 liter of O_2 from FRC and then expired to RV, the single-breath N_2 test was widely used in clinical studies. It was found satisfactory in terms of reproducibility and capacity to differentiate between smokers and nonsmokers (Stanescu et al., 1968a).

The estimate of alveolar gas inhomogeneity from ΔN_2 assumed complete washout of the dead space. Indeed, Fowler (1949) had found that during quiet breathing the expired volume required to wash out the dead space did not exceed 500 ml and chose 750 ml because it represented "approximately the mean normal washout volume plus 2 standard deviations." However, breaths performed at constant inspiratory and expiratory flow rates without any end-inspiratory breath holds frequently demonstrate a steeper slope at the 750-ml expired volume point than later in expiration (Cumming et al., 1967). More important, physiological variables (e.g., preinspiratory lung volume, flow, and inspired volume) may have inconsistent effects on ΔN_2 due to varying contributions from phase II and phase III. This effect may be particularly marked at high lung volumes (when dead space is greatest), in patients with airflow obstruction, and/or when inert gas tracers with low diffusivity are used.

Anthonisen et al. (1969-1970), using the VC maneuver proposed by Comroe and Fowler (1951), quantified the slope of the linear portion of the alveolar plateau. In addition to overcoming the technical objections described above, the test made it possible for several other measurements to be made simultaneously (Buist and Ross, 1973). Subsequent investigators, using smaller inspired volumes (from FRC), also favored a measurement of the linear portion of the alveolar plateau obtained during expiration to RV. Factors influencing these tests and the information obtained from them are presented in the following two sections.

C. "Tidal" Single-Breath Tests

Although the slope of the alveolar plateau has been used as an index of ventilation inhomogeneity for many years (Fowler, 1949; Kjellmer et al., 1959), the physiological variables involved in the performance of the test and their effects on the slope and other features of the single-breath washout have not been clarified. The proposed volume of inspired O_2 was initially 1 liter (Fowler, 1949) and higher inspired volumes were reported to decrease the slope (Fowler, 1949) or increase it (Kjellmer et al., 1959). Recently, Meyer et al. (1983) were unable to demonstrate any significant change in the slope of He or SF_6 alveolar plateaus when tidal volume was doubled in dogs. Similarly, Makowska, Crawford, and Engel (unpublished observations) saw no change in slope when inspired volume was varied between 1 and 2 liters in normal subjects. However, a significant decrease has been demonstrated after an inspiratory capacity of O_2 (Paiva et al., 1984). In contrast, most investigators agree on the influence of preinspiratory lung volume when a constant volume of tracer is inhaled. As the preinspiratory lung volume increases, the slope decreases (Fowler, 1949; Cumming et al., 1967), whereas at starting volumes below FRC the slopes are steeper (Jones, 1967). However, a reversed relationship between lung volume and alveolar slope has also been reported (Mills and Harris, 1965; Kjellmer et al., 1959), although this was probably due to measurement artefact (see above).

During the performance of a single-breath test flow rates are generally kept low and constant. However, the influence of flow is not without conflicting observations. Increasing inspiratory flow has been shown to steepen the N_2 slope (Kjellmer et al., 1959) as well as the SF_6 slope (Lacquet and Van Muylem, 1982), but a recent study in dogs showed a definite inverse relationship between inspiratory flow and slope for both He and SF_6 (Meyer et al., 1983). Similarly, although earlier studies failed to show any influence of expiratory flow on the slope of the N_2 plateau (Kjellmer et al., 1959; Mills and Harris, 1965), Meyer et al. (1983) showed an inverse relationship between expiratory flow and the slope of He and SF_6 plateaus in dogs. In contrast, a definite positive relationship for both gases was observed by Lacquet and Van Muylem (1982) in humans.

All investigators have observed that the slope of the alveolar plateau flattens if a breath hold is interposed between inspiration and expiration. However, the magnitude of this effect and the relationship to breath-hold duration is not clear. Fowler noted that the effect of breath holding is greatest for the first second and progressively diminishes thereafter. Kjellmer et al. (1959) noted a decrease after the first 3 sec of breath holding, with little further effect after longer periods. In contrast, the recent studies of Meyer et al. (1984) in dogs showed a relatively small effect of breath holding, and more surprisingly, a relatively constant rate of change over a period of 10 sec. The magnitude of this change averaged less than 2% of the initial slope per second. A possible explanation for this observation may be the relatively low expiratory flow rates used. The lower the flow, the more the first part of the expiration is analogous to an end inspiratory breath hold. Makowska, Crawford, and Engel (unpublished observations) observed a 7-10% per second change in He and SF_6 slopes during a 5-sec breath hold in humans, and the rate of change in slope with breath-hold time was such that a single exponential was not adequate to account for the curvilinearity. These different observations could not be due to species differences because measurements of slope changes in the trachea of anesthetized dogs have previously been shown to be exponential in time course, falling from 7.5% of the initial slope during the first 2 sec to 2.5% per second between 4 and 10 sec of breath holding (Engel et al., 1974). Of interest is the fact that simultaneous measurements within a peripheral airway, 3.2 mm in diameter, showed a slightly lower initial slope which decreased by 12.3% per second during the first 2 sec and by 3.3% of the initial slope per second between 4 and 10 sec of breath holding. The relatively greater initial rate of decrease presumably reflects the greater diffusion dependence of the slope emanating from small peripheral lung units.

D. Vital Capacity Single-Breath N_2 Test

The test originally proposed by Comroe and Fowler (1951) was modified by Anthonisen et al. (1969-1970) and became more generally accepted clinically as well as being used as a tool in epidemiological studies. The subject inhales a vital capacity (VC) of O_2 followed by full exhalation to RV; both inspiratory and expiratory flows are maintained approximately constant and less than 0.5 liter/sec, and the measurement of the slope is made over the linear portion of the alveolar plateau. As mentioned previously, an important technical advantage of this test is the clear distinction between phase II and phase III, as the FE_{N_2} within the first liter of expired volume may be "contaminated" by the "shoulder" of the curve, making the computed value of the slope very sensitive to several physiological variables. This is particularly true near TLC, where anatomic dead space is greatest. Another potential advantage of this test is that in contrast to a fixed inspired volume of 1 liter, the VC inspiration effectively normalizes the test for differences in lung volume. One of the chief interests, when first introduced, was the measurement of phase IV, which indicates the lung volume at which a marked increase in airways closure of dependent lung regions takes place. In addition, absolute lung volume can be estimated from the total amount of N_2 expired following the inspiration of a known volume of O_2 using dilution principles. This allows the calculation of closing capacity when equipment for measuring lung volumes may not be available. The potential for obtaining a measurement of closing volume or closing capacity as well as the slope of phase III makes the VC single-breath test particularly useful both in epidemiological and clinical studies.

Although subjects may be discouraged from breath holding at end inspiration, it is difficult to ensure a sharp transition from inspiration to expiration at TLC. Since at that lung volume all dimensions are at their maximum, equilibration of gas concentration differences within the lung periphery is likely to be greater than at lower lung volumes, where airway cross sections are smaller and end-inspiratory breath holds may be more successfully minimized. Not surprisingly, therefore, the range of normal values for the phase III slope measured in the VC test is substantially lower (Buist and Ross, 1973) than in maneuvers with smaller inspired volumes. This is associated with better reproducibility and a slope which is less influenced by minor physiological variables. Furthermore, if the increased slope in disease is due to structural abnormalities and differences in mechanical properties, the detection of these may be enhanced by the possible homogenization of intra-acinar concentration differences at TLC.

Factors Influencing the Slope of the Alveolar Plateau

Physiological

Breath holding at end inspiration diminishes the slope of phase III, presumably due to equilibration of gas concentrations among units ventilated in parallel both within and between acini. Increasing expiratory flow systematically flattens the slope (Baschoff et al., 1967). This effect must be due to a different mechanism than breath holding, as the effective time for mixing is decreased. A possible explanation is a reduction of the gravity-dependent sequential emptying of vertically distributed lung regions which empty synchronously during rapid expiration (Millette et al., 1969) in contrast to their sequential emptying at slow flow rates (Anthonisen et al., 1970). A corollary of this reasoning is that during a slow expiration the vertically distributed inhomogeneity in gas concentrations, which itself is due to the inequality of regional RV/TLC ratios, contributes significantly to the slope of the N_2 phase III. Evidence supporting this hypothesis is conflicting. Reversals of posture during brief breath holds at end inspiration measurably decrease the slope of N_2 phase III (Anthonisen et al., 1970). However, the effect is very much smaller than that on ^{133}Xe slopes, which, following inhalation of a bolus at RV, reflect predominantly interregional differences. Cortese et al. (1976) failed to see any significant differences between the slope of phase III measured in the standard manner and that obtained after tilting normal subjects from the standing to the supine, lateral, or prone postures at end inspiration. They concluded that the slope of phase III appears to depend more on the emptying pattern of small regions with widely varying volume-to-ventilation ratios than on gravity-dependent sequences of emptying. Nevertheless, they found that the slope was higher when subjects were in the supine and lateral positions than when in the upright posture.

Convincing evidence against an important interregional contribution to the slope in the upright posture was provided by the elegant experiments of Michels and West (1978), who performed single-breath tests in a Lear Jet whose flight path allowed them to simulate 0, 1, or 2*g* gravity fields. From washouts of argon boluses inhaled at RV the authors concluded that virtually all the topographical inequality of ventilation is abolished during short periods of 0*g*. However, the slope of the N_2 plateau did not differ between maneuvers performed at 0, 1, or 2*g*, or when inspiration and expiration were each performed in different gravity fields. The average breath-hold period of 6.5 sec interposed between inspiration and expiration in these studies should have favored any interregional contribution, as concentration differences among small units could have partly equilibrated. The fact that no slope differences were observed under the different conditions constitutes strong evidence that non-gravity-dependent intraregional inhomogeneity is the major determinant of the VC single-breath N_2 slope of phase III.

An alternative explanation for the flow-dependent flattening of the alveolar slope is a shift from compliance determined to resistance determined emptying of units within lung regions. Provided that the resistances and compliances of units are not inversely related, an increased influence of resistance should diminish sequential emptying and therefore the alveolar slope.

Because the R value decreases progressively during expiration (Kim et al., 1966), the N_2 in the alveolar gas is progressively concentrated. Thus, merely as a consequence of continuing gas exchange, a rising slope of the N_2 alveolar plateau is predictable. Recently, Cormier and associates investigated this phenomenon extensively and determined that gas exchange was responsible for 10% of the slope of phase III (Cormier and Belanger, 1983). It is pertinent that in tests using inspired inert gas tracers, with resulting negative slopes, gas exchange will flatten the slope by the same proportion. Therefore, when this effect is ignored, slope differences of 20% may be obtained between N_2 and inhaled inert gases even when there is no difference in gas distribution.

Pathological Factors

The VC single-breath N_2 test has attracted much attention because of its potential for identifying early lung abnormality in the development of chronic airflow obstruction. For this reason, numerous investigators compared the slope in normal nonsmoking subjects with that in healthy cigarette smokers. In all cases, the mean value in cigarette smokers was higher than in nonsmokers and a varying proportion of cigarette smokers had abnormal values (Buist and Ross, 1973). Similarly, some patients with asymptomatic bronchial asthma have increased slopes, but the degree of airflow obstruction is not well correlated with the slope of phase III (Siegler et al., 1976; Stanescu et al., 1968b).

Several studies attempted to define the anatomical and/or pathological abnormality related to an abnormal slope of phase III in cigarette smokers. Cosio et al. (1977) were the first to demonstrate a steeper slope in patients with minor airway pathology in surgically removed lobes compared to a group with relatively normal airways. The authors considered inflammation of airways to be the most important variable. However, a subsequent similar study did not show any correlation between the slope of phase III and the degree of bronchial narrowing among a group of cigarette smokers (Berend et al., 1979). Studies of excised human lungs do show a correlation with mural inflammation and with an increase in musculature of nonalveolated small airways (Petty et al., 1980). There is also a negative correlation with mean peripheral airways diameter (Salmon et al., 1982).

Although inequality of airway narrowing in the lung periphery may be the basis for a steep slope of phase III in disease, in normal lungs inhomogeneity of static mechanical properties may constitute the principal mechanism responsible for the slope of the N_2 phase III after a VC breath of O_2. An interesting observation has recently been reported by Berend and Grunstein (1983), who noted that the slope of phase III, in relatively normal excised human lungs, correlated positively with lung distensibility, or the exponent (K) derived from a monoexponential fitting of the deflation pressure volume curve. In emphysematous lungs there was no correlation. The authors suggested that in normal lungs an increased K represents a greater dispersal of static mechanical properties, which in turn accounts for the steeper slope.

E. Bolus Studies

Inhalation of a small volume of a foreign gas allows one to trace the distribution of gas inhaled at a particular lung volume or time interval during inspiration. Studies utilizing a bolus of radioactive gas have been extremely fruitful in clarifying the topographical or interregional distribution of inspired gas as a function of lung volume, flow rate, or body posture (Chap. 5). Because of the vertical gradient of closed airways at RV a bolus of tracer gas inhaled from RV results in a large vertical concentration gradient, so that, on expiration, the slope of the alveolar plateau reflects predominantly sequential emptying of topographically distributed lung regions (Engel and Macklem, 1977). The gravity determined basis of this slope is demonstrable in studies in which posture is reversed at end inspiration prior to expiration, when almost a mirror-image reversal of the slope is obtained (Anthonisen et al., 1970). Studies during brief periods of zero gravity have shown complete flattening of slopes following inhalation of an argon bolus at RV (Michels and West, 1978).

When a bolus of tracer gas is inhaled at a lung volume above closing volume, the vertical concentration gradient is much reduced. In the original studies by Dollfus et al. (1967) vertical distribution was thought to remain unchanged when the ^{133}Xe bolus was inhaled at lung volumes between 26 and 90% of VC. In this volume range distribution was noted to be preferentially to lung bases with a vertical gradient of approximately 2:1. Later, Anthonisen et al. (1978) showed a progressive change in the vertical distribution of an inhaled bolus at lung volumes above closing volume and demonstrated a relationship between the vertical concentration gradient and the slope of the alveolar plateau obtained at the mouth.

These studies indicated the presence of sequential filling and emptying of topographically distributed regions at lung volumes above closing volume, but they did not exclude the presence of sequential volume changes within regions. To examine these, Fukuchi et al. (1980) studied single-breath washouts after inhalation of a bolus of He in seated human subjects, prone dogs with the chest intact or widely open, and within single lobes of open-chested dogs. Boluses inhaled at 20, 40, 60, and 80% of VC, followed by air up to TLC, produced, on expiration, a range of slopes that was similar in the human subjects, in the dogs, and within a single lobe. Because the pattern of emptying must have been constant for each maneuver, the fan of curves (Fig. 6) reflects the degree of sequential filling. The results convincingly showed that the pattern of sequential filling and emptying demonstrable in seated human subjects could have an entirely intralobar or intraregional basis. Assuming a convective sequence as a possible mechanism for the findings, the authors studied a two-compartment model comprising two units with different monoexponential P-V relationships (Fig. 1) and found, by optimization techniques, the combination of exponents and compartmental volumes that would reproduce both the set of lobar washouts and the lobar P-V curves. The results suggested that the experimental findings could be

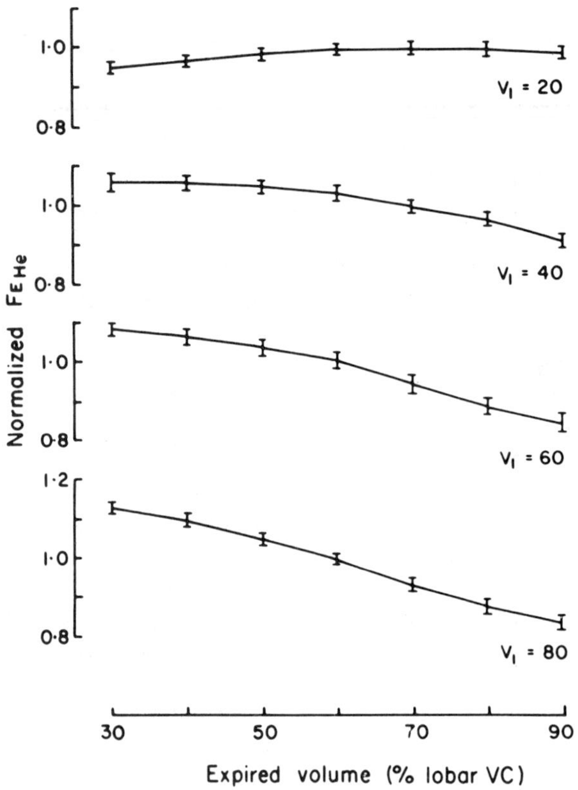

Figure 6 Normalized alveolar plateaus from single-breath helium washouts within single lobes of open-chested dogs. Inhalation of helium bolus at different percentage of lobar vital capacity (VI = 20, 40, 60, 80) produces a range of slopes. See the text for details. (From Fukuchi et al., 1980.)

explained if only 12% of the lobe had mechanical properties which differed sufficiently from the remainder.

Although experimental evidence suggests that sequential filling and emptying of both topographically distributed regions and relatively small intraregional units may contribute to the slope of the alveolar plateau, model analyses of simultaneous convection and diffusion within the lung acinus show yet another mechanism which must be present (Luijendijk et al., 1980; Engel and Paiva, 1981) (Chap. 6). It is likely that all three mechanisms contribute to the slope of the alveolar plateau and that the relative contributions may vary depending on the specific details of the breath studied.

F. Multiple Tracer Studies

Since the work of Georg et al. (1965), numerous investigators have utilized two or more inert gases with different diffusivities to study the diffusion dependence of gas mixing within the lung. The consistent observation that Fowler dead space for He is less than that for a less diffusible gas (e.g., SF_6) is predictable on the basis of analyses of simultaneous convection and diffusion even within a symmetrical lung model (Chap. 6).

All studies in human subjects and most animal studies have shown that the slope of the alveolar plateau is steeper for a less diffusible gas (e.g., SF_6) than for a lighter gas (e.g., He). Although initially the different slopes were interpreted as evidence in favor of longitudinal or series concentration gradients within acini (Georg et al., 1965; Cumming et al., 1967), recent model analyses make it clear that the results could be produced equally well by diffusion-dependent inhomogeneity among parallel units (Chap. 6).

A notable exception to the results noted above is the study of Meyer et al. (1983), in which very similar slopes for both gases were obtained in dogs. Under some experimental conditions (e.g., changes in flow rate and inspired volume) significant differences were observed, but these were not systematic in relation to the variables studied. The authors concluded that the relative magnitude of the slopes of the two gases depends on the experimental conditions alone. It is difficult to explain these anomalous findings. One possible explanation is the relatively long time scale of the single-breath maneuvers. Slopes were measured between 60 and 95% of the expired volume, which in the standard maneuver was equivalent to a time interval of 8-13 sec. It is possible that diffusion equalized concentration differences among small units, so that the slopes reflected predominantly sequential emptying of larger, unequally ventilated, and relatively diffusion independent lung units. The remarkably small effects of breath holding on the slopes of either He or SF_6 alveolar plateaus (see Sec. V.C) would be consistent with this explanation. Indeed, a similar explanation was suggested by De Vries and Luijendijk (1982) to account for the similar slopes of He, argon, and SF_6 during a maneuver in which expiration was very slow. Simulation of intra-acinar inhomogeneity under these experimental conditions predicts a horizontal or flat alveolar plateau.

Recent model analyses, incorporating the effect of intra-acinar branching asymmetry, have contributed greatly to the understanding of diffusion dependent inhomogeneity of gas concentrations. Pathways of different length and capacitance (subtended volume) offer substantially different resistances to diffusion. Consequently, relatively large concentration differences may exist between small lung units separated by relatively short distances (Chap. 6). Similarly, unequal airway narrowing in small airways, where convective velocities are so low that flow-resistive pressure drops are negligible, may be responsible for substantial gas concentration inhomogeneity because of differences in their diffusive resistances. Experimental findings tend to support these predictions. In pigs, unlike in dogs, the slope of the alveolar plateau was found to be the same for He and SF_6 despite being steeper (Kelly et al., 1982a). This diffusion-independent ventilation inhomogeneity was thought to reflect a relatively symmetrical porcine acinus. However, on inhalation of a methacholine aerosol the slopes of both gases became steeper, that for He exceeding that for SF_6 (Kelly et al., 1982b). It is possible that the bronchoconstrictor produced unequal airway narrowing extending into the acinus, thus introducing a basis for diffusion-dependent inhomogeneity of gas distribution. The relatively steeper He slope could be due to the more proximal position of the He diffusion front, where the effect of the bronchoconstrictor may have been relatively greater.

Studies of patients with pulmonary emphysema show greater separation of He and SF_6 than found in normal subjects (Georg et al., 1965). This was thought to be due to larger concentration gradients within the abnormally dilated air spaces. However, Siegler, Fukuchi, and Engel (unpublished) observed greater separation between He and SF_6 in cigarette smokers with relatively normal pulmonary function tests. Since advanced emphysema was unlikely in these patients, the greater separation between the two tracer gases could not be interpreted in terms of dilated air spaces. Because of diffusion-convection interaction, unequal airway narrowing in the lung periphery could enhance the difference between alveolar plateau slopes for the two gases (Kelly et al., 1982b).

If the slope of the alveolar plateau were due mainly to diffusion-dependent mechanisms, breath holding should flatten the He slope more than the SF_6 slope. This is what happens in normal lungs. Convective mechanisms may steepen the alveolar plateau for both gases. If differences in static mechanical properties are responsible, breath holding may still be expected to flatten the He slope more than the SF_6 slope. However, if differences in dynamic mechanical properties are involved (see Sec. IV.A) breath holding at end inspiration will allow convective pendelluft to equilibrate pressure differences, reducing gas concentration inhomogeneity to the same extent for both gases. Indeed, Magnussen and Smidt (1981) measured very similar large reductions in He and SF_6 slopes during breath holding in patients with chronic obstructive lung disease. Although both slopes were steeper and differed more than in healthy subjects, there was little change in the difference between the two slopes as a function of breath-hold time. The authors concluded that in such patients a relatively large separation of the tracer gases occurs during the passage of the inspirate through a lung of altered geometry. A high diffusive resistance in the lung periphery slows diffusive mixing at end inspiration, resulting in the persistent difference between the slopes of the two gases.

VI. Multiple-Breath Inert Gas Washout

Single-breath studies give a comprehensive picture of gas mixing only in a lung that is perfectly homogeneous. In such a lung, alveolar gas has a uniform composition, determined by the volume of the inspirate ($V_T - V_D$) in relation to the FRC. A second breath of inspirate results in an identical washout with the alveolar gas composition reduced by the same proportion. When the inspired gas is unevenly distributed within the lung, resulting in an inequality of alveolar gas concentrations (F_A), the expirate of the first breath is weighted by the better ventilated units. The second and subsequent breaths reflect to a progressively lesser degree the better ventilated units and progressively more the poorly ventilated units of the lung. The greater the inhomogeneity of gas distribution, the greater the number of breaths required to obtain an overall description of the inhomogeneity of gas distribution within the lung.

Although any inert gas may be used after equilibration within the lung, the most common method of study consists of the washout of resident N_2 by breathing pure O_2. The principle of the method, established by Cournand et al. (1941), is based on a lung model with cyclic ventilation such that

$$F_{A_n} = F_{A_0} x \omega^n \tag{1}$$

where F_{A_0} and F_{A_n} are fractional concentrations of N_2 at time zero and after n inspirations of O_2. At each breath F_A is decreased by a factor ω, which is the alveolar dilution factor equivalent to $V_0/(V_0 + V_T - V_D)$ (Darling et al., 1944), where V_0 is the end-expiratory volume. Equation (1) may be written in the logarithmic form

$$\log F_{A_n} = F_{A_0} + n \log \omega \tag{2}$$

Since $\log F_{A_0}$ and $\log \omega$ are constants, $\log F_{A_n}$ should be a linear function of n; that is, a plot of $\log F_{A_n}$ against breath number should constitute a straight line (Fig. 7A). Because of the difficulty of identifying the true alveolar gas concentration, it is preferable to use mean expired concentration for each breath ($\bar{F}_E$). By rearrangement from the Bohr equation ($V_T = V_D + V_A$),

$$\bar{F}_{E_n} = F_{A_n} \frac{V_T - V_D}{V_T} \tag{3}$$

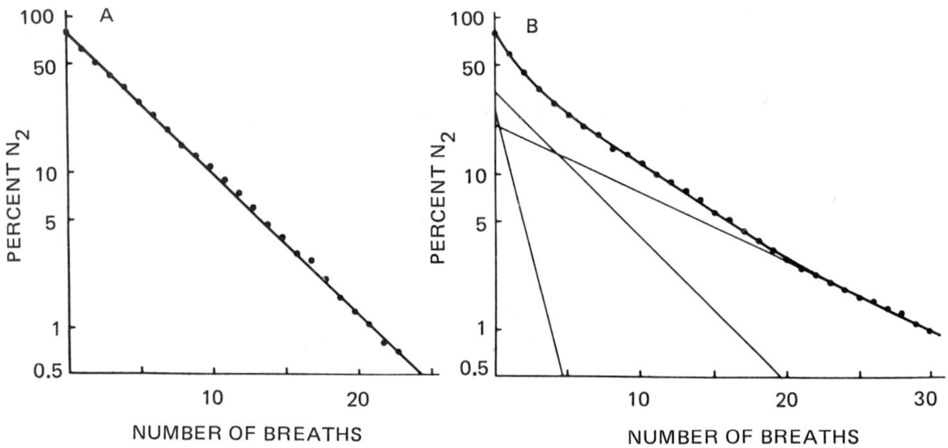

Figure 7 Logarithmic plot of alveolar N_2 concentration for consecutive breaths during O_2 breathing: (A) monoexponential washout of a uniformly ventilated lung; (B) multiexponential washout curve illustrates "exponential stripping" into three monoexponential washout rates. (From Bouhuys et al., 1956.)

The fraction $(V_T - V_D)/V_T$ is the dilution factor due to dead space. By substitution,

$$\log \bar{F}E_n = \log FA_0 \frac{V_T - V_D}{V_T} + n \log \omega \tag{4}$$

Thus log $\bar{F}E$ plotted against n yields a straight line, the value of which at n = 0 is log FA_0 $(V_T - V_D)/V_T$ and the slope of which is log ω.

In practice, many experimentally obtained curves in normal subjects, and most curves from patients with abnormal lungs, cannot be described by the single exponential function of Eq. (4). The interpretation of such N_2 washout curves was first studied by Robertson et al. (1950) and is based on the theory that the curve corresponds to the sum of two or more exponential functions representing two or more lung compartments. When n reaches a certain value, the contribution of the first exponential to $\bar{F}E_{N_2}$ becomes negligible and the plot of log $\bar{F}E_{N_2}$ becomes a straight line as n increases beyond this value. A slope of the straight portion of the curve represents the washout of the poorly ventilated compartment or the one with the highest alveolar dilution factor. When a straight line is drawn through this last portion of the experimental curve, with extrapolation to the ordinate, the other exponential component can be determined by subtraction from the original curve (Fig. 7B). In most cases the result is a straight line which represents the better ventilated compartment of the lung. If the resultant curve is not linear, the subtraction process may be repeated. This "exponential stripping" of the experimental data constitutes a mathematical representation of the N_2 washout on the basis of a lung model consisting of two (or three) spaces independently ventilated at different rates.

An alternative handling of the washout data was proposed by Cumming (1967), who plotted the quantity of N_2 per liter of lung volume remaining in the lung against the number of turnovers of the original volume. This lung N_2 decay curve is identical to the conventional washout curve in a homogeneously ventilated lung. Departure from the line of perfect mixing reflects the series or Fowler dead space in both cases. If the line is curved, however, the identity between the two curves disappears. The initial rapid fall seen in the washout curve, reflecting the "fast space," is seen in the decay curve to represent only a small quantity of N_2. Furthermore, whereas washout curves lie on either side of the line of perfect mixing, a decay curve always lies to the right of it. The extent to which the decay curve is displaced from the line of perfect mixing indicates the degree of inefficiency of gas mixing.

A. Simple Indices of Ventilation Inhomogeneity

To quantify the inhomogeneity of ventilation distribution represented by the N_2 washout a variety of simple indices have been utilized in the past. The simplest consists of the measurement of the alveolar N_2 concentration after 7 min of O_2 breathing (Cournand et al., 1941). In normal lungs this is usually less than 2% and is equivalent to a single point on the curve relating alveolar N_2 concentration to the number of breaths of O_2. The lung clearance index (LCI) is the ventilation required to wash out N_2 down to a given low value (usually 1.5% or 2%) divided by lung volume. Prolongation of N_2 clearance by unequal ventilation distribution or added dead space increases the LCI, whereas prolongation due to hyperinflation is eliminated by dividing the cumulative ventilation by the lung volume (Table 1).

A moment analysis of the washout curve formed by the sequence of end-tidal N_2 concentrations was proposed by Saniie et al. (1979) as a useful quantification of washout dynamics. The ratio of first to zeroth moment is the mean; from the ratio of the second to zeroth moment the variance can be derived. Inasmuch as moments are computed from all the points of the washout curve, they include more information and are less affected by measurement error than are the above-mentioned indices, which are derived from only two points. However, none of the above indices differentiates between the effect of an enlarged dead space and that of unequal gas distribution.

Table 1 Indices of Ventilation Inhomogeneity

Subjects	Age (yr)	Number	Mean	SE	Reference
		(a) Lung clearance index (LCI, %)			
Normal	18–34	6	8.5		Bouhuys and van Lennep (1962)
Normal	24–34	19	9.1	0.2	Bouhuys (1963)
Normal	35–44	24	9.0	0.3	Bouhuys (1963)
Normal	45–54	22	9.6	0.3	Bouhuys (1963)
Normal	55–65	15	10.0	0.6	Bouhuys (1963)
Normal	20–40	28	8.8	0.1	Edelman et al. (1968)
Normal	41–60	51	9.7	0.2	Edelman et al. (1968)
Normal	>61	38	10.8	0.3	Edelman et al. (1968)
Normal	20–48	9	5.0	0.1	Prowse and Cumming (1973)
Normal	33 ± 4	6	8.4	0.2	Fleming et al. (1980)
Normal	34 ± 3.5	14	7.9	0.4	Cutillo et al. (1981)
COPD patients	63 ± 3	14	13.1	3.5	Cutillo et al. (1981)
		(b) Mixing ratio			
Normal	20–40	28	1.57	0.04	Edelman et al. (1968)
Normal	41–60	51	1.76	0.04	Edelman et al. (1968)
Normal	>61	38	1.96	0.05	Edelman et al. (1968)

Normal	20-48	9	1.26	0.07	Prowse and Cumming (1973)
Normal	33 ± 4	6	1.50	0.04	Fleming et al. (1980)
Normal	34 ± 3.5	14	1.58	0.07	Cutillo et al. (1981)
COPD patients	63 ± 3	14	2.55	0.19	Cutillo et al. (1981)
		(c) Pulmonary N_2 clearance delay (%)			
Normal	22-35	10	21	4	Fowler et al. (1952)
Normal	53-81	7	46	13	Fowler et al. (1952)
Normal	24-34	19	29	5	Bouhuys (1963)
Normal	35-44	24	33	6	Bouhuys (1963)
Normal	45-54	22	41	7	Bouhuys (1963)
Normal	55-65	15	70	12	Bouhuys (1963)
Normal	25-52	4	55	14	Cutillo et al. (1972)
Normal	34 ± 3.5	14	38	10	Cutillo et al. (1981)
COPD patients	58-70	5	197	25	Fowler et al. (1952)
COPD patients		16	252	59	Cutillo et al. (1972)
COPD patients	63 ± 3	14	219	30	Cutillo et al. (1981)

Because the LCI depends on the magnitude of tidal volume and dead space, Edelman et al. (1968) proposed an index consisting of the ratio of the observed to the ideal number of breaths required to reduce end tidal N_2 to 2%. By estimating dead space from body height and relating the measured value of LCI to the ideal value for a uniformly ventilated space, an index, independent of tidal volume, lung volume, and dead space, is obtained. Curve fitting is not required and only the washout to the point of 2% end tidal N_2 is considered. To the degree that the estimated anatomical dead space is correct, an increased mixing ratio (MR) reflects greater maldistribution of inspired gas (Table 1).

The pulmonary N_2 clearance delay (PNCD) also expresses the nonuniform distribution of inspired gas quantitatively in a single figure and is independent of the size of the anatomical dead space (Table 1c). It is based on the calculation of the average number of breaths during which N_2 molecules remain in the lung before being washed out. In the presence of nonuniform distribution N_2 molecules will, on the average, be washed out more slowly than under homogeneous conditions. Thus inequality of ventilation distribution increases the "actual average number of breaths" during which N_2 molecules remain in the lung. This is compared to the "ideal average breath number" derived from the alveolar dilution factor for a homogeneously ventilated lung of the same volume and with the same $V_T - V_D$. In uniformly ventilated lungs the ideal and actual average number of breaths are equal. In nonuniformly ventilated lungs the actual value is larger. The PNCD is calculated from the expression

$$\left[\frac{\text{Actual average breath number}}{\text{Ideal average breath number}} - 1\right] \times 100$$

The average number of breaths during which N_2 molecules remain in a system having two components, each with different dilution factors (ω_1, ω_2) and in which the fraction of the total lung volume occupied by each compartment is, respectively, f_1 and f_2, is equivalent to $f_1/(1 - \omega_1) + f_2/(1 - \omega_2)$. It can be shown that $f_1/\omega_1 + f_2/\omega_2 = 1/W$, where W is the value of the alveolar dilution factor that would obtain in a uniformly ventilated system having the same total volume and $V_T - V_D$ as the two components. The ideal average breath number is therefore $1/(1 - W)$. This index is similar to the one initially proposed by Robertson et al. (1950).

A compartmental analysis introduced by Briscoe and Cournand (1959) became widely used in clinical studies and describes the lung inhomogeneity by two (or more) washout rates and the corresponding fractional volumes of the lung compartments. Instead of dilution factors for each exponential component the authors calculated the ratio of alveolar ventilation to the volume of each compartment ($\dot{V}_A/L$). In 18 studies on six normal subjects the authors found that in nonmonoexponential washout curves, $\dot{V}_A/L$ of the poorly ventilated compartment ranged from 2.38 to 0.92 min^{-1} with a mean of 1.38 min^{-1}. The percentage volume of lung so ventilated ranged from 21 to 94%, with a mean of 62%. They concluded that the average normal lung is unevenly ventilated in such a way that about half the lung is only half as well ventilated as the other half. In contrast, in patients with emphysema there was a wide scatter in the findings, but in a typical case three-fourths of the lung was only one-fifth or one-tenth as well ventilated as the remaining one-fourth. In some curves in which three exponential components were identifiable, the difference in $\dot{V}_A/L$ between compartments may have been as great as 45:1. These observations were the first attempts at quantifying the order of magnitude of the uneven specific ventilation in emphysematous lungs.

A series of studies by C. J. Martin and co-workers specifically dealt with the magnitude of the dispersal of specific ventilation in different lungs, the physiological factors that can alter these, and the sequence of compartmental contributions during a single expiration. End-expiratory N_2 concentrations from each of the first 18 breaths of O_2 were used to construct a N_2 washout curve. This was simulated on an analog computer that provided the alveolar dilution ratios [$\omega = V_0/(V_0 + \Delta V)$, where $\Delta V = (V_T - V_D)/6$ in a six-compartment model] (Hashimoto et al., 1967). The results of such analyses showed a surprisingly wide dispersion of $V_0/\Delta V$ even in normal subjects. In patients with airflow obstruction the dispersal was even greater, although it did not correlate with the degree of obstruction. Breathing with increased tidal volume or increased inspiratory flow rate enhanced the dispersion (Young et al., 1968).

Tsunoda et al. (1972) described a lung model made up of four compartments, derived from end tidal N_2 concentrations of an 18-breath washout. Using alveolar dilution ratios and N_2 concentrations measured at specific points during each expiration, the authors calculated the fraction of total flow at that volume from each compartment. The dead space volume (V_D) was treated as one of the compartments with a dilution ratio of zero. At the beginning of expiration 100% of the expired gas was from V_D. This contribution diminished rapidly but continued beyond a volume equal to twice the measured volume of dead space, persisting further into expiration in older than in younger subjects. In none of the normal subjects did the dead-space contribution continue beyond 600 ml of the expiration. The sloping alveolar plateau was reflected in a progressive increase in contribution from the poorly ventilated compartment, whereas the best-ventilated compartment made its greatest contribution early in expiration. Surprisingly, in patients with airflow obstruction, all the compartments increased their contribution in the course of expiration, except for the dead-space compartment, whose contribution progressively diminished (Martin et al., 1974). The authors concluded that the N_2 rise on the alveolar plateau in patients with airflow obstruction was principally a function of dead-space delivery.

Most indices of ventilation inhomogeneity indicate greater ventilation maldistribution in older age groups (Tables 1 and 2). However, at least some of the effects of age observed in earlier studies must have been due to the concomitant effect of smoking. Bouhuys (1963) found a correlation between smoking and LCI in patients aged 45 years or more. The variability of the PNCD between subjects and the poor reproducibility within subjects limits its usefulness in assessing small differences. In young subjects no correlation was seen between PNCD and LCI in one study (Bouhuys, 1963), probably due to the fact that 35% of the curves were treated as monoexponential, so that the PNCD may have underestimated the unevenness of ventilation distribution.

Increasing ventilation by addition of an instrumental dead space (260 and 480 ml) decreased the PNCD from 35% to 6% (Bouhuys et al., 1957). In fact, in most cases the semilogarithmic N_2 washout plot was converted to a straight line, so that no inhomogeneity was apparent. This was interpreted to mean that the additional dead space served as a mixing chamber slowing down the washout of the better-ventilated units more than that of the poorly ventilated units. Although the LCI increased from 7.4 to 12.2 in the presence of additional dead space, when the latter was accounted for, the efficiency of ventilating the lung proper was uninfluenced. Inhalation of epinephrine by normal subjects caused a slight increase in the LCI (Bouhuys and Van Lennep, 1962). This could not be explained by changes in tidal volume or breathing rate and presumably was due to an increase in anatomical dead space which was not measured.

One of the few studies attempting to relate the indices of ventilation maldistribution to lung anatomy was that of Lillington et al. (1959), who measured N_2 clearance rates and the dead space of individual lungs of five normal men in the supine and both lateral decubitus positions by using bronchospirometric catheters. Multiple exponential clearance curves indicated the presence of uneven ventilation within individual lungs in all positions. In the supine posture the clearance rates and relative magnitudes of slowly and rapidly ventilated compartments of both lungs were similar. However, the clearance rates of both compartments of one lung were only half as great when the lung was in the superior position as they were in the same lung when the subject was supine. The authors concluded that the slow clearance rates of the superior lung appear to be largely responsible for the observed retardation of N_2 clearance from subjects in the lateral decubitus posture. These results were among the first to show a regional unevenness of alveolar ventilation.

In contrast to the physiological factors discussed above, lung pathology can easily be shown to affect all indices of ventilation distribution, sometimes to such a degree that it makes a test useful diagnostically despite a relatively poor reproducibility in normal subjects. An example is the PNCD (Table 2), which in patients with a variety of cardiopulmonary disorders ranges from 115 to 248% (Fowler et al., 1952).

Practical Limitations

Computation of compartmental washout rates and volumes from multiple-breath inert gas washouts is partly dependent on the accuracy and reproducibility of the data. In practice, variability in tidal volume, FRC, and frequency may influence the pattern of N_2 elimination by introducing "noise." In addition, the accuracy of the data depends on that of the analyzer, the normally used N_2 analyzer being sensitive to the fluctuations in water vapor pressure when dry O_2 is breathed. Respiratory mass spectrometers, which measure the N_2 concentration as a fraction of total dry gas, overcome this problem but may have a poorer signal-to-noise ratio.

Although for theoretical reasons it is desirable to continue the washout for as long as possible, practical limitations mitigate against prolonging the washout down to very low values of expired N_2. As alveolar N_2 tension decreases, N_2 diffuses out of the blood and tissues. Elimination of N_2 from the tissues depends on local circulation rates and it takes several hours before tissue N_2 becomes negligible. During the first minutes of the washout, tissue N_2 elimination is quantitatively smaller than pulmonary N_2 washout, so that the two processes can be separated with sufficient accuracy. However, as the alveolar N_2 concentration decreases, the contribution of N_2 from the blood becomes substantial. Thus in normal subjects after 5 min of washout, when the expired N_2 drops below 1%, the contribution from the blood may constitute more than 20% (Robertson et al., 1950). Conventionally, the correction for blood and tissue N_2 appearing in the expired gas is obtained from the total amount of N_2 eliminated, which in turn is estimated by the formula of Cournand et al. (1941). Errors in this correction are probably small early in the procedure, but later, as alveolar N_2 concentration becomes low, the correction may become increasingly inaccurate (Fowler et al., 1952).

Recently, the reproducibility of the various indices derived from a multiple-breath N_2 washout was systematically examined in a group of normal subjects and patients with chronic airflow obstruction (Cutillo et al., 1981). In two consecutive washouts in which the difference in tidal volume was less than 10% and variation in frequency did not exceed two to three breaths per minute, analysis of variance showed that intersubject variation of LCI, mixing ratio, pulmonary clearance delay (PNCD), and the specific ventilation of the slow space ($\dot{V}A_S/L$) were significantly greater than the intrasubject variation for both normal subjects and patients with chronic airflow obstruction. The average percent magnitude of the difference between repeated measurements was 8.4% for LCI, 10.1% for MR, and 15.5% for $\dot{V}A_S/L_S$. The latter appeared to be the most reproducible measurement obtained from graphic analysis of the N_2 washout curve according to a multicompartment lung model. In contrast, the correlation between duplicate measurements of the specific ventilation of the fast space and the fractional volume of the slow space were very poor, suggesting that the practical usefulness of these variables may be limited. The authors concluded that although the reproducibility of the N_2 washout data was generally acceptable, the variation of measurements repeated under comparable experimental conditions is not negligible and should be taken into consideration when the significance of experimental N_2 washout changes is to be evaluated in individual subjects. The intrasubject variability of the moment ratio (M_1/M_0) has been claimed to be smaller than that of most other indices of ventilation inhomogeneity obtainable from a N_2 washout (Fleming et al., 1980).

Theoretical Limitations

Briscoe and Cournand (1959) addressed the question of whether a washout curve analyzable into two components could not, in fact, be representative of the summated effect of more than two different components. They summed the washout of five compartments, the ventilation of which was distributed normally, and then analyzed the summed curves in the conventional manner. They found that the curve synthesized from five components was in fact analyzable into only two components. The authors pointed out that this would not be the case if the washout had been followed for a long time to a lower gas concentration and if measurements were sufficiently accurate to make certain that small deviations from linearity were significant. Both the specific ventilation and the relative volume of the least ventilated units are overestimated when the summed curve is interpreted in terms of two compartments only.

It is important to note that the two-compartment analysis does not necessarily reflect a bimodal distribution of specific ventilation. Indeed, it was pointed out by Van Liew (1962) that addition of up to 20 compartments with a unimodal continuous distribution of ventilation will produce a washout curve analyzable into two (or three) compartments. A detailed analysis of the theoretical limits to measurement of uneven ventilation was published by Nye (1961b). He addressed the anomaly that the lungs of normal subjects either manifest a monoexponential washout or behave as though half their volume, or more, were less that half as well ventilated as the remainder (Briscoe and Cournand, 1959). Milder degrees of unevenness were seldom reported. He investigated to what extent this sudden transition from apparent evenness to apparent gross unevenness may be an artifact imposed by the limitations of the technique employed. He emphasized that for accurate analysis of the two-component N_2 washout curve it is essential to obtain the slope and y-axis intercept of the terminal straight portion. If for any reason the curve is not plotted far enough down to establish this, the available portion of the curve will be forced into a fit either with a straight line or with another curve composed of two different exponential processes. Assuming that a two-component curve reaches its asymptote when the fast component has fallen to two logarithmic cycles below the slow component, Nye (1961b) stressed that if the graphical analysis of the curve is to be correct, the curve must be plotted at least to this point and a short distance beyond. The ordinate value at this point (y_a) depends on the evenness ratio (ratio of turnover rate of poorly ventilated to that of well-ventilated compartments) and on the relative size of the poorly ventilated compartments. Thus if a slow space that is only one-third as well ventilated as the remainder of the lung occupies half the lung volume, y_a will be reached when the washout is continued down to 1% of the initial value. However, if the compartment is half as well ventilated as the rest of the lung, the washout needs to continue down to 0.1% for accurate analysis.

Simulation of N_2 washout curves from two compartments ventilating asynchronously, such that inspired gas for one compartment is partly derived from the expired gas from the other, can also be shown to produce only two exponential components (Nye, 1961b). The curve will resemble that furnished by a synchronously ventilated two-compartmental model with different characteristics, and a unique solution will be possible only in terms of the latter model. The distortions induced in the initial model were found to be like those of dead-space mixing: The volume and tidal volume of the well-ventilated region appeared smaller than they actually were, and the volume and usually the tidal volume of the poorly ventilated region appeared larger. In the presence of marked unevenness, asynchrony introduced little distortion. When ventilation was more even, distortion became more marked.

The net result of all the distortions and limitations described above is additive. Thus instrumental limitations (due to tissue N_2 elimination and fluctuations in FRC) obscure the presence of mild unevenness of ventilation and overestimate the size of the poorly ventilated space. This overestimate is further enhanced by the mixing effect of dead space and the presence of asynchrony.

All analyses of multiple-breath N_2 washout, whether they result in exponential functions derived from graphical analysis of clearance curves or in continuous distributions of $\Delta V/V_0$ (see below), implicitly assume the lung to be composed of a variable number of independently and unequally ventilated units. Yet these units are only the result of a method of analysis that attempts to explain the experimentally found washout behavior of the lungs according to the properties of an oversimplified model with the same washout behavior as the lungs under study. Indeed, it may be shown that for any combination of series and parallel units an equivalent model consisting of a collection of parallel units exists and behaves in a manner indistinguishable with respect to the washout test (Evans, 1970). All factors that contribute to nonuniform distribution enter into the nonlinearity of the plot and the resultant indices of distribution. Thus the compartments or units must not be conceived of as having a particular anatomical or physiological reality. Although numerous authors have emphasized this point in the past, some investigators have been unable to resist the temptation to attempt to identify such units anatomically (Hashimoto et al., 1967; Lewis and Martin, 1979).

B. Continuous Distributions

Because of the structural inhomogeneity of the lung, indices of ventilation maldistribution based on an arbitrary selection of two, four, or six compartments necessarily constitute a gross oversimplification of the maldistribution. Theoretically, a continuous distribution of parameters reflecting the gas mixing inequality should more accurately represent the functional behavior of the lung. The first attempts to measure this were made by Gomez et al. (1964), who analyzed the end-tidal data from a multiple breath N_2 washout by fitting a continuous function of four parameters. The authors obtained continuous distribution functions of specific tidal volumes ($\Delta V/V_0$) and quantified several parameters to describe them. These included the maximal amplitude of the function, its modal value ($\Delta V/V_0$ at the maximal amplitude), the half-width of the curve (i.e., the distance along the abscissa between points at which the ordinate was half of maximum), and the first moment of the function (mean $\Delta V/V_0$). Although improving on the previous analyses, this approach suffered from the fact that the distribution sought may not have been adequately described by the parametric function. For example, the latter did not allow for the bi- or trimodal patterns observed by others using more sophisticated analyses.

Nakamura et al. (1966) and Okubo and Lenfant (1968) both used a direct inversion of the Laplace transform performed on curves fitted by hand to mixed expired data collected at 15 to 30-sec intervals. The distribution of lung volume and ventilation was computed as a function of clearance time constants. In normal subjects the authors found that the frequency distribution of both parameters was symmetrical with a relatively narrow base. Maximum frequency was observed at time constants ranging from 0.35 to 0.60

min in normal subjects, whereas in patients with chronic airflow obstruction the highest frequency was shifted substantially to the right and the range of distribution was much larger. In neither group of subjects did the ventilation and lung volume distribution function correspond exactly. The mathematical technique used in this method made it exquisitely sensitive to small variations either in the data or in the curve fitted to the data prior to analysis. In addition, the use of data collected at intervals rather than computed on a breath-by-breath basis restricted the ability to resolve the faster components. Therefore, the dead space may not have been well described in subjects with chronic airflow obstruction.

To overcome some of these problems, Lewis et al. (1978) described a new technique for recovering a continuous distribution of ventilation as a function of specific ventilation ($\Delta V/V_0$) from the N_2 washout. The technique is similar to that utilized to recover distributions of ventilation/perfusion ratios, yielding a distribution represented as fractional ventilations of 50 compartments plus dead space (Fig. 8). From mixed expired N_2 data, obtained using an apparatus to control the subject's tidal volume and FRC, the following observations were made: (1) the distributions in young, nor-

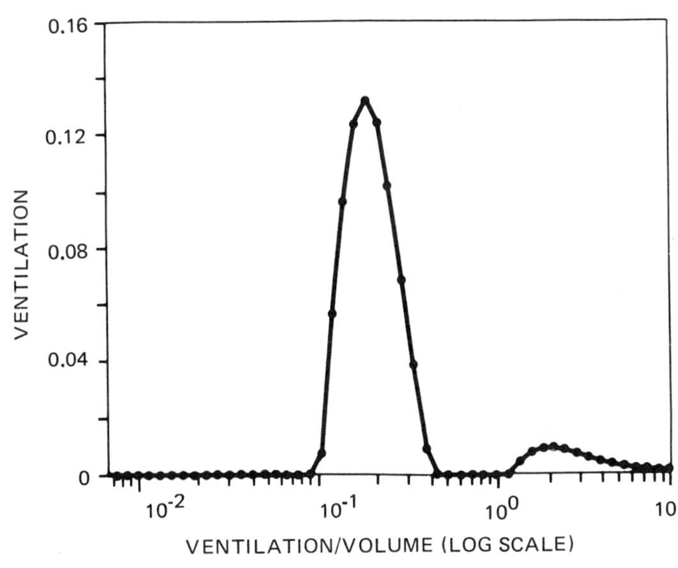

Figure 8 Continuous distribution of ventilation recovered from a multiple-breath N_2 washout in a normal subject. Note relatively narrow, unimodal pattern. Small amount of ventilation in the very high ventilation/volume regions may represent noise. (From Lewis et al., 1978.)

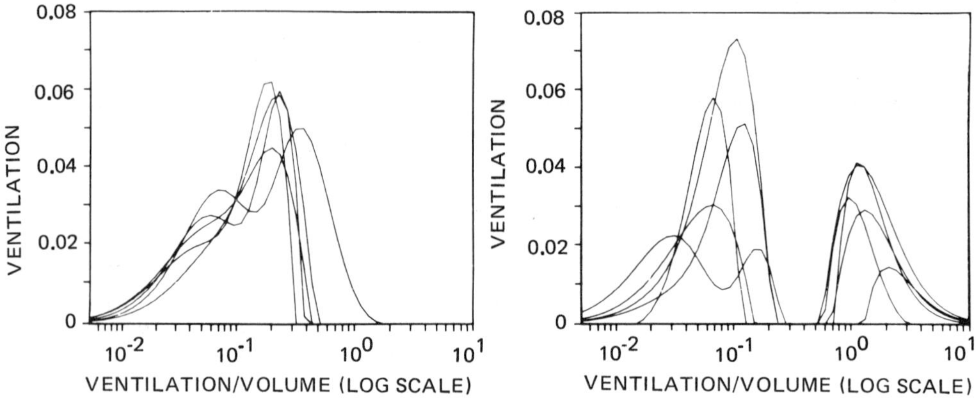

Figure 9 Ventilation distribution patterns in patients with chronic airflow obstruction. Left: Asymmetrical unimodal distribution. Right: Bimodal distribution. (From Lewis et al., 1978.)

mal subjects were narrow and unimodal with a mean ln standard deviation of 0.56 ± 0.13; (2) those of subjects over age 40 were broader (ln SD 0.86 ± 0.19) with more poorly ventilated units; (3) patients with pulmonary disease of all descriptions showed an enlarged dead space; and (4) patients with chronic airflow obstruction had a variety of distributions which were broader and, in some cases, bimodal (Fig. 9).

The criticisms leveled at the uniqueness of the recovered distribution of ventilation/perfusion ratios apply to some degree to the results of N_2 washout analyses. Although in the latter at least 18 data points are used (instead of 6) and N_2 concentrations may be measured more accurately than the retentions used in ventilation/perfusion studies, the potential number of lung units greatly exceeds the number of breaths measured and many distributions are compatible with a given set of washout data. Wagner (1979) addressed this question using the technique of linear programming to evaluate the variability among all such compatible distributions. He found that using the first 20 breaths of the washout, narrow distributions of $\Delta V/V_0$ could be specified. Distributions with up to four distinct modes could also be well specified, but for broad distributions the shape could not be adequately defined. Good resolution in the region of high $\Delta V/V_0$ was critically dependent on measuring accurately the first few breaths of the washout. In general, the resolution of a N_2 washout test depends on the particular case. The more complex a distribution, the less resolution is possible from the same number of breaths. Although fine detail is rarely recoverable from a

20-breath washout, the physiologically more important major features can usually be specified. Provided that on repeated testing a given individual manifests similar distributions, a significant change in the recovered distribution can be attributed to a change in the subject's lungs. As emphasized by Lewis et al. (1978), "significant" changes involve alterations in the shape of the entire distribution rather than in the flow to a given compartment.

All the foregoing analyses of ventilation maldistribution utilized the data derived from a progressive washout of an inert gas (usually N_2) present in the lung at the onset of the washout. The latter consisted of breathing a gas mixture not containing the specific tracer gas. Recently, an ingenious modification of this procedure was proposed by Lewis et al. (1982). It consists of having the subject inspire breaths of air at predetermined points during the standard N_2 washout. The rationale for this is that information about a specific compartment is obtained only while the N_2 concentration in that compartment is changing. The fast spaces in the lung are rapidly cleared and over the bulk of the washout contain no N_2. If several breaths of tracer are added late in the test, the fast space fills again with tracer and additional information is obtained. The washout of the slow space is relatively unaffected by this maneuver. If the dynamics of the fast space are better defined, it should be possible to characterize more accurately the contribution of the slow compartment to the N_2 decay. An optimal input is the sequence of breaths, alternating between O_2 and air, that causes the maximal changes in tracer concentration in all compartments of the system. In engineering terms this is called the principle of maximal excitation. Since the optimal input pattern depends on the features of the lung under study (as well as the noise in the system), they cannot be determined until the washout test is completed. However, Lewis et al. (1982) examined nominal inputs which, although not optimal for any particular lung model, could increase the information recovered from the washout of models with characteristics spanning the physiological and pathological range. These were shown to substantially increase the information recovered from the washout simulations. Although experimental studies in normal subjects have not as yet validated this technique, possibly due to the additional noise introduced into the system when delivering the nominal inputs, this innovative approach is promising and may constitute an important step in the direction of better characterizing the ventilation maldistribution in normal and abnormal lungs.

C. Dead Space

The understanding and measurement of dead space has been characterized by persistent confusion due to differences (often subtle) in semantics, conceptualization, and methodology. Although early in this century the difficulty in defining and measuring "alveolar" gas was at the center of disputes (Haldane, 1915; Krogh and Lindhard, 1917), recent developments in the estimation of dead space have contributed to the variety of measurements and their interpretation. This section will review the different measurements of dead space, focusing on those derived from the multiple-breath washout. Their interpretation will be discussed in the context of current theories of intra-acinar mixing.

The *anatomical dead space* refers to the volume of the airways from the mouth to the respiratory bronchioles. Since the end of the nineteenth century morphological measurements using casts and other techniques have indicated that the volume of the conducting airways increases with increasing lung distention, ranging from 144 ml in collapsed lungs to 260 ml after maximal inspiration (Loewy, 1894). Approximately 50% of the anatomical dead space volume is located in the upper airways.

The single-breath estimation of dead space popularized by Fowler (1948) is the functional equivalent of the anatomical dead space. It differs from the latter insofar as the peripheral boundary is not morphologically determined but consists of a diffusion front whose position at end inspiration is a function of flow, gas diffusivity, and lung volume (see Sec. V.A and Chap. 6). The accurate measurement of the *Fowler dead space* (V_{DF}) requires that the alveolar plateau represents a flow weighted mean of the alveolar gas concentrations and that any changes in flow with expired volume be linear for all compartments. In abnormal lungs where these prerequisites are not met, Fowler dead space may be underestimated.

Bohr (1891) defined a functional dead space using a mass transport equation

$$P_E V_T = P_I V_D + P_A V_A$$

where the tidal volume (V_T) was partitioned into an alveolar volume (V_A) and an effective dead space (V_D). P_I, P_A, and P_E were the partial pressures of inspired, alveolar, and mixed expired gases, respectively. Rearranging, when $P_I = 0$, yields

$$\frac{V_D}{V_T} = \frac{P_A - P_E}{P_A}$$

Inferring P_A from end tidal gas allows for the calculation of the *Bohr dead space* (V_{DB}). The difficulty in defining P_A of respiratory gases, particularly when distribution of inspired gas is uneven, has led to the use of arterial instead of alveolar values for P_{CO_2}, based on the assumption of complete equilibration between the alveolus and end capillary. This defines the *physiological dead space* (V_{Dp}), which is given by

$$\frac{V_{Dp}}{V_T} = \frac{Pa_{CO_2} - PE_{CO_2}}{Pa_{CO_2}} \tag{5}$$

To a variable extent the calculated V_{Dp} will be influenced by the distribution of ventilation and perfusion. In the presence of a ventilation/perfusion mismatch, V_{Dp} includes the volume in the gas exchanging zone that reflects the ventilation/perfusion inhomogeneity as well as the anatomical dead space. The volume may be thought of as a zone which is ventilated but not perfused and is referred to as the *alveolar* or *parallel dead space* (Folkow and Pappenheimer, 1955). V_{Dp} may be determined during the elimination of any gas from the lungs under steady-state conditions. However, the value of V_{Dp} depends also on the blood-gas partition coefficient of the gas.

The first calculations of dead space from monoexponential multiple-breath washouts were performed by Bateman (1950). Fowler et al. (1952) treated the non-monoexponential curve as a sum of a series of exponentials, each with its own alveolar dilution ratio. By comparing these to an ideal alveolar dilution ratio which described washout from lungs with the same volume and the same total (V_T - V_D), the washout dead space (V_{Dw}) could be calculated. More sophisticated computer-assisted analyses of the washout curve as a sum of four exponentials were subsequently used extensively to study V_{Dw} (Lewis and Martin, 1979; Martin et al., 1979). The dead space was defined as a compartment having an infinite specific ventilation. In practice this was computed as a ventilation not represented in the other compartments. This definition of dead space is sensitive to noise in the early breaths. If the measured N_2 on the first few breaths is erroneously high, it can be interpreted as indicating a very well ventilated compartment, which would contribute N_2 only on the first one or two breaths. The ventilation of this compartment would otherwise be assigned to the dead space.

Although in many studies the magnitude of the washout dead space was found to be similar to that of V_{DF}, in a N_2 washout in which lung volumes, flow rates, and frequency were controlled, V_{Dw} consistently exceeded V_{DF}, obtained from the first three breaths, by approximately 40 ml (Martin et al., 1979). The difference was present at all lung volumes and at breathing frequencies ranging from 15 to 60 breaths per minute. Since in the parallel model dead space is defined as that portion which contains no N_2 at end inspiration, and hence includes the series dead space (V_{DF}), the additional volume must necessarily be derived from the "alveolar" compartment. (This conclusion presupposes an accurate estimation of series dead space, which may not always be possible.) Lewis and Martin (1979) speculated that the difference between V_{Dw} and V_{DF} may reflect the volume of alveoli on respiratory bronchioles which are swept clear of N_2 during inspiration. Alternatively, they postulated units that collapsed during expiration and opened during inspiration. Neither of these explanations is plausible. Alveoli on respiratory bronchioles swept clear of N_2 during inspiration would necessarily be located mouthward of the diffusion front and hence would contribute to the Fowler dead space. The fact that $V_{Dw} - V_{DF}$ is constant over the whole lung volume range argues against the existence of units which open during inspiration and close on expiration. Their mechanical properties would need to be rather strange, so that their existence in normal lungs would seem to be highly improbable.

One of the difficulties with the conventional parallel model used to explain N_2 washouts is the observation that, when measured end tidal N_2 concentration is plotted for each breath, the extrapolation to the ordinate frequently falls below the alveolar N_2 value prior to washout. Even when large tidal volumes are utilized to ensure a nearly monoexponential washout, the intercept on the ordinate is too low (Roos et al., 1955). The low intercept can be attributed to dead space in end tidal gas but is incompatible with the conventional parallel model without gross asynchrony of emptying.

In a lung model consisting of a single perfectly mixed compartment and an anatomical dead space, washout of the tracer will follow a single exponential pattern (Fig. 10A). A plot of end tidal N_2 concentration ($F_{ET_{N_2}}$) will run parallel to and above a plot of mixed expired N_2 ($\bar{F}_{E_{N_2}}$). Extrapolation of the monoexponential to the ordinate will correspond to the value of $F_{A_{N_2}}$ prior to the washout ($F_{A_0N_2}$). For $\bar{F}_{E_{N_2}}$, from Eq. (4), the value at n = 0 ($F_{E_0N_2}$) is log $F_{A_0N_2}(V_T - V_D)/V_T$. Rearranging, the *washout dead space* obtained in this way (V_{Dw}) is given by

$$\frac{V_{Dw}}{V_T} = 1 - \frac{F_{E_0N_2}}{F_{A_0N_2}} \tag{6}$$

Because of the extrapolation of the linear regression the accuracy of the intercept on the ordinate should be greater than any measurement derived from a single breath, and V_{Dw} will be the same as V_{DF}.

In a lung model consisting of two independently and unequally ventilated compartments a sloping alveolar plateau may be obtained if the poorly ventilated compartment contributes more later in expiration. A plot of the logarithm of $F_{ET_{N_2}}$ against breath number is now curvilinear, reflecting the sum of two exponentials (Fig. 10B). However, provided that the asynchrony of emptying is not extreme, extrapolation to the ordinate still corresponds to the initial alveolar concentration prior to washout. A plot of mean expired concentration runs approximately parallel to that of $F_{ET_{N_2}}$. In this model the value of $V_{Dw} - V_{DF}$ is a measure of the retarding effect of the inequality in ventilation distribution on lung clearance. It is important to note that in nonuniform lungs with sequential emptying, end-tidal concentra-

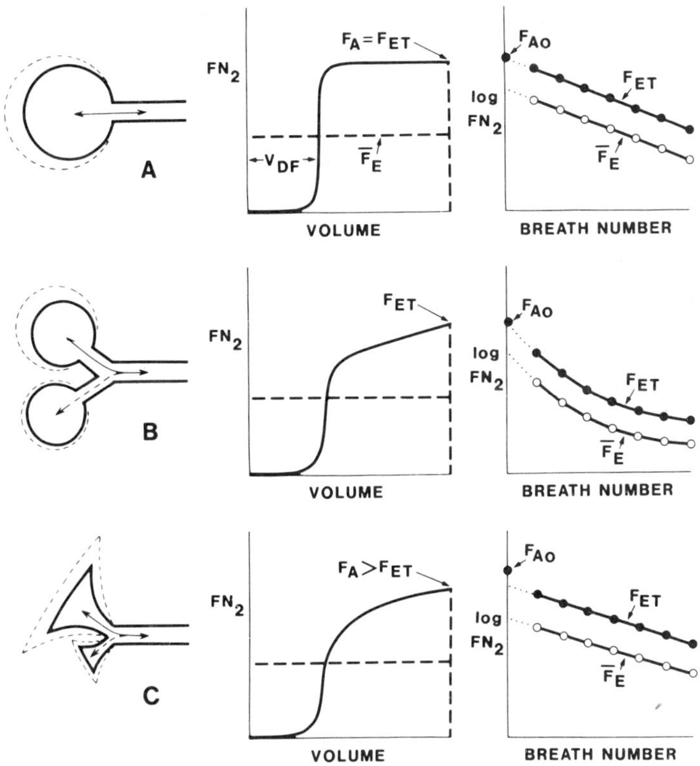

Figure 10 Relationship between lung model, single- and multiple-breath washouts. (A) Single alveolar compartment with dead space (VDF) giving rise to horizontal alveolar plateau so that end-tidal (FET) and alveolar (FA) concentrations are equivalent. Multibreath washout on semilog plot is linear for FET, extrapolating to initial FA (FA_0). Extrapolation of linear plot of mean expired concentration ($\overline{F}E$) allows the calculation of dead space (VDw where VDw = VDF). (B) Sequential filling and emptying of two unequally ventilated compartments giving rise to sloping alveolar plateau. Multibreath washout is curvilinear (biexponential) for FET, which extrapolates to FA_0. Curves $\overline{F}E$ and FET are approximately parallel. (C) Uniformly expansile two-trumpet model giving rise to sloping alveolar plateau such that FET < FA. Multibreath washout is linear for FET, which extrapolates below FA_0. Measurement of VDw from extrapolation of $\overline{F}E$ curve shows that VDw > VDF.

tion, which constitutes a flow-weighted mean of alveolar concentrations, may not correspond to the volume-weighted mean that would be the best choice for alveolar concentration.

If "the air in the air sacs is not at the end of an inspiration of the same composition throughout, because the inspired air is incompletely mixed with the air previously contained" (Krogh and Lindhard, 1917), the effect will simulate a further increase in dead space, so that the value of V_{DW} - V_{DF} will increase. The effect of such a diffusion (or time) dependent inhomogeneity in alveolar gas concentrations may be represented by the two-trumpet model (Chap. 6) and gives rise to an essentially monoexponential washout (Fig. 10C), but extrapolation of the $F_{ET_{N_2}}$ curve to the ordinate falls below the value of $F_{A_{0}N_2}$. In abnormal lungs, where inequality of airway diameter rather than asymmetry of branching is the main basis for the diffusion-dependent inhomogeneity, the latter may give rise to a non-monoexponential washout (see Sec. VI.D).

The concept of diffusive interdependence between parallel units within the acinus has been discussed in detail in Chapter 6. In the presence of asymmetrical branching or inequality of airway lumena, differences in inspired gas concentrations will be established even if volume expansion is homogeneous. These differences persist throughout the respiratory cycle, although diffusive pendelluft during expiration reduces them. Because the initial boundary conditions for the second breath differ from the homogenous alveolar concentrations existing prior to the first breath, the increase in the relative intra-acinar concentration differences during the second breath is smaller (Fig. 11). Within several breaths a quasi-steady state is reached in normal lungs, and the intraacinar concentration differences relative to the inspired concentration remain constant (Paiva et al., 1982). It is the apparent discontinuity of the first few breaths which results in the extrapolated F_{ET} values falling below the initial alveolar concentration (Fig. 10C). Using the Bohr formulation, it is possible to estimate the effective dead space (V_{DW}') related to this diffusion-dependent inhomogeneity. Thus $V_{DW}'/V_T = (1 - F_{ET_0}/F_{A_0})$.

In their informative paper Roos et al. (1954) described the pattern of N_2 concentrations in gas fractions examined at different points of the expired breath during a multiple-breath washout (Fig. 12). The relative concentration differences between these gas fractions increased during the first few breaths, reaching a maximum by about the fourth breath, following which they remained relatively constant. This is consistent with the rapid establishment of a quasi-steady state during the first few breaths of a N_2 washout. Similarly, intra-acinar diffusion during the time of a respiratory cycle may be reflected in the more curvilinear washout of gas fractions expired early in the breath, when intra-acinar inhomogeneity is greater, than those expired near end expiration (Fig. 12). It is noteworthy that this wash-

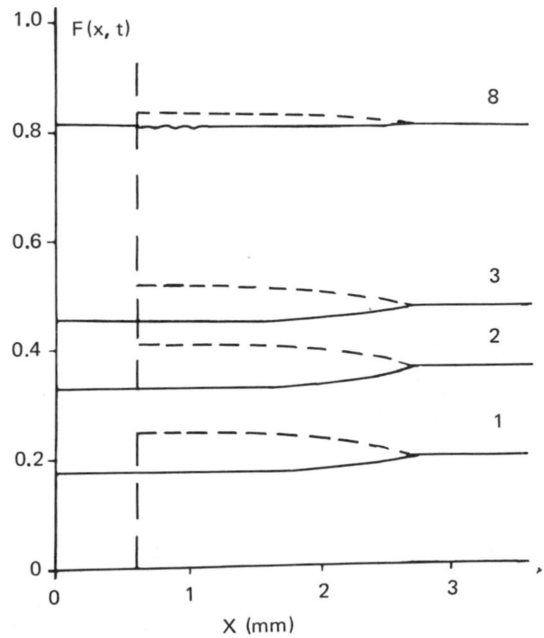

Figure 11 Fractional end-expiratory concentrations of inspired gas in an asymmetrical two-trumpet model for breath numbers 1, 2, 3, and 8. Dashed lines are concentrations in the smaller unit. The abscissa is the distance from the alveolar end of the larger unit. The branch point is located at x = 2.7 mm. Note the increase in concentration difference between the two units for breath 2. (From Paiva et al., 1982.)

out pattern may represent a fast-time-constant component in the conventional multiexponential fit. The intra-acinar diffusion-dependent component of dead space is additive to the Fowler dead space as well as to an effective component representing the mixing impairment due to the ventilation inequality of independently ventilated parallel units. The influence of this component, calculated using a mass balance approach, is illustrated in Figure 13, where a V_T of 1 liter is partitioned among two lung compartments of 1.5 liters each. Depending on the specific ventilation ratio, mixing efficiency and the ventilatory dead space vary markedly.

Dead Space Interrelationships

The alveolar component of dead space given by (V_{DW} - V_{DF}) is greater in patients with chronic airflow obstruction than in normal subjects (Lewis

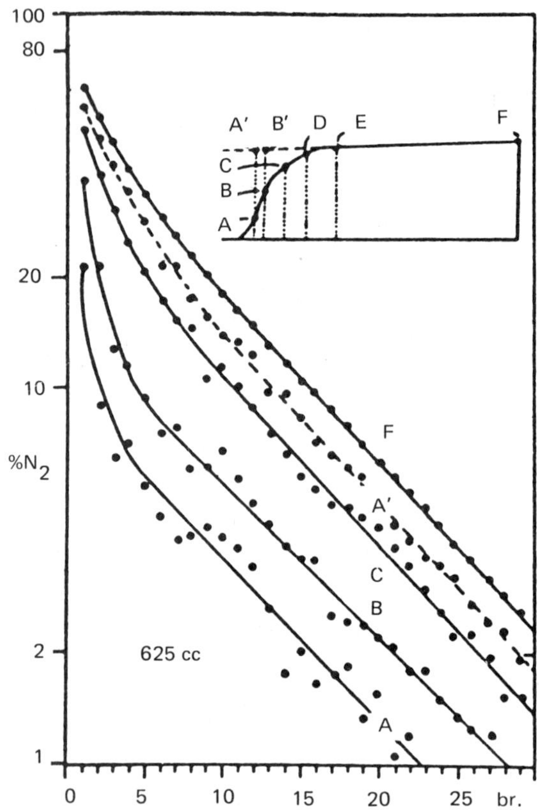

Figure 12 Logarithmic plot of N_2 concentration of gas fractions at different points of the expired breath (A-F) during multiple-breath washout. Note the greater initial curvilinearity of the gas fractions measured earlier within each breath and the approximately parallel plots of all gas fractions after the first six to eight breaths. (From Roos et al., 1954.)

and Martin, 1979). A similar conclusion is reached when the fraction of V_{DW} delivered in the expirate after the first 400 ml is measured in patients and normals. In contrast, increases in lung volume and/or breathing frequency in normal subjects increase V_{DW} to the same extent as they increase V_{DF} (Martin et al., 1979). In fact, most of the change is seen in the phase I of the single-breath washout. Similarly, the increase in V_{DW} after atropine also consists predominantly of an increase in V_{DF}, especially the phase I component. From these observations one may infer that changes in lung volume and bronchomotor tone affect dead space predominantly by virtue of changes in the volume of conducting airways without substantially influencing the in-

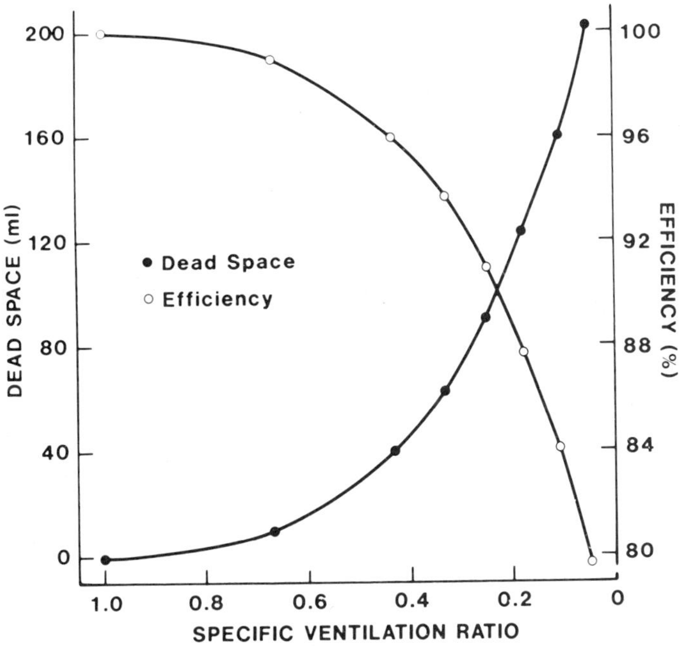

Figure 13 Mixing efficiency and effective respiratory dead space computed for two lung compartments (1.5 liter each) ventilated with a total tidal volume of 1 liter and no anatomical dead space. Note the progressive fall in efficiency and increase in effective dead space as the relative ventilation of the poorly ventilated compartment decreases.

homogeneity within alveolar gas. Increases in breathing frequency increase dead space by displacing the diffusion front further into the acinus, thus increasing Fowler dead space, but here, too, alveolar gas inhomogeneity does not appear to be enhanced. In contrast, in obstructive lung diseases and to some degree with aging, the inhomogeneity within alveolar gas is increased.

Of particular interest is the relationship between V_{Dw} and tidal volume. Bouhuys et al. (1957) observed a good correlation between V_{Dw} and V_T in normal subjects, the V_{Dw} constituting approximately 20% of V_T. The authors puzzled over this relationship and concluded that it was not likely to be due to changes in end inspiratory volume since correlation with the latter was not as good. Lacquet et al. (1975) observed that dead space, calculated by parameter fitting of washout curves, differed for He and SF_6. At a constant breathing frequency (40 breaths per minute) V_{Dw} for SF_6 increased from 190 ml at a V_T of 400 to 400 ml at a V_T of 1800 ml, (i.e., 15 ml per 100 ml increase in V_T). For the same change in V_T the V_{Dw}

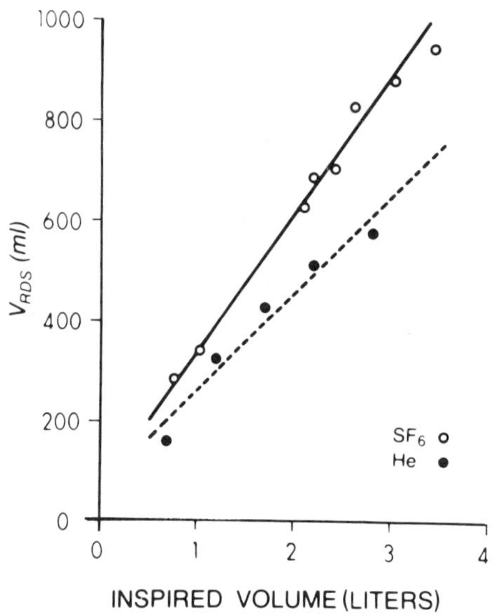

Figure 14 Rebreathing dead space (VRDS) measured with He and SF_6 at different inspired volumes in a normal subject. Duration of first breath was 4 sec. Note the greater increase in VRDS with SF_6 than with He for a given increment in tidal volume. (From Petrini et al., 1982.)

for He increased from 180 ml to 250 ml, an increment of 5 ml per 100 ml VT. Since these increments were much greater than the change in VDF with lung volume and differed for the two gases, they could not have represented dilatation of conducting airways. Similarly, during closed-circuit equilibration of an inert gas (see Sec. VII.A) a rebreathing dead space (VRDS), analogous to VDW, greatly exceeds the predicted Fowler dead space (Petrini et al., 1982). The increase in VRDS with tidal volume is also much steeper than that of VDF and differs for He and SF_6 (Fig. 14).

Gray et al. (1956) conceptualized dead space to be a "virtual cylindrical space which if filled with inspired air at the beginning of expiration and then washed out by laminar flow would yield the observed expired dead air volume." A relationship with tidal volume would therefore reflect a variable degree of washout of the anatomical dead space. Although this concept may be useful to explain measurements with small tidal volumes (at physiological frequencies), it is unlikely to explain the relationship at tidal volumes above 500 ml. Measurements of F_{N_2} in small airways of excised lungs during single breaths of O_2 show a complete washin of the dead space relatively early in inspiration (Engel et al., 1973b). An alternative explanation is that breathing with greater tidal volumes enhances ventilation maldistribution among independently ventilated units with differing curvilinear pressure-volume relationships. In addition, the higher tidal volumes, and therefore higher flow rates, enhance the diffusion-dependent intra-acinar inhomogeneity. Only in part is this due to a more peripheral displacement of the diffusion front which is reflected in a larger Fowler dead space. Recent simulations of the intra-acinar distribution of ventilation predict an increased inhomogeneity when breathing at a ventilation corresponding to that seen during moderate exercise (Paiva and Engel, 1984).

Calculation of the Bohr dead space (V_{DB}) from end tidal samples of alveolar air also shows a correlation with tidal volume. Although initially the large dead space calculated during muscular exercise was attributed to enhanced gas exchange, similar results were obtained when hyperpnea was induced by breathing hypercapnic gas mixtures or during eupnea when tidal volume and breathing frequency were varied (Haldane, 1915). Indeed, Haldane's observations on V_T dependence of V_{DB} using CO_2 were qualitatively similar to those made more recently by investigators using inert gases. It is now clear that the differences between the size of dead space obtained by the Oxford group and that by Krogh and Lindhard (1917) were not due primarily to the difference between inert and respiratory gases but to the concept of the dead space underlying the measurements (Bouhuys, 1964). Although the spatial localization of alveolar gas inhomogeneity proposed by Krogh and Lindhard was somewhat simplistic, these authors clearly understood that a diffusion nonuniformity of gas concentrations must exist within the acinus. However, whereas Krogh and Lindhard measured a dead space analogous to what is currently referred to as Fowler dead space, Haldane's dead space included the diffusion-dependent inhomogeneity of alveolar gas concentration.

The dead space obtained from inert gas washout (V_{Dw}) and the conventionally measured V_{Dp}, using arterial P_{CO_2}, would be similar if the volume of inspired air subjected to dilution were coextensive in time and space with the volume subjected to gas exchange (Gray et al., 1956). Although in reality this may not be the case, it is tempting to compare the tidal volume dependence of V_{Dp} with that of V_{Dw}.

When breathing at constant tidal volumes, V_{Dp} increases only slightly with lung volume (Lifshay et al.,1971), probably less than the V_{DF}, resulting in a decrease in alveolar dead space (Severinghaus and Stupfel, 1957). In contrast, with increases in V_T, V_{Dp} increases substantially both in normal subjects (Rossier and Buhlman, 1955) and in patients with chronic airflow obstruction (Read and Lee, 1969). Expressions relating V_{Dp} to V_T generally indicate that the former equals a constant plus a fraction varying with V_T. If perfusion distribution does not change with V_T, the fraction of V_T going to relatively underperfused or overventilated areas (i.e., alveolar dead-space volume) should increase in proportion to (alveolar) tidal volume. To a variable degree this increase may correspond to a greater inhomogeneity within the gas phase represented by the increase in V_{Dw}.

D. Gas Mixing Efficiency

The ventilatory or gas mixing efficiency of the lung (E) is a measure of the adequacy with which inspired gas is mixed with that already present in the lung. The calculation of ventilatory efficiency is intimately related to that of dead space and utilizes a mass balance approach. During a single breath of O_2, measurement of the Fowler dead space (V_{DF}) as well as $\bar{F}E_{N_2}$ allows the latter to be compared with a predicted value based on perfect mixing in a lung of the same volume (V_L) and V_{DF} given by $0.79\ V_L/(V_L + V_T - V_{DF})$. The ratio is an index of mixing efficiency for that breath (Cumming and Guyatt, 1982) and reflects the impairment in mixing within the "alveolar" compartment (distal to the diffusion front) due to both the ventilation maldistribution among diffusion independent units and the diffusion-dependent inhomogeneity in gas concentrations. In 10 normal subjects Cumming and Guyatt (1982) found this single-breath mixing efficiency to be approximately 89%.

A single-breath washout is weighted by the better-ventilated units and the derived mixing efficiency therefore overestimates that of the whole lung. A more complete approach requires the analysis of a multiple-breath washout of a resident inert gas during tidal breathing and many of the indices described in the preceding sections of this chapter are also measures of ventilatory efficiency. Conventionally, 100% efficiency represents perfect mixing in an ideal lung model incorporating the physical characteristics of the lung under study. The pulmonary N_2 clearance delay (PNCD) of Fowler et al. (1952) was expressed as an efficiency [equivalent to 100/(1 + PNCD)] which was relatively independent of breathing frequency and $(V_T - V_D)/V_L$ ratio. It averaged 83% in 10 young normal subjects. The lung clearance index (LCI) has also been used to calculate efficiency, as reflected in the mixing ratio of Edelman et al. (1968). When Fowler dead space was estimated from the subject's height, a mixing efficiency of 56% was obtained from N_2 washout studies in 117 normal men breathing with a V_T of 0.82 liter.

A systematic study of alveolar gas mixing efficiency was performed by Cumming and Guyatt (1982) from N_2 washouts in normal subjects and patients with chronic airflow obstruction. They measured the ratio of theoretical lung turnover number/experimental turnover number at 90% clearance and calculated a washout dead space (V_{DW}) from $V_T \times$ (1 - turnover ratio). A multibreath alveolar mixing efficiency (E_{90}) could then be obtained from $100\ [1 - (V_T - V_{DW})/(V_T - V_{DF})]$. In five normal subjects E_{90} was 75% at a V_T of 492 ml and 72% at a V_T of 758 ml. On another occasion E_{90} in 10 normal subjects, breathing with a V_T of 675 ml, was 70% (Kox et al., 1982). In contrast, in 10 patients with severe airflow obstruction, the first-breath efficiency and E_{90} at a mean V_T of 673 ml were 73% and 40%, respectively.

The reasons for the low alveolar mixing efficiency are probably complex. Even in the presence of perfect intra-acinar mixing, unequal expansion of different acini or larger lung units constitutes an impairment in mixing (Fig. 13). A sixfold difference in specific ventilation will give rise to an 89% alveolar mixing efficiency. Since interregional ventilation differs by a factor of 2, intraregional differences need to be only of the order of 3:1 to account for the single-breath efficiency measured in normal subjects. However, the lower efficiency obtained from multibreath washouts reflects a greater inhomogeneity present even in normal subjects. An 80% efficiency requires a specific ventilation ratio of 20:1 (Fig. 13). Predictions of intra-acinar mixing efficiency are limited by our ignorance of acinar anatomy, but one estimate is 99% (Paiva and Engel, 1984). Even in the presence of extreme branching asymmetry, intra-acinar mixing efficiency should not be less than 95% (Bowes et al., 1982).

The effect of lung volume on ventilatory efficiency is apparent when normal subjects are made to breathe near residual volume (RV) or near total lung capacity. At both lung volumes E_{90} is lower than at FRC (Prowse and Cumming, 1973). Furthermore, the N_2 decay curves obtained near RV are more curvilinear than those at FRC. The authors attributed this to the greater interregional inhomogeneity near RV. However, the fact that a 5-sec end-inspiratory breathhold abolished the increase in curvature suggests an intraregional mechanism, possibly related to an inhomogeneous distribution of airway closure (Engel et al., 1976).

Estimates of true alveolar mixing efficiency in patients with airflow obstruction are difficult because of the uncertainty surrounding the measurement of V_{DF}. However, unequal narrowing of small airways could substantially lower the efficiency due to more marked diffusion-dependent inhomogeneity. Whereas in normal lungs abolition of bronchomotor tone makes little difference (Kox et al., 1982), in abnormal lungs fixed airway narrowing and occlusion probably further impair the mixing process and delay the establishment of a quasi-steady state during a multiple-breath washout. This delay results in a non-monoexponential curve which may be identical to one produced by simultaneous washout of two or more unequally ventilated diffusion-independent, parallel units (Fig. 15B). In contrast, due to the tidal nature of ventilation, a series inhomogeneity (e.g., Fowler dead space) is reconstituted in an identical manner during each breath, resulting in a steady state which gives rise to a monoexponential washout (Fig. 15A). Evidence supporting this diffusion-dependent impairment of gas mixing in patients with severe airflow obstruction has been provided by Von Nieding et al. (1977) using two gases with different diffusivities (Sec. VI.E). The analysis above makes it clear that attempts to distinguish between series and parallel inhomogeneity on the basis of linearity or curvilinearity of washout (or decay) curves (Cumming, 1967) are of questionable validity.

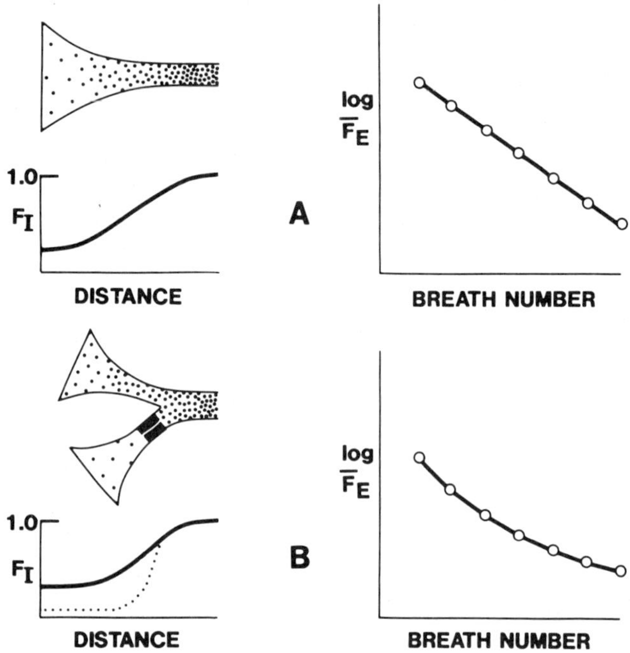

Figure 15 Diffusion-dependent concentration gradients and multiple-breath washout. (A) Concentration of inspirate (FI) after first inspiration within symmetrical trumpet model (left) and the logarithm of mixed expired concentration ($\bar{F}E$) plotted against breath number (right). Note the linear washout. (B) Distribution of FI after first inspiration within two-trumpet model with marked inequality of airway cross sections (left) and the curvilinear semilogarithmic plot of $\bar{F}E$ against breath number (right).

E. Dual Inert Gas Washouts

When the lung is equilibrated with a gas containing tracer quantities of two gases with different diffusivities, the multiple-breath washout of the two gases differs (Okubo and Piiper, 1974; Von Nieding et al., 1977). The lighter gas is washed out more rapidly than the denser one. This is predictable, as the Fowler dead space for the two gases is not the same (Lacquet et al., 1975). Kawashiro et al. (1976) quantified the different washout rates of He and SF_6 in normal subjects and concluded that only about half of the difference can be attributed to different Fowler dead spaces, the remainder being due to a diffusion limitation within the alveolar space. Unfortunately, technical uncertainties surrounding the response-time correction of the mass spectrometer used render the validity of this partitioning uncertain.

When end-tidal or mean expired concentrations of both gases are plotted during a multiple-breath washout, the He concentration is initially greater than that for SF_6. However, after a variable number of breaths a crossover point (COP) occurs following which the relationship is reversed (Lacquet et al., 1975). The factors influencing the COP were studied in detail by Von Nieding et al. (1977), who found that, in normal subjects breathing with tidal volumes of 700 to 750 ml, the COP occurred after four to six breaths. Breathing at high lung volumes delayed it slightly, whereas breathing below FRC advanced it a little. Surprisingly, the COP was relatively frequency independent. Patients with bronchial asthma in remission demonstrated a COP in the range of that seen in healthy subjects. When asthma was induced, the position of the COP did not change significantly, although the overall washout was delayed substantially both in time and with respect to the cumulative expired volume. In marked contrast, the COP in patients with severe emphysema was not reached before a mean of 60 breaths. Despite the somewhat greater age of this population and smaller tidal volumes, this radical difference in diffusion dependence suggested real differences in the pattern of gas mixing within the lung periphery. Von Nieding et al. (1977) correctly inferred that the observation was due to diffusion-dependent inhomogeneity present in emphysematous lungs, although the model used to quantify this was oversimplified. A plausible explanation for these observations, based on a two-trumpet model, is that the delayed COP is due to diffusion interaction within an acinus or small lung unit in which gross inequality of airway diameter is present (De Vries et al., 1981). If units are almost completely obstructed during tidal breathing, their contribution to the expirate will be almost entirely by diffusion. This may even entail diffusion across alveolar walls into the better-ventilated units. Only a gross degree of gas transport asymmetry could simulate the experimental data, indicating that inequality of Fowler dead space or asymmetry of branching alone is not sufficient.

F. Slope of the Alveolar Plateau

Sequential emptying of unequally ventilated units results in a sloping alveolar plateau. If the better-ventilated unit contributes more to the early part of expiration, the N_2 slope is always positive. Paiva (1975) analyzed the behavior of a two-compartment model representing such a system. He showed that during a multiple-breath washout both the slope (S) and the mean expired concentration ($\bar{F}_E$) fall progressively, but that the ratio ($S/\bar{F}_E$) or the normalized slope (S_n) progressively increases. After a variable number of breaths the value of S_n approaches an asymptote whose magnitude is a function of the inequality of ventilation and the degree of sequential emptying of the two units. The increase in S_n is based on the fact that the concentration difference between the two compartments increases progressively in relation to $\bar{F}_E$ until the better ventilated unit is completely washed out. Beyond this point a relative equilibrium is achieved and S_n does not rise further.

The diffusion-dependent inhomogeneity within the lung periphery, as modeled by two trumpets subtended at a branch point, also gives rise to a sloping alveolar plateau as a consequence of interaction between diffusion and convection during inspiration and expiration (Fig. 10C). After the first breath a concentration difference is established between the two trumpets, serving as the initial condition for the second breath. Despite greater dilution, the concentration difference in relation to $\bar{F}_E$ increases during the first few breaths (Fig. 11), but even in the presence of extreme branching asymmetry, a relative equilibrium is quickly established. Thus the normalized slope of the alveolar plateau (S_n) rises for only the first few breaths and then remains constant. Recently, several investigators examined experimental data in relation to the foregoing two models. Paiva et al. (1982) studied eight young nonsmoking subjects during quiet breathing, computing S_n from the terminal 30% of the expired volume in each breath. The slope was normalized by dividing it by the end expiratory N_2 concentration. The authors could not detect a significant increase in S_n between breath numbers 2 and 10 and concluded that diffusion-dependent inhomogeneity best accounts for the results obtained. However, there was a large scatter in the data and there were technical difficulties with the measurement of the slope during normal tidal breathing. Zwart et al. (1982) studied He washout after equilibration in 20 normal subjects breathing at different frequencies and tidal volumes. The authors attempted to differentiate between a diffusion-dependent and a diffusion-independent basis for the sloping alveolar plateau by measuring the He Bohr dead space for consecutive breaths. A sequentially emptying diffusion-independent model should result in progressively increasing V_{DB} during a multiple-breath washout, whereas the diffusion-dependent model should result in a rapid achievement of the steady state with no further changes in V_{DB}. The authors concluded that indeed in most of their subjects there was no evidence for progressive increase and that the experimental results could best be accounted for by the diffusion-dependent mechanism. However, here too the experimental data were noisy, partly due to the large range in V_T. The authors attempted to overcome this problem by subtracting the CO_2 Bohr dead space from the He Bohr dead space and

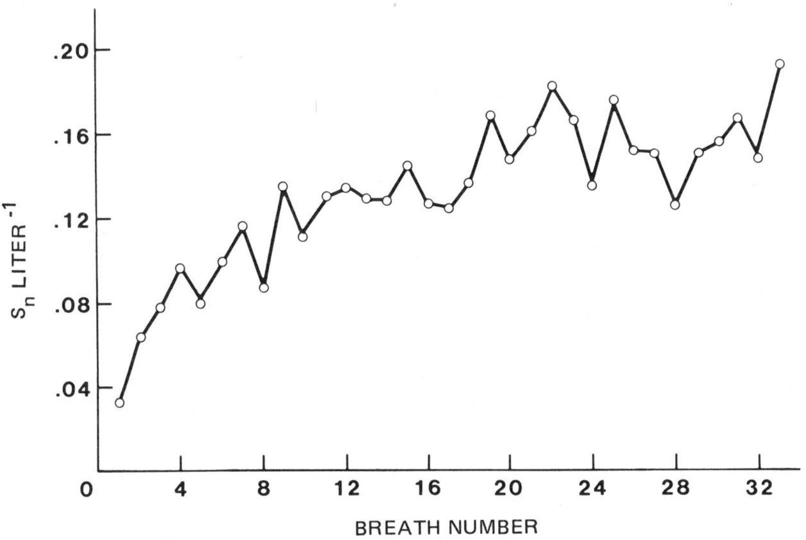

Figure 16 Slope of the alveolar plateau normalized by the mean expired concentration of each breath (S_n) during a multiple-breath N_2 washout. Each point is the mean of two runs in one subject. Note the initially rapid and subsequently gentler rise in S_n. (From Crawford et al., 1985.)

plotting the difference for consecutive breaths. No significant change as a function of breath number was seen but relative scatter was even greater.

More recently, Crawford et al. (1985) performed multiple-breath N_2 washouts in six normal subjects with rigorous control of tidal volume and frequency. The slope of the alveolar plateau was computed from the last quarter of each 1-liter expiration. The normalized slope (S_n) increased rapidly during the first four breaths and then rose more slowly. Although in some subjects an asymptote was reached, the mean data showed progressive increase in S_n over the 25-30 breaths examined (Fig. 16). The authors suggested that the initial rapid rise represents the additive effect of diffusion-dependent inhomogeneity and sequential emptying of unequally ventilated units, whereas the more gradual rise during the subsequent breaths is relatively diffusion independent. This analysis can potentially quantify the contributions of the two mechanisms under specific experimental conditions.

Kaethner et al. (1984) measured the normalized slope of the alveolar plateau during washout of He and SF_6 in dogs previously equilibrated with these gases and found the value of S_n for both gases to increase progressively as a function of lung washout. In expirograms obtained after different degrees of washout, achieved by high-frequency ventilation instead of conventional ventilation, S_n increased only slightly or not at all as a function of N_2 clearance. This is consistent with the conclusion that the inequality of ventilation among units which empty sequentially during conventional ventilation is due to differences in relative volume expansion.

VII. Other Experimental Approaches

A. Closed-System Gas Equilibration

Equilibration of lung gas with an inert gas of different composition in a closed system has been studied for nearly two centuries. A bag or spirometer of known volume and containing a known gas concentration is equilibrated by rebreathing with the lung gas whose concentration is also known. The number of breaths required to obtain equal gas concentrations in all parts of the closed lung-bag system depends on the volume of the lungs, the volume of the bag, the dead space and initial concentration difference between them, the tidal volume, and the distribution of inspired gas. As in the open-system lung washout, a number of indices of gas mixing efficiency has been derived from the pattern of inert gas concentrations. Indeed, the mathematical treatment of the data is similar and the mixing process can usually be described as the sum of two exponentials (Nye, 1961a). Theoretically, the open-circuit method may be considered as a closed-circuit method in which the bag is of infinite size (Rauwerda, 1946).

Recently, Hughes et al. (1982) reexamined the relationship between the rebreathing technique and the classical open-circuit washout after prior equilibration. The logarithm of the difference between the gas concentration in the bag and the equilibrium value was plotted against breath number (Fig. 17). Both in normal subjects and patients with airflow obstruction the curve consisted of an initial rapid phase and a second phase which was slower and virtually monoexponential. Indeed, the latter characteristic allowed estimation of an equilibrium value even when a final plateau was not reached. The diffusion dependence of gas mixing was illustrated by the different behavior of helium and SF_6. Whereas during lung washout this difference was very small and similar to that found in other studies, during closed-circuit equilibration a substantial separation was observed. The interpretation of this interesting observation in terms of gas mixing mechanisms is not yet clear.

B. Gas Exchange

Elimination of an inert gas from the blood by the lung is dependent on the balance between ventilation and perfusion and the blood-gas partition coef-

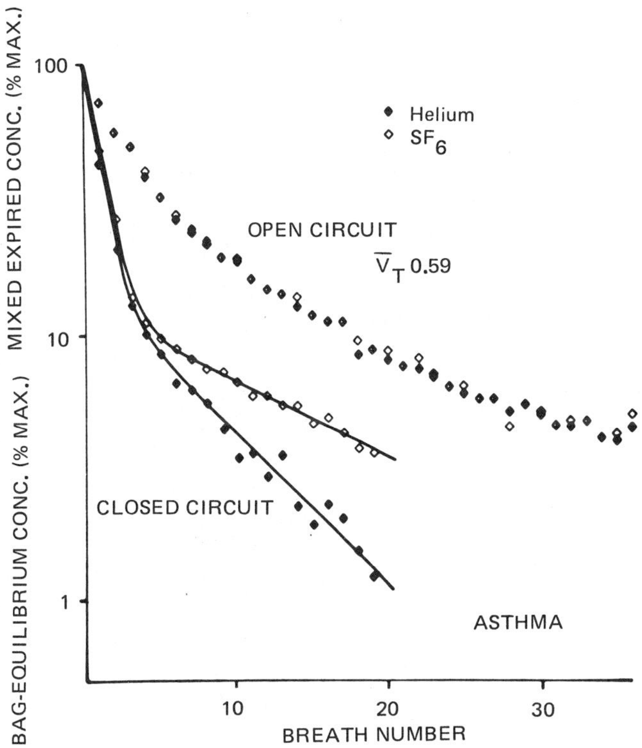

Figure 17 Comparison of open-circuit washout with closed-circuit washin of He and SF_6 tracer gases in a subject with mild asymptomatic asthma. Mean tidal volume ($\bar{V}_I$) was 0.59 liter in open circuit and 0.65 liter in closed circuit. Note the greater difference between He and SF_6 in the closed-circuit washin. (From Hughes et al., 1982.)

ficient of the gas. This concept also applies to a part of the lung and has been utilized extensively in recent years to estimate the distribution of ventilation/perfusion ratios in normal subjects and patients with lung disease. An implicit assumption of this analysis is that gas mixing within each alveolar "compartment" is complete and not diffusion limited. Yet experimental data incompatible with this model have been published. If two gases of similar solubility but different diffusivity are infused intravenously, their relative retentions and excretions should be influenced by any inefficiency of gas mixing. Conversely, if a difference in the retention and/or excretion of the two gases is observed, it can be said that incomplete gas mixing constitutes a measurable limitation to gas exchange. A formal theoretical analysis of this phenomenon has been published by Scheid et al. (1981). Computing physiological dead space from retention and excretion data, Hlastala et al. (1982) demonstrated a greater dead space for Freon 22 than for acetylene (molecular weight 86.5 and 26, respectively). Although the heavier gas had only a 5% greater physiological dead space, this could represent a substantial difference in gas concentrations within the acinus, as most of the dead-space volume is constituted by anatomical dead space in the conducting airways and is identical for both gases. A similar observation was made previously by Adaro and Farhi (1971). Ohta and Farhi (unpublished observations) showed that following a single breath of a gas mixture containing acetylene and Freon, successive arterial blood samples during breath holding at end inspiration showed a higher percentage of acetylene than of Freon during the early periods of breath holding, and the relation was reversed later. All these studies suggested that diffusion-dependent inhomogeneity plays a significant role in gas exchange within the alveolar compartment of the lung. However, this conclusion cannot be accepted without reservation. In none of the studies was V_{DF} measured for the two gases. Because of the difference in diffusivity, the V_{DF} for acetylene would be smaller, and hence alveolar concentrations higher, during inspiration (lower during infusion) than that of the heavier gas. This alone would result in a separation of the two gases with a better exchange of the lighter gas. Whether a proportion of the demonstrable difference in gas exchange is due to a difference in the alveolar dead space cannot be ascertained from the results provided. Similarly, theoretical analyses aiming to estimate an effective diffusive resistance or conductance cannot differentiate between the effects of different Fowler dead spaces and an additional diffusion-dependent inhomogeneity peripheral to the diffusion front. Oversimplified models in which the diffusion-dependent inhomogeneity is represented by a "gas film" with a finite diffusive resistance (Scheid et al., 1981) are particularly difficult to interpret, as Adaro and Piiper (1981) have shown that this leads to an overestimation of diffusive resistance when comparing the behavior of two gases with differing molecular weights.

A different approach to the study of alveolar gas mixing was taken by Bondi and Van Liew (1973), who measured arterial blood pH continuously in anesthetized-paralyzed dogs. During breath holding at end inspiration there was often a rise in pH or a "hump" before the fall brought on by CO_2 accumulation. When the carrier gas was changed from N_2 to He, the hump in the breath-holding curve was more rounded and higher, as would be expected if diffusive gas mixing at end inspiration would normally be incomplete. An alternative explanation, however, could be that continued diffusive exchange between the alveolar gas and dead space may be favored in the presence of He, even if alveolar gas were homogeneous. The observation that the hump did not differ when N_2 was replaced by SF_6 further complicated the explanation. In subsequent studies continuous arterial PO_2 measurements indicated a 14% more rapid fall of Pa_{O_2} during end expiratory breath holds on N_2 than on He (Johnson and Van Liew, 1974). This led the authors to conclude that diffusion limitation to O_2 transport existed in the lung gas in the absence of convection. When convection was included by resuming ventilation, the washin of O_2, as judged by the rate of rise of Pa_{O_2}, was 13% faster with N_2 than with He. Switching from He to N_2 during the breath hold resulted in an even faster washin and the opposite switch produced the slowest O_2 washin of all. Finally, the steady-state difference in PO_2 between inspired air and arterial blood was 6% smaller with N_2. Although the authors attempted to explain their observations in terms of Taylor dispersion, it is most unlikely that this mechanism could be responsible for significantly altering gas exchange (see Chap. 3). However, an alternative explanation of these results is not apparent.

An account of alveolar gas mixing in relation to gas exchange would not be adequate if it did not mention the paradoxical effect of the carrier gas on O_2 exchange. Several investigators have demonstrated a decrease in the alveolar-arterial O_2 difference in both animals (Martin et al., 1972) and in humans (Wood et al., 1976) when the carrier gas density is increased either by increasing ambient pressure or by replacing N_2 by SF_6. Similarly, the uptake of CO is enhanced when N_2 is replaced by SF_6 as compared with He (Kvale et al., 1975). In contrast, arterial PCO_2 and the V_{Dp}/V_T ratio may increase or remain unchanged, suggesting that gas density acts differently on the pulmonary exchange of O_2 and CO_2. A change in ventilation-perfusion matching obtained in some way could explain these results. However, Christopherson and Hlastala (1982) confirmed the paradoxical effect of gas density in dogs breathing a He-O_2 mixture but could not demonstrate any change in $\dot{V}_A/Q$ distribution using a multiple inert gas elimination technique. The adequacy of sampling alveolar gas is not at issue, as at least in some of the studies the reduction in (A-a) D_{O_2} was clearly due to a change in arterial PO_2. Until now these interesting observations remain unexplained. Finally, despite the considerable number of studies showing similar trends, a recent one, apparently carried out with no less rigor, failed to show any influence of gas physical properties on gas exchange in healthy humans (Nemery et al., 1983).

C. Frequency Dependence of Compliance

When the lung is modeled as consisting of independently ventilated units, each with a different compliance (C) and resistance (R), the product of these (RC) determines the rate of entry of gas into each lung unit (Otis et al.,

1956). Units whose RC product or time constant is low should fill and empty faster than regions with a high RC. According to the time constant theory, changes in gas flow at different breathing frequencies may be reflected in changes in dynamic compliance (C_{dyn}). In normal subjects aged 30-49 years, C_{dyn}, when corrected for pulmonary inertance, is frequency independent up to 90 breaths per minute (bpm) (Macklem, 1971). In older subjects C_{dyn} decreases significantly. However, the frequency independence of C_{dyn} in young normal subjects does not necessarily imply synchronous or homogeneous gas flow distribution. Using a two-compartment model, Bake et al. (1974) calculated that when C_{dyn} decreased by 7% at 100 bpm, the distribution of tidal volume could change by 30%. When the difference in resistance was increased so that time constants differed 10-fold and a detectable fall in C_{dyn} was simulated (25% at 100 bpm), the tidal volume ratio changed by 100%. In fact, it is implicit in the analysis of Otis et al. (1956) that gas flow and ventilation distribution may be quite frequency dependent when C_{dyn} is not. Furthermore, differences in time constants must exceed a factor of 2.5-3.0 before C_{dyn} falls abnormally. Yet prediction of frequency dependence of C_{dyn} from a compartmental analysis of a multibreath N_2 washout, performed at a single frequency, showed a good correaltion with measurements in healthy smokers and in normal subjects after carbachol-induced bronchoconstriction (Wanner et al., 1974). Furthermore, differences between N_2 washouts performed at different breathing frequencies roughly matched the change in C_{dyn} (Ingram and Schilder, 1967). Assuming values for regional compliance and resistance, derived from the gradient of regional expansion, Bake et al. (1974) calculated that interregional differences in time constants could account for only a 7% reduction in C_{dyn} at 100 bpm. In fact, there is good evidence that regional ventilation distribution remains unchanged in subjects who increase their breathing frequency from 12 to 57 bpm even when C_{dyn} can be shown to fall by 35% (Forkert et al., 1978). The basis for this fall must therefore lie within rather than between lung regions.

D. Regional Clearance Studies

In a homogeneously ventilated region a plot of expired gas concentration against breath number is similar to that using alveolar gas concentrations. In contrast, in an inhomogeneously ventilated region, the concentration of gas leaving is weighted initially by the better-ventilated units, whereas that within the region is weighted by the poorly ventilated units. Thus the washout at the exit of such a region will differ from the decay of gas within the region. In keeping with the foregoing analysis, frequency dependence of intraregional gas flow distribution is demonstrable by comparing multiple-breath washouts of a radioactive inert tracer gas, measured at the mouth, with decay curves obtained by external counting over the chest. During quiet breathing at 10-12 bpm a multiple-breath washout of ^{133}Xe recorded at the mouth corresponds to that measured over the whole lung (Forkert et al., 1978). The expired curve constitutes an average of regional washout rates, weighted by the better-ventilated dependent region. However, at 60 bpm all the regional washouts are delayed relative to that at the mouth, requiring a greater alveolar ventilation to halve the initial gas concentration ($VA_{0.5}$). Hence the $VA_{0.5}$ of all regions is greater (washout is slower) than the $VA_{0.5}$ recorded at the mouth. These observations clearly indicate frequency-dependent maldistribution within lung regions, not easily detectable by analysis of expired gas. Indeed, numerous studies have shown little effect of breathing frequency on multiple-breath inert gas washouts recorded at the mouth (Bouhuys et al., 1961; Ingram and Schilder, 1967; Young et al., 1968).

Forkert et al. (1978) examined the possible mechanisms responsible for the difference between regional and mouth washouts at high breathing frequencies. They concluded that intraregional frequency dependence of ventilation distribution is due primarily to parallel time constant inequalities, which may differ by about a factor of 10! The fall in dynamic compliance with breathing frequency correlated with the increase in chest/mouth $VA_{0.5}$ ratio. However, whereas frequency dependence of C_{dyn} is enhanced when subjects breathe a denser gas mixture (Forkert et al., 1975), the increase in regional chest/mouth $VA_{0.5}$ ratios was unchanged. Hence the correlation between the two sets of observations does not necessarily point to a single underlying mechanism.

E. Inhomogeneity of Breath Sounds

An ingenious approach to the measurement of intraregional ventilation maldistribution is that of recording breath sounds with two identical microphones at the same horizontal level over the chest (Ploysongsang, 1984). Two microphone-amplifier systems were calibrated and adjusted to have identical sensitivity and frequency response to vesicular breath sound intensity. After adequate compensation for sound transmission, phase differences in the sound envelopes recorded over the two parts of the chest wall reflected a sequence in inspiratory flow to the two regions.

In 34 volunteers, consisting of 19 nonsmokers and 15 smokers with minimal symptoms, the outputs of the two microphones were plotted in an X-Y mode during small breaths of 200-300 ml at flow rates of 1-5 liters/sec. The resultant loops could be analyzed and quantified in terms of phase angles. The nonsmokers tended to have smaller phase angles of about 2-4°, whereas smokers had phase angles of about 7-9°. The direction of looping was consistent between any two positions at the same horizontal level. The phase angle (θ) was found to correlate with the frequency dependence of C_{dyn} but not with the slope of phase III during a single-breath N_2 test. Since similar measurements of breath intensity were previously shown to indicate the distribution of regional ventilation (Ploysongsang et al., 1978), it is likely that the results do indeed reflect sequences of inspiratory flow within the same horizontal lung slice. The fact that even in normal nonsmoking subjects a small but significant degree of looping was observed at flows of 1-5 liters/sec is consistent with the presence of intraregional differences in static and/or dynamic mechanical properties.

VIII. Summary

Distribution of inspired gas is not uniform even in normal lungs. Both in terms of localization and mechanism the nonuniformity is determined at a series of branch points extending from the carina to the lung periphery, and subtending alveolated lung units of progressively decreasing size. Nonuniform distribution of the inspirate at the most proximal branch points (subtending lobar and sublobar bronchi) relates to regional differences in pulmonary compliance and resistance as well as in pleural pressure (Chap. 5). At the proximal branch points within lung regions, when flow-resistive pressure drops are substantial, dynamic factors related to the time constants of the subtended units contribute to the distribution of bulk flow and/or inspired volume. More peripherally, where axial flow velocities are low, interaction between convection and molecular diffusion determines the inflow and outflow of the inspired gas species. Intra-acinar asymmetry of path lengths as well as inequality of airway cross sections may result in marked parallel inhomogeneity of gas concentrations even in the presence of homogeneous lung expansion. In addition, however, nonuniform pressure-volume relationships of different units probably contribute to the inequality of ventilation distribution at most levels of the branch point hierarchy.

The concepts discussed above have been inferred from experimental data which consist predominantly of studies in which inert gases are breathed and expired gas is analyzed. Single inspirates and/or washouts of inert gas provide some information about the dead space of the lung and the unequal distribution of inspired gas. However, results from single-breath tests are weighted by the better-ventilated units. The more nonuniform the lung, the less well represented is its behavior by a single breath. Multiple-breath washouts of an equilibrated gas offer the potential for a more comprehensive description of the dead space, mixing efficiency, and gas distribution in the lung. Advances in computer technology and modeling techniques hold out exciting possibilities for a more accurate representation of ventilation inequality in the form of continuous distributions of specific ventilation of lung units. At the same time, comparison of the experimental data with predictions from sophisticated models based on well-defined physical mechanisms and anatomy should help to elucidate and quantify the factors responsible for the inhomogeneity of ventilation distribution and impairment in gas mixing in normal subjects and in patients with different lung diseases.

References

Adaro, F., and Farhi, L. E. (1971). Effects of intra lobular gas diffusion on alveolar gas exchange. *Fed. Proc.*, **30**:437.

Adaro, F., and Piiper, J. (1981). Interpretation of simultaneous intrapulmonary equilibration of gases of differing diffusivities. *Prog. Respir. Res.*, **16**:68-72.

Anthonisen, N. R., Danson, J., Robertson, P. C., and Ross, W. R. D. (1969-70). Airway closure as a function of age. *Respir. Physiol.*, **8**:58-65.

Anthonisen, N. R., Robertson, P. C., and Ross, W. R. D. (1970). Gravity-dependent sequential emptying of lung regions. *J. Appl. Physiol.*, **28**: 589-595.

Anthonisen, N. R., Peress, L. J., Siegler, D. M., and Dhingra, S. (1978). Lung volume, volume history, and the distribution of inhaled boluses. *Respir. Physiol.*, **33**:279-288.

Bake, B., Wood, L., Murphy, B., Macklem, P. T., and Milic-Emili, J. (1974). Effect of inspiratory flow rate on regional distribution of inspired gas. *J. Appl. Physiol.*, **37**:8-17.

Bashoff, M. A., Ingram, R. H. Jr., and Schilder, D. P. (1967). Effect of expiratory flow rate on the nitrogen concentration vs. volume relationship. *J. Appl. Physiol.*, **23**(6):895-901.

Bateman, J. B. (1950). Studies of lung volume and intrapulmonary mixing. Nitrogen clearance curves: apparent respiratory dead space and its significance. *J. Appl. Physiol.*, **3**:143-160.

Berend, N., and Grunstein, M. J. (1983). Determinants of maldistribution of ventilation in excised human lungs. *Aust. N.Z. J. Med.*, **13**:554.

Berend, N., Woolcock, A. J., and Marlin, G. E. (1979). Correlation between the function and structure of the lung in smokers. *Am. Rev. Respir. Dis.*, **119**:695-705.

Birath, G. (1959). Respiratory dead space measurements in a model lung and healthy human subjects according to the single breath method. *J. Appl. Physiol.*, **14**(4):517-520.

Bohr, C. (1891). Ueber die Lungenathmung. *Skand. Arch. Physiol.*, **2**:236-268.

Bondi, K. R., and Van Liew, H. D. (1973). Fluxes of CO_2 in the lung gas studied by continuously recorded arterial pH. *J. Appl. Physiol.,* **35**: 42-46.

Bouhuys, A. (1963). Effect of posture in experimental asthma in man. *Am. J. Med.,* **34**:470-476.

Bouhuys, A. (1964). Distribution of inspired gas in the lungs. In *Handbook of Physiology,* Sec. 3: *Respiration,* Vol. I. Edited by W. O. Fenn and H. Rahn. Washington, D.C., American Physiological Society, pp. 715-733.

Bouhuys, A., and Van Lennep, H. J. (1962). Effect of body posture on gas distribution in the lungs. *J. Appl. Physiol.,* **17**(1):38-42.

Bouhuys, A., Hagstam, K. E., and Lundin, G. (1956). Efficiency of pulmonary ventilation during rest and light exercise. *Acta Physiol. Scand.,* **35**:289-304.

Bouhuys, A., Jonsson, R., and Lundin, G. (1957). Influence of added dead space on pulmonary ventilation. *Acta. Physiol. Scand.,* **39**:105-120.

Bouhuys, A., Lichtneckert, S., Lundgren, C., and Lundin, G. (1961). Voluntary changes in breathing pattern and N_2 clearance from lungs. *J. Appl. Physiol.,* **16**:1039-1042.

Bowes, C., Cumming, G., Horsfield, K., Loughhead, J., and Preston, S. (1982). Gas mixing in an asymmetrical model of the pulmonary acinus with asymmetrical alveolar ducts. *J. Appl. Physiol.,* **52**:624-633.

Briscoe, W. A., and Cournand, A. (1959). Uneven ventilation of normal and diseased lungs studied by an open-circuit method. *J. Appl. Physiol.,* **14**:284-290.

Buist, A. S., and Ross, B. B. (1973). Quantitative analysis of the alveolar plateau in the diagnosis of early airway obstruction. *Am. Rev. Respir. Dis.,* **108**:1079-1089.

Christopherson, S. K., and Hlastala, M. P. (1982). Pulmonary gas exchange during altered density gas breathing. *J. Appl. Physiol. Respir. Environ. Exercise Physiol.,* **52**(1):221-225.

Comroe, J. H., Jr., and Fowler, W. S. (1951). Lung function studies: VI. Detection of uneven alveolar ventilation during a single breath of oxygen. *Am. J. Med.,* **10**:408-413.

Cormier, Y., and Belanger, J. (1983). Quantification of the effect of gas exchange on the slope of phase III. *Bull. Eur. Physiopathol. Respir.,* **19**:13-16.

Cortese, D. A., Rodarte, J. R., Rehder, K., and Hyatt, R. E. (1976). Effect of posture on single-breath oxygen test in normal subjects. *J. Appl. Physiol.,* **41**:474-479.

Cosio, M., Ghezzo, H., Hogg, J. C., Corbin, R., Loveland, M., Dosman, J., and Macklem, P. T. (1977). The relations between structural changes in small airways and pulmonary-function tests. *N. Engl. J. Med.*, **298**: 1277-1281.

Cournand, A., Baldwin, R., Darling, R. C., and Richards, D. W. (1941). Studies on intrapulmonary mixture of gases: IV. The significance of the pulmonary emptying rate and a simplified open circuit measurement of residual air. *J. Clin. Invest.*, **20**:681-689.

Crawford, H., Makowska, M., Paiva, M., and Engel, L. A. (1985). Convection and diffusion dependent ventilation maldistribution in normal subjects. *J. Appl. Physiol. Respir. Environ. Exercise Physiol.* (submitted).

Cumming, G. (1967). Gas mixing efficiency in the human lung. *Respir. Physiol.*, **2**:213-224.

Cumming, G., and Guyatt, A. R. (1982). Alveolar gas mixing efficiency in the human lung. *Clin. Sci.*, **62**:541-547.

Cumming, G., Horsfield, K., Jones, J. G., and Muir, D. C. F. (1967). The influence of gaseous diffusion on the alveolar plateau at different lung volumes. *Respir. Physiol.*, **2**:386-398.

Cutillo, A., Omboni, E., and Delgrossi, S. (1972). Effects of respiratory frequency on distribution of inspired gas in normal subjects and in patients with chronic obstructive lung disease. *Am. Rev. Respir. Dis.*, **105**:756-767.

Cutillo, A., Perondi, R., Turiel, M., Egger, J., Watanabe, S., and Renzetti, A. (1981). Reproducibility of multibreath nitrogen washout measurements. *Am. Rev. Respir. Dis.*, **124**:505-507.

Darling, R. C., Cournand, A., and Richards, D. W. (1944). Studies on intrapulmonary mixture of gases: V. Forms of inadequate ventilation in normal and emphysematous lungs, analyzed by means of breathing pure oxygen. *J. Clin. Invest.*, **23**:55-67.

De Vries, W. R., and Luijendijk, S. C. M. (1982). Shape of single breath washout curves of gases with different diffusion coefficients and blood solubilities. *Bull. Eur. Physiopathol. Respir.*, **18**:215-227.

De Vries, W. R., Luijendijk, S. C. M., and Zwart, A. (1981). Helium and sulphur hexafluoride washout in asymmetrical lung models. *J. Appl. Physiol.*, **51**:1122-1130.

Dollfuss, R. E., Milic-Emili, J., and Bates, D. V. (1967). Regional ventilation of the lung, studied with boluses of ^{133}xenon. *Respir. Physiol.*, **2**:234-246.

Edelman, N. H., Mittman, C., Norris, A. H., Shock, N. W. (1968). Effects of respiratory pattern on age differences in ventilation uniformity. *J. Appl. Physiol.*, **24**:49-53.

Engel, L. A., and Macklem, P. T. (1977). Gas mixing and distribution in the lung. *International Review of Physiology*, Vol. 14: *Respiratory*

Physiology II. Edited by J. G. Widdicombe. Baltimore, University Park Press, pp. 37-82.

Engel, L. A., and Paiva, M. (1981). Analyses of sequential filling and emptying of the lung. *Respir. Physiol.,* **45**:309-321.

Engel, L. A., Menkes, H., Wood, L. D. H., Utz, G., Joubert, J., and Macklem, P. T. (1973a). Gas mixing during breathholding studied by intrapulmonary gas sampling. *J. Appl. Physiol.,* **35**:9-17.

Engel, L. A., Wood, L. D. H., Utz, G., and Macklem, P. T. (1973b). Gas mixing during inspiration. *J. Appl. Physiol.,* **35**:18-24.

Engel, L. A., Utz, G., Wood, L. D. H., and Macklem, P. T. (1974). Ventilation distribution in anatomical lung units. *J. Appl. Physiol.,* **37**:194-200.

Engel, L. A., Grassino, A., and Anthonisen, N. R. (1975). Demonstration of airway closure in man. *J. Appl. Physiol.,* **38**:1117-1125.

Engel, L. A., Landau, L., Taussig, L., Martin, R. R., and Sybrecht, G. (1976). Influence of bronchomotor tone on regional ventilation distribution at residual volume. *J. Appl. Physiol.,* **40**:411-416.

Evans, J. W. (1970). The gas washout determination under a symmetry assumption. *Bull. Math. Biophys.,* **32**:59-63.

Fleming, G. M., Chester, E. H., Saniie, J., Saidel, G. M. (1980). Ventilation inhomogeneity using multibreath nitrogen washout: comparison of moment ratios and other indexes. *Am. Rev. Respir. Dis.,* **121**:789-794.

Folkow, B., and Pappenheimer, J. R. (1955). Components of the respiratory dead space and their variation with pressure breathing and with bronchoactive drugs. *J. Appl. Physiol.,* **5**:102-110.

Forkert, L., Wood, L. D. H., and Cherniack, R. M. (1975). Effect of gas density on dynamic pulmonary compliance. *J. Appl. Physiol.,* **39**:906-910.

Forkert, L., Anthonisen, N. R., and Wood, L. D. H. (1978). Frequency dependence of regional lung washout. *J. Appl. Physiol.,* **45**:161-170.

Forkert, L., Dhingra, S., and Anthonisen, N. R. (1979). Airway closure and closing volume. *J. Appl. Physiol. Respir. Environ. Exercise Physiol.,* **46**:24-30.

Fowler, W. S. (1948). Lung function studies: II. The respiratory dead space. *Am. J. Physiol.,* **154**:405-416.

Fowler, W. S. (1949). Lung function studies: III. Uneven pulmonary ventilation in normal subjects and in patients with pulmonary disease. *J. Appl. Physiol.,* **2**:283-299.

Fowler, W. S., Cornish, E. R., and Ketty, S. S. (1952). Lung function studies: VIII. Analysis of alveolar ventilation pulmonary N_2 clearance curves. *J. Clin. Invest.,* **31**:40-50.

Fukuchi, Y., Cosio, M., Kelly, S., and Engel, L. A. (1977). Influence of pericardial fluid on cardiogenic gas mixing in the lung. *J. Appl. Physiol.,* **42**:5-12.

Fukuchi, Y., Cosio, M., Murphy, B., and Engel, L. A. (1980). Intraregional basis for sequential filling and emptying of the lung. *Respir. Physiol.,* **41**:253-266.

Georg, J., Lassen, N. A., Mellemgaard, K., and Vinther, A. (1965). Diffusion in the gas phase of the lungs in normal and emphysematous subjects. *Clin. Sci.,* **29**:525-532.

Gomez, D. M., Briscoe, W. A., and Cumming, G. (1964). Continuous distribution of specific tidal volume throughout the lung. *J. Appl. Physiol.,* **19**(4):683-692.

Gray, J. S., Grodins, S., and Carter, E. T. (1956). Alveolar and total ventilation and dead space problem. *J. Appl. Physiol.,* **9**:307-320.

Greifenstein, F. E., King, R. M., Latch, S. S., and Comroe, J. M. (1952). Pulmonary function studies in healthy men and women 50 years and older. *J. Appl. Physiol.,* **4**:641-648.

Haldane, J. S. (1915). The variation in the effective dead space in breathing. *Am. J. Physiol.,* **38**:20-28.

Hashimoto, T., Young, A. C., and Martin, C. J. (1967). Compartmental analysis of the distribution of gas in the lungs. *J. Appl. Physiol.,* **23**: 203-209.

Hlastala, M. P., McKenna, H. P., Middaugh, M., and Robertson, H. T. (1982). Role of diffusion-dependent gas inhomogeneity in gas exchange in the dog. *Bull. Europ. Physiopath. Resp.,* **18**:373-380.

Horsfield, K., and Cumming, G. (1968). Functional consequences of airway morphology. *J. Appl. Physiol.,* **24**:384-390.

Horsfield, K., Gabe, I., Mills, C., Buckman, M., and Cumming, G. (1982). Effect of heart rate and stroke volume on gas mixing in dog lung. *J. Appl. Physiol.,* **53**(6):1603-1607.

Hughes, J. M. B., Jones, H. A., and Davies, E. E. (1982). Applications of multi-breath washin measurements in closed circuit using a mass spectrometer. *Bull. Eur. Physiopathol. Respir.,* **18**:309-317.

Ingram, R. H., Jr., and Schilder, D. P. (1967). Association of a decrease in dynamic compliance with a change in gas distribution. *J. Appl. Physiol.,* **23**:911-916.

Johnson, L. R., and Van Liew, H. D. (1974). Use of arterial pO_2 to study convective and diffusive gas mixing in the lungs. *J. Appl. Physiol.,* **36**:91-97.

Jones, J. G. (1967). The effect of preinspiratory lung volume on the result of the single breath O_2 test. *Resp. Physiol.,* **2**:375-385.

Kaethner, T., Kohl, J., and Scheid, P. (1984). Gas concentration profiles along the airways of dog lungs during high-frequency ventilation. *J. Appl. Physiol. Respir. Environ. Exercise Physiol.,* **56**:1491-1499.

Kawashiro, T., Sikand, R. S., Adaro, F., Takahashi, H., and Piiper, J. (1961). Study of intrapulmonary gas mixing in man by simultaneous washout of helium and sulfur hexafluoride. *Resp. Physiol.*, **28**:261-275.

Kelly, S., Cohen, C., Powell, E., Paiva, M., and Engel, L. A. (1982a). Gas mixing in the lungs of dogs and pigs. *Respir. Physiol.*, **47**:341-349.

Kelly, S., Paiva, M., and Engel, L. A. (1982b). Bronchoconstriction and gas mixing in canine and pig lungs. *Bull. Eur. Physiopathol. Respir.*, **18**:229-237.

Kim, T. S., Rahn, H., and Farhi, L. E. (1966). Estimation of true venous and arterial pCO_2 by gas analysis of a single breath. *J. Appl. Physiol.*, **21**:1338-1344.

Kjellmer, I., Sandqvist, L., and Berglund, E. (1959). Alveolar plateau of the single breath nitrogen elimination curve in normal subjects. *J. Appl. Physiol.*, **14**(1):105-108.

Kox, W., Langley, F., Horsfield, K., and Cumming, G. (1982). Effect of atropine on alveolar gas mixing in man. *Clin. Sci.*, **62**:549-551.

Krogh, A., and Lindhard, J. (1917). The volume of the dead space in breathing and the mixing of gases in the lungs of man. *J. Physiol.*, **51**:59-90.

Kvale, P. A., Davis, J., and Schroter, R. C. (1975). Effect of gas density and ventilatory pattern on steady-state CO uptake by the lung. *Respir. Physiol.*, **24**:385-398.

Lacquet, L. M., and Van Muylem, A. (1982). He and SF_6 single-breath expiration curves. Comparison with the Paiva-Engel model. *Bull. Eur. Physiopathol. Respir.*, **18**:239-246.

Lacquet, L. M., Van der Linden, L. P., and Paiva, M. (1975). Transport of H_2 and SF_6 in the lungs. *Respir. Physiol.*, **25**:157-173.

Lewis, S., and Martin, C. J. (1979). Characteristics of the washout dead space. *Respir. Physiol.*, **36**:51-36.

Lewis, S., Evans, J. W., and Jalowayski, A. A. (1978). Continuous distribution of specific ventilation recovered from inert gas washout. *J. Appl. Physiol.*, **44**:416-423.

Lewis, S. M., D'Argenio, D. Z., Bekey, G. A., and Mittman, C. (1982). Optimal inputs for parameter determination of inert gas washout from the lung. *Respir. Physiol.*, **50**:111-127.

Lifshay, A., Fast, C. W., and Glazier, J. B. (1971). Effects of changes in respiratory pattern on physiological dead space. *J. Appl. Physiol.*, **31**: 478-483.

Lillington, G. A., Fowler, W. S., Miller, R. D., and Helmolz, H. F., Jr. (1959). Nitrogen clearance rates of right and left lungs in different positions. *J. Clin. Invest.*, **38**:2026-2034.

Loewy, A. (1894). Ueber die Bestimmung der Grösse des "Schädlichen

Luftraumes" im Thorax und der alveolaren Sauerstoffspannung. *Arch. Ges. Physiol.,* **58**:416-427.

Luijendijk, S. C. M., Zwart, A., De Vries, W. R., and Salet, W. M. (1980). The sloping alveolar plateau at synchronous ventilation. *Pfluegers Arch.,* **384**:267-277.

Macklem, P. T. (1971). Airway obstruction and collateral ventilation. *Physiol. Rev.,* **51**:368-436.

Magnussen, H., and Smidt, U. (1981). Intrapulmonary gas transport of He and SF_6 in healthy subjects and patients with chronic obstructive lung disease. *Respiration,* **41**:73-81.

Martin, R. R., Zutter, M., and Anthonisen, N. R. (1972). Pulmonary gas exchange in dogs breathing SF_6 at 4 Atm. *J. Appl. Physiol.,* **33**:86-92.

Martin, C. J., Tsunoda, S., and Young, A. C. (1974). Lung emptying patterns in diffuse obstructive pulmonary syndromes. *Respir. Physiol.,* **21**:157-168.

Martin, C. J., Das, S., and Young, A. C. (1979). Measurements of the dead space volume. *J. Appl. Physiol. Respir. Environ. Exercise Physiol.,* **47**(2):319-324.

Meyer, M., Hook, C., Rieke, H., and Piiper, J. (1983). Gas mixing in dog lungs studied by single breath washout of He and SF_6. *J. Appl. Physiol. Respir. Environ. Exercise Physiol.,* **55**:1795-1802.

Michels, D. B., and West, J. B. (1978). Distribution of pulmonary ventilation and perfusion during short periods of weightlessness. *J. Appl. Physiol.,* **45**:9876-998.

Millette, B., Robertson, P. C., Ross, W. R. D., and Anthonisen, N. R. (1969). Effect of expiratory flow rate on emptying of lung regions. *J. Appl. Physiol.,* **27**:587-591.

Mills, R. J., and Harris, P. (1965). Factors influencing the concentration of expired nitrogen after a breath of oxygen. *J. Appl. Physiol.,* **20**:103-109.

Nakamura, T., Takishima, T., Okubo, T., Sasaki, T., and Takahashi, H. (1966). Distribution function of the clearance time constant in lungs. *J. Appl. Physiol.,* **21**:227-232.

Nemery, B., Nullens, W., Veriter, C., Brasseur, L., and Frans, A. (1983). Effects of gas density on pulmonary gas exchange of normal man at rest and during exercise. *Pfluegers Arch.,* **397**:57-61.

Nye, R. E. (1961a). Closed circuit method for measuring uneven ventilation. *J. Appl. Physiol.,* **16**:1109-1114.

Nye, R. E. (1961b). Theoretical limits to measurement of uneven ventilation. *J. Appl. Physiol.,* **16**:1115-1123.

Okubo, T., and Lenfant, C. (1968). Distribution function of lung volume and ventilation determined by lung N_2 washout. *J. Appl. Physiol.,* **24**:658-667.

Okubo, T., and Piiper, J. (1974). Intrapulmonary gas mixing in excised dog lung lobes studied by simultaneous wash-out of two inert gases. *Respir. Physiol.,* **21**:223-239.

Olsen, H. C., and Gilson, J. C. (1960). Respiratory symptoms, bronchitis and ventilatory capacity in men. *Br. Med. J.,* **1**:45-46.

Otis, A. B., McKerrow, C. B., Bartlett, R. A., Mead, J., McIlroy, M. B., Selverstone, N. J., and Radford, E. P., Jr. (1956). Mechanical factors in distribution of pulmonary ventilation. *J. Appl. Physiol.,* **8**:427-443.

Paiva, M. (1973). Gas transport in the human lung. *J. Appl. Physiol.,* **35**(3):401-410.

Paiva, M. (1975). Two new pulmonary functional indexes suggested by a simple mathematical model. *Respiration,* **32**:389-403.

Paiva, M., and Engel, L. A. (1982). Influence of bronchial asymmetry on cardiogenic gas mixing in the lung. *Respir. Physiol.,* **49**:325-338.

Paiva, M., and Engel, L. A. (1984). Model analysis of gas distribution within the human lung acinus. *J. Appl. Physiol.,* **56**.

Paiva, M., Van Muylem, A., and Engel, L. A. (1982). The slope of phase III in multibreath N_2 washout and washin. *Bull. Eur. Physiopathol. Respir.,* **18**:273-280.

Palmieri, G. G. (1949). La petite respiration cardiaque et les dyskinésies cardio-pulmonaires. *Bull. Schweiz. Akad. Med. Wiss.,* **5**:55-68.

Petrini, M. F., Peterson, B. T., Hyde, R. W., Lam, V., Utel, M. J., and Kallay, M. C. (1982). Uneven gas mixing during rebreathing assessed by simultaneously measuring dead space. *J. Appl. Physiol. Respir. Environ. Exercise Physiol.,* **53**(4):930-939.

Petty, T. L., Silvers, G. W., Stenford, R. E., Baird, M. D., and Mitchell, R. S. (1980). Small airway pathology is related to increased closing capacity and abnormal slope of phase III in excised human lungs. *Am. Rev. Respir. Dis.,* **121**:449-456.

Ploysongsang, Y. (1983). The lung sounds phase angle test for detection of small airway disease. *Respir. Physiol.,* **53**:203-214.

Ploysongsang, Y., Macklem, P. T., and Ross, W. R. D. (1978). Distribution of regional ventilation measured by breath sounds. *Am. Rev. Respir. Dis.,* **117**:657-664.

Power, G. G. (1969). Gaseous diffusion between airways and alveoli in the human lung. *J. Appl. Physiol.,* **27**:701-709.

Prowse, K., and Cumming, G. (1973). Effects of lung volume and disease on the lung nitrogen decay curve. *J. Appl. Physiol.,* **34**:23-33.

Rauwerda, P. E. (1946). Unequal ventilation of different parts of the lung. Ph.D. thesis, University of Groningen, Groningen, The Netherlands.

Read, J., and Lee, J. (1969). Effect of changes of tidal volume on dead space in obstructive lung disease. *J. Appl. Physiol.*, **26**:105-110.

Robertson, J. S., Siri, W. E., and Jones, H. B. (1950). Lung ventilation patterns determined by analysis of nitrogen elimination rates; use of the mass spectrometer as a continuous gas analyzer. *J. Clin. Invest.*, **29**:577-590.

Roelsen, E. (1938). Fractional analysis of alveolar air after inspiration of hydrogen as a method for the determination of the distribution of inspired air in the lungs. *Acta Med. Scand.*, **95**452-482.

Roos, A., Dahlstrom, H., and Murphy, J. P. (1954). Distribution of inspired air in the lungs. *J. Appl. Physiol.*, **7**:645-659.

Rossier, P. H., and Buhlman, A. (1955). The respiratory dead space. *Physiol. Rev.*, **35**:860-876.

Ruff, F., Martin, R. R., and Milic-Emili, J. (1981). Previous volume history of the lung and regional distribution of residual volume. *J. Appl. Physiol.*, **51**:313-316.

Salmon, R. B., Saidel, G. M., Inkley, S. R., and Niewoehner, D. E. (1982). Relationship of ventilation inhomogeneity to morphologic variables in excised human lungs. *Am. Rev. Respir. Dis.*, **126**:686-690.

Saniie, J., Saidel, G. M., and Chester, E. H. (1979). Real-time moment analysis of pulmonary nitrogen washout. *J. Appl. Physiol.*, **46**:1184-1190.

Scheid, P., Hlastala, M. P., and Piiper, J. (1981). Inert gas elimination from lungs with stratified inhomogeieity. Theory. *Respir. Physiol.*, **44**:299-309.

Severinghaus, J. W., and Stupfel, M. (1957). Alveolar dead space as an index of distribution of blood flow in pulmonary capillaries. *J. Appl. Physiol.*, **10**:335-348.

Siebeck, R. (1911). Ueber den Gasaustausch zwischen Aussenluft und Alveolen. 2e Mitteilung. Ueber die Bedeutung and Bestimmung des "Schädlichen Raumes" bei der Atmung. *Skand. Arch. Physiol.*, **25**:81-95.

Siegler, D. I. M., Fukuchi, Y., and Engel, L. A. (1976). Influence of bronchomotor tone on ventilation distribution and airway closure in asymptomatic asthma. *Am. Rev. Respir. Dis.*, **114**:123-130.

Slutsky, A. S. (1981). Gas mixing by cardiogenic oscillations. A theoretical, quantitative analysis. *J. Appl. Physiol.*, **51**:1287-1293.

Stanescu, D., Teculescu, D., and Pacuraru, R. (1968a). Reproducibility and normal values of the single breath nitrogen test. *Scand. J. Respir. Dis.*, **49**:322-330.

Stanescu, D. C., Teculescu, D. B., Pacuraru, R., and Popa, V. (1968b). Effect of bronchoconstrictor aerosol on the alveolar plateau of the single breath O_2 test. *Thorax*, **23**:628.

Tsunoda, S., Young, A. C., and Martin, C. J. (1972). Emptying pattern of lung compartments in normal man. *J. Appl. Physiol.,* **32**:644-649

Van Liew, H. D. (1962). Semilogarithmic plots of data which reflect a continuum of exponential processes. *Science,* **138**:682-683.

Von Nieding, G., Lollgen, H., Smidt, U., and Linde, H. (1977). Simultaneous washout of helium and sulfur hexafluoride in healthy subjects and patients with chronic bronchitis, bronchial asthma, and emphysema. *Am. Rev. Respir. Dis.,* **116**:649-659.

Wagner, P. D. (1979). Information content of the multibreath nitrogen washout. *J. Appl. Physiol.,* **46**:579-587.

Wanner, A., Zarzecki, S., Atkins, N., Zapata, A., and Sackner, M. A. (1974). Relationship between frequency dependence of lung compliance and distribution of ventilation. *J. Clin. Invest.,* **54**:1200-1213.

Wei, J. H., Hoffman, E. A., Ritman, E. L., and Wood, E. H. (1985). Cardiogenic motion of the right lung parenchyma in anesthetized intact dogs. *J. Appl. Physiol.* (in press).

West, J. B., and Hugh-Jones, P. (1961). Pulsatile gas flow in bronchi caused by the heart beat. *J. Appl. Physiol.,* **16**:697-702.

Wood, L. D. H., Bryan, A. C., Bau, S. K., Weng, T. R., and Levison, H. (1976). Effect of increased gas density on pulmonary gas exchange in man. *J. Appl. Physiol.,* **41**:206-210.

Worth, H., and Smidt, U. (1982). Phase II of expiratory curves of respiratory and inert gases in normals and in patients with emphysema. *Bull. Eur. Physiopathol. Respir.,* **18**:247-253.

Young, A. C., Martin, C. J., and Hashimoto, T. (1968). Can the distribution of inspired gas be altered? *J. Appl. Physiol.,* **24**:129-134.

Zuntz, N. (1882). Physiologie der Blutgase und des respiratorischen Gaswechsels. In *Handbook der Physiologie,* Vol. 4. Edited by L. Hermann. Leipzig, Voge.

Zwart, A., Jansen, J. R. C., and Luijendijk, S. C. M. (1982). Bohr dead space during helium washout. *Bull. Eur. Physiopathol. Respir.,* **18**: 261-272.

8

Distribution and Mixing in Gas-Exchange Organs of Nonmammalian Vertebrates

PETER SCHEID

Institut für Physiologie
Ruhr-Universität
Bochum, Federal Republic of Germany

JOHANNES PIIPER

Max-Planck-Institut für experimentelle Medizin
Göttingen, Federal Republic of Germany

I. Introduction

When each alveolar portion of the mammalian lung receives an equal share of ventilation and blood flow, and when mixing in alveolar gas is complete, the alveolar lung may be referred to as homogeneous or ideal. In fact, gas partial pressures will be identical throughout the alveolar region, and the gas exchange efficiency will be the highest possible for this lung. Thus regional variation of alveolar gas composition is indicative of heterogeneity and of a state of impaired gas exchange efficiency of the mammalian alveolar lung.

This situation is, in general, fundamentally different in nonmammalian vertebrates. Due to strikingly different structures of the gas exchange organs, variations in gas composition in the region of gas exchange may well occur in the face of ideal matching of ventilatory and perfusive flows. In fact, these variations may indicate a peculiarly high gas exchange efficiency. Also, these gas exchange organs may be charged with heterogeneities, like mismatch of flows, which would impair their efficiency for gas transfer; however, unlike in the alveolar lung, regional variability of gas composition is not necessarily indicative of functional heterogeneity.

It is the aim of this chapter to show the relationship between the structure of the gas exchange organ and the distribution and mixing of the respired medium (air or water) and to describe the resulting features of gas exchange performance. The study will be confined to two vertebrate classes, birds and fishes, because their gas exchange organs are structured in a particularly characteristic manner which allows a simple model analysis, and because there exist both theoretical and experimental bases on which to rest this analysis. Moreover, on species of the other vertebrate classes, there are only few studies which are relevant to the topic of this study (on snakes: Read and Donnelly, 1972; Donnelly and Woolcock, 1978; Gratz et al., 1981; on turtles: Burggren et al., 1978; Spragg et al., 1980; on the distribution of skin blood flow in frogs: Moalli et al., 1980). Experimental findings related to ventilation distribution in fishes, amphibians, reptiles, and birds have been reviewed by Hughes (1973). Problems that may arise for oxygen uptake in aquatic animals from incomplete mixing of the ambient water have recently been considered by Piiper and Scheid (1981).

II. Birds

A. Anatomy of the Lung-Air Sac System

The avian respiratory system comprises two components (Duncker, 1971, 1972, 1974): the parabronchial lung, in which gas exchange takes place, and the air sacs, which allow the volume changes required for tidal ventilation (Fig. 1A) (see Scheid, 1979, 1982). The gas volume of the parabronchial lung is small and appears to change little during the respiratory cycle. On the other hand, no significant gas exchange occurs in the air sacs (Magnussen et al., 1976). This division of labor is distinct from the situation in the mammalian lung, where the alveoli provide both gas exchange and tidal volume changes.

In most birds there exist nine air sacs, four paired and one unpaired, which are, from cranial to caudal: the cervical, the clavicular (unpaired), the cranial thoracic, the caudal thoracic, and the abdominal air sacs (Fig. 1). According to their connections to the bronchial system and to their function in ventilation, it is useful to distinguish two groups of air sacs: the cranial air sacs (cervical, clavicular, and cranial thoracic), and the caudal air sacs (caudal thoracic and abdominal).

The trachea divides into two primary bronchi or main bronchi, one for each body side. Each primary bronchus gives rise to four medioventral secondary brochi (ventrobronchi) which ramify on the ventral surface of the lung. Further caudal, a variable number of mediodorsal secondary bronchi (dorsobronchi) originate from the primary bronchus and ramify on the laterodorsal surface of the lung.

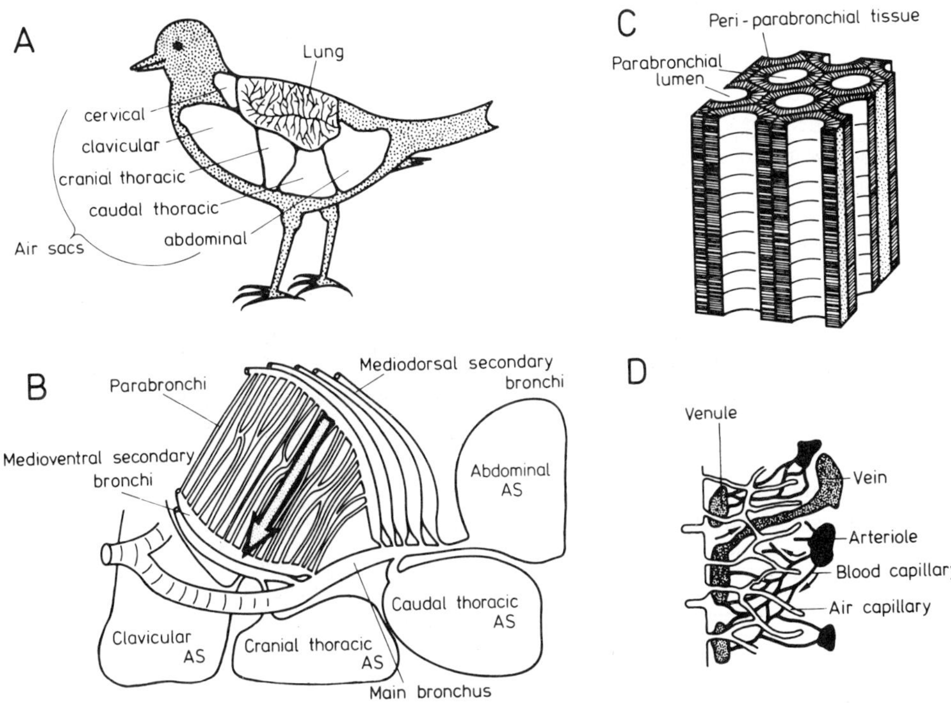

Figure 1 Anatomy of the respiratory system in birds. (A) Location of lungs and air sacs in the body. (B) Bronchial system and its connection with the air sacs. Arrow in the parabronchial lung indicates direction of (unidirectional) ventilatory flow. (C) Section from the parabronchial lung. (D) Relation between air capillaries and blood capillaries in the periparabronchial tissue. Blood flow from arterioles through blood capillaries into venules and veins indicated by arrows.

These two sets of secondary bronchi, ventrobronchi and dorsobronchi, are connected by a number of tertiary bronchi, or parabronchi (300-500 in both lungs of a chicken), which are arranged in a regular parallel array and show only little anastomosing (Fig. 1B). These parabronchi constitute the main portion of the lung which is present in all birds and has been termed paleopulmo by Duncker (1971). In addition, there exists an additional network of parabronchi, the neopulmo (Duncker, 1971), which extends, to a variable degree among different bird species, from the main bronchus and dorsobronchi to the caudal air sacs.

The diameter of the parabronchial lumen is about 1 mm, and the surrounding mantle of periparabronchial tissue is about 200-500 μm thick, with variability among species (Fig. 1C). In this tissue there is an interwoven tubular network of very fine (10-20 μm in diameter) air capillaries, which depart in radial direction from the parabronchial lumen, and the blood capillaries, in which blood flows from arterioles in the periphery of the mantle to collecting venules near the parabronchial lumen (Fig. 1D). It is in this meshwork of air capillaries and blood capillaries where gas exchange takes place.

B. Distribution of Airflow to Air Sacs

Tidal changes in the volume of the respiratory system are largely determined by changes in air sac volume with only small fluctuations in the volume of the parabronchial lung. This is not only due to the larger compliance of the air sacs (Scheid and Piiper, 1969) compared with the lung (Macklem et al., 1979), but is mainly a result of the much smaller lung gas volume compared with that of the air sacs (Scheid et al., 1974b; Scheid, 1978a). In addition, rhythmic innervation, in phase with respiration, of the costodiaphragmatic muscles appears to minimize respiratory changes of the parabronchial gas volume. Thus the lung behaves like a rigid flow-through system that is ventilated by action of the bellows-like air sacs (see Scheid, 1979).

The compliance of the air sacs is probably largely determined by the elasticity of the body wall and the muscle tone. Generally, both inspiration and expiration are active, brought about by action of striated muscles (see Fedde, 1976). Birds lack a diaphragm, and the air sacs extend throughout the thoracoabdominal cavity.

Since all air sacs are ventilated synchronously, the sum of air sac ventilation must equal total ventilation. Scheid et al. (1974b) measured volume and ventilation of the individual air sacs in ducks by dilution and washout of helium. They found in spontaneously breathing ducks that the volume and the ventilation of caudal and cranial air sac groups was about equal (Fig. 2). In relaxed, artificially ventilated ducks, the caudal group contained a larger share of the volume and received a larger share of ventilation, probably due to increased compliance in parts of the thoracoabdominal cavity not covered by the rib cage.

The air sacs send extended outgrowths into spaces between muscles, ligaments, and bones, and even into bones (femur, humerus, vertebrae, cranium). Such diverticula are certainly not ventilated and their gas content probably equilibrates with surrounding tissues. They may contribute to reducing the specific gravity of the bird by enlarging the body dimensions at constant body mass, and to increasing thermal insulation, particularly of the brain (Warncke and Stork, 1977). But also the main, ventilated portions of the air sacs show a considerable degree of stratified inhomogeneity, as

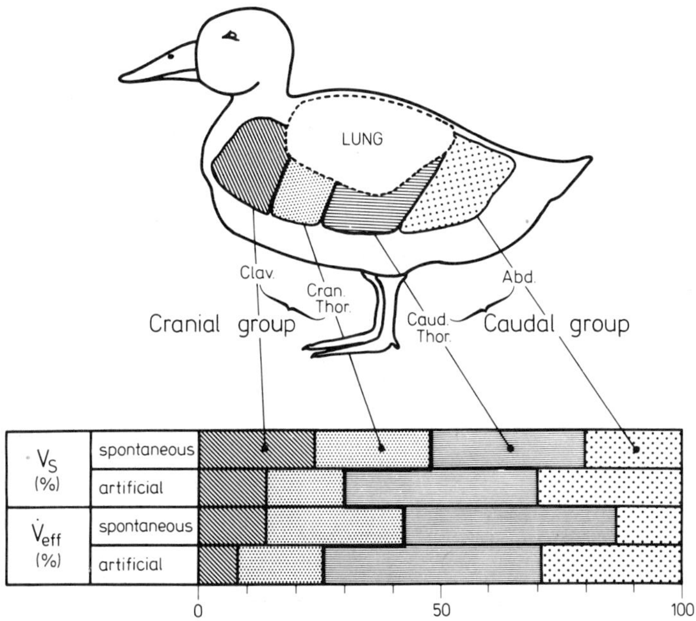

Figure 2 Distribution of volume (V_S) and effective ventilation ($\dot{V}_{eff}$) to the air sacs during spontaneous breathing and artificial ventilation. (Modified from Scheid et al., 1974b.)

shown by Torre-Bueno et al. (1980). This effect is of importance when the relationships between gas concentrations and effective ventilation are quantitatively analyzed.

C. Direction and Pattern of Airflow

Air reaches the alveoli of mammalian lungs after passing through a number of branching bronchiolar tubes, the airways thus forming a dead end, to-and-fro system for airflow. The flow of air in the avian lung, on the other hand, cannot easily be predicted from structural considerations. Since the parabronchial tubes of the avian lung are open at both ends, air can flow through them in either direction, and the path taken by the air between the trachea and the air sacs is likewise unpredictable. In fact, this problem has long been a matter of controversy and imaginative speculation (see Scheid, 1979).

In recent years, several investigators attempted to apply direct techniques to measure airflow in the avian respiratory tract. Bretz and Schmidt-Nielsen (1970, 1971) devised a flow-sensitive catheter probe incorporating two thermistors as sensing elements. This probe could be advanced through the main bronchus into a ventrobronchus or dorsobronchus. They observed flow in awake ducks during rest and thermal panting, as well as in anesthetized birds.

Scheid and Piiper (1970b, 1971a) devised a flowmeter tube containing a heat source and a thermocouple element which they could implant through the lateral body wall into the larger dorsobronchi of the duck. Recordings were made in awake animals at rest and during heat-induced panting, and also in pump-ventilated birds after relaxation.

Brackenbury (1971) constructed small tubes in which flow could be measured manometrically. He implanted the tube from the lateral body wall into the major dorsobronchi in geese, and observed airflow in anesthetized, spontaneously breathing animals.

All of these authors observed air to flow in the dorsobronchi during both inspiration and expiration, flow direction being the same in these bronchi in both respiratory phases (i.e., from the main bronchus into the dorsobronchi) (Fig. 3). This implies, with the given anatomy of the bronchial connections, that airflow through the parabronchi of the paleopulmo is also in the same direction during inspiration and expiration, from dorsobronchi toward ventrobronchi. This pattern is usually referred to as unidirectional airflow in the avian parabronchial lung. Support for the unidirectional flow thesis was also obtained by observations of inert or respiratory gases at various sites in the respiratory system after bolus injections of the gases at key sites (Schmidt-Nielsen et al., 1969; Bouverot and Dejours, 1971; Bretz and Schmidt-Nielsen, 1972).

Although the unidirectional flow through the parabronchi appears to have been demonstrated beyond a reasonable doubt, there are still controversies about the pattern of flow in other parts of the respiratory system. In particular, the direction of inspiratory flow across the ventrobronchial orifices into the main bronchus is much debated. Of particular interest is the "inspired loop hypothesis" of Hazelhoff (1943) by which, during inspiration, parabronchial gas flows from ventrobronchi into the main bronchus and thus more than once over the parabronchi. Debate also exists about whether all flow from caudal air sacs during expiration is directed into the (paleopulmonic) lung or whether some gas passes the direct way out through the main bronchus.

These questions have recently been tackled by measurement of gas concentration profiles, using a mass spectrometer, along ventrobronchi and main bronchi in awake spontaneously breathing ducks (Powell et al., 1981). Figure 4 summarizes the results. During inspiration, fresh air is measured along the main bronchus, even caudal to the ventrobronchial orifices, suggesting that there exists no "inspired loop." But the reversed flow upon inspiration, from main bronchus into ventrobronchi, is similarly excluded since there is

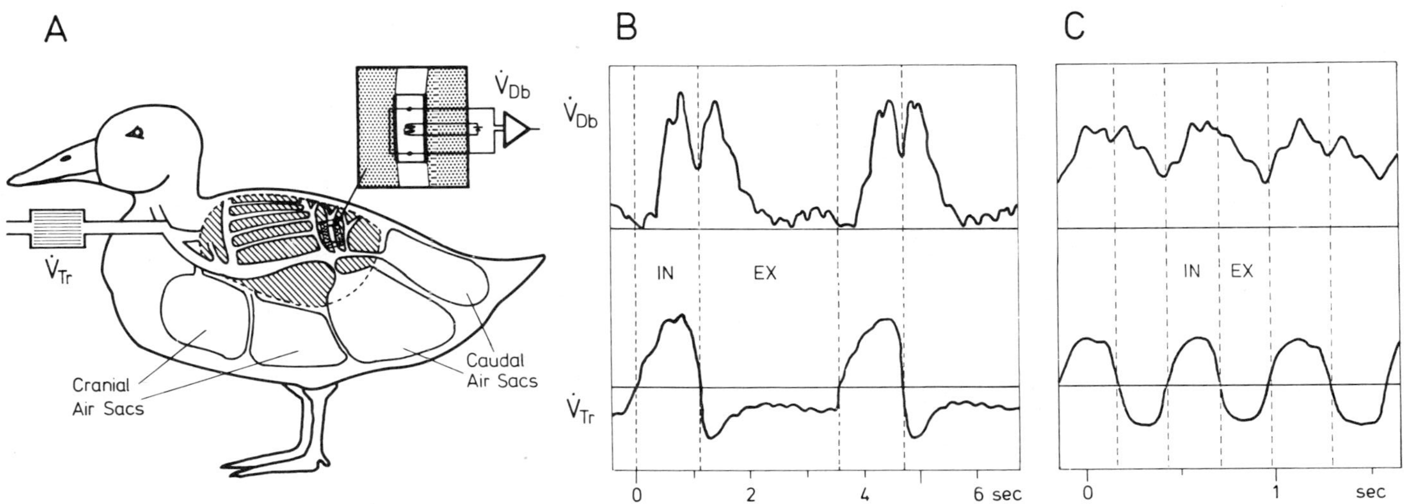

Figure 3 Measurement of dorsobronchial airflow ($\dot{V}_{Db}$) in the duck. (A) Experimental situation with a direction-sensitive flowmeter implanted in the dorsobronchus, and with a pneumotachometer to measure tracheal flow ($\dot{V}_{Tr}$). (B) $\dot{V}_{Db}$ and $\dot{V}_{Tr}$ during inspiration (IN) and expiration (EX). Note that $\dot{V}_{Db}$ is positive, that is, in the direction from main bronchus toward parabronchi, during both respiratory phases. (C) Measurements during panting (note the expanded time scale). $\dot{V}_{Db}$ is still unidirectional with attenuated flow fluctuations (partial rectification). (Modified from Scheid and Piiper, 1971a.)

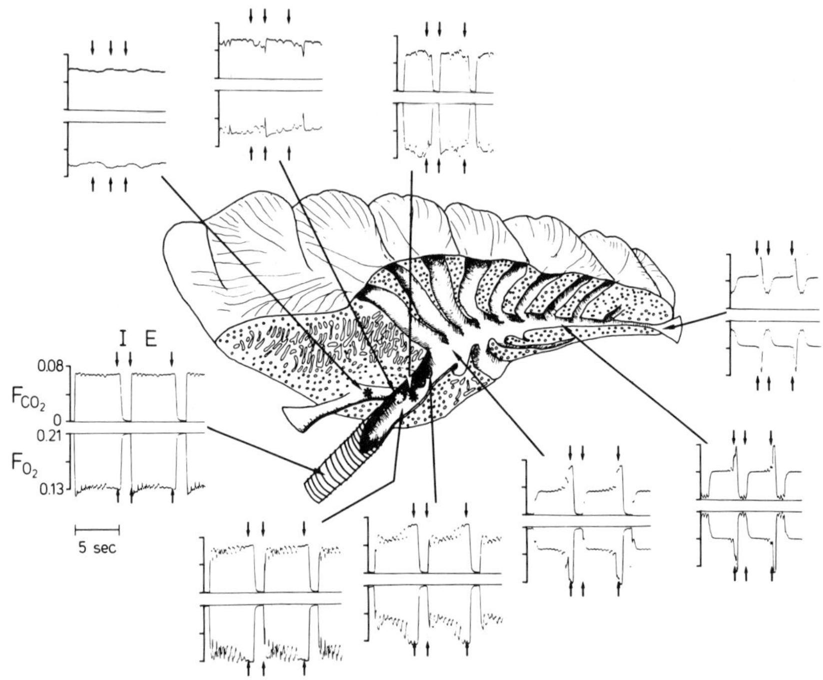

Figure 4 Measurement of respiratory cyclic variations of CO_2 and O_2 fractions at various sites in the bronchial system of spontaneously breathing ducks, obtained by mass spectrometry. See the text for an explanation. (Modified from Powell et al., 1981.)

no fresh gas phase observed in the ventrobronchi. Thus the ventrobronchial orifices act like a functional valve that is closed during inspiration. Comparison of the expiratory levels of gas concentration in ventrobronchi, caudal main bronchus, and trachea suggests that there is only a small fraction of expired air leaving caudal air sacs directly through the main bronchus, thereby bypassing the lung. These results agree with those of Bretz and Schmidt-Nielsen (1971), obtained by flow measurements. Figure 5 is a diagram of airflow in the resting bird according to the results outlined above.

The simplest explanation for the unidirectional airflow would be the existence of anatomic valves, opened and closed in phase with breathing. Although claimed by a number of authors in the past (see Scheid, 1979), valves or similar anatomic elements that would cause unidirectional airflow have never been found by anatomists (King and Payne, 1960).

Scheid et al. (1972) have shown that the unidirectional dorsobronchial

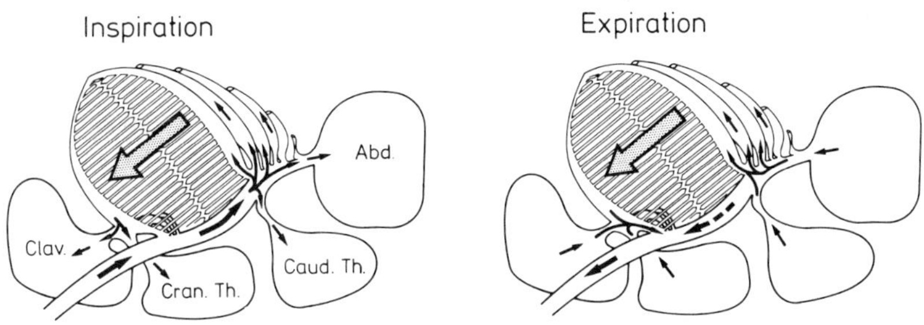

Figure 5 Schema of gas flow in the avian bronchial system during inspiration (left) and expiration (right). For details, see the text. (Modified from Scheid, 1979.)

flow persists in the paralyzed, pump-ventilated (and even in the dead) animal. These authors have also experimented with isolated parts of the bronchial system excised from a duck that was fixed by glutaraldehyde. They concluded that some aerodynamic mechanisms, such as boundary layer detachment, local jet formation, and/or the Bernoulli effect, may be involved in producing the respiratory airflow rectification. A similar conclusion was reached by Brackenbury (1972). There is certainly more work to be done in this field, which appears to call for cooperation between physiologists and fluid dynamicists.

Recently, Molony et al. (1976) found airflow resistance across the ventrobronchial orifices into the main bronchus to be CO_2-dependent—high at low CO_2, and vice versa. The anatomic correlate of such a CO_2-dependent flow resistance is not identified. The authors suggested that this dependence could provide part of a functional valving mechanism.

It is tempting to assume that the unidirectional air flow in the parabronchi is of benefit for gas exchange with blood. This would, in fact, be the case if the parabronchial lung operated as a countercurrent system, as had been proposed earlier (Schmidt-Nielsen, 1971). However, the actual arrangement of blood flow and gas flow in the parabronchi suggests a different model for gas exchange, the crosscurrent model, the efficiency of which does not depend on the direction of flow (see below). Thus rectification of parabronchial gas flow is not required for the functioning of the gas exchange system.

Piiper and Scheid (1973) have suggested that flow reversal would create a functional breath-holding situation during the time required for flow reversal. They have indicated that the rates of drop in P_{O_2} and rise in P_{CO_2} could be intolerably high due to the small parabronchial gas volume. However, direct evidence shows that gas exchange with intermittent ventilatory flow is only little impaired compared with gas exchange during continuous ventilatory flow, probably because parabronchial gas is mixed during breath holding with that in the adjoining airways by way of convection and diffusion (Scheid et al., 1977). Hence the functional residual volume in the gas exchange region appears to be larger than the combined volume of the parabronchial air spaces (Scheid, 1978a).

During panting, airflow in the dorsobronchi, and thus in the lung, is still unidirectional (Bretz and Schmidt-Nielsen, 1971; Scheid and Piiper, 1971a). In fact, the oscillations in flow rate within a respiratory cycle appear to be largely attenuated at high breathing rates. Reversal of flow at the extremely high respiratory rates during panting could indeed be detrimental, as suggested by Piiper and Scheid (1973).

It is interesting to note that intrapulmonary CO_2 receptors, the activity of which affects breathing, seem to be located at the caudal (inflow) end of the parabronchus (Scheid et al., 1974a; see also Fedde, 1976; Bouverot, 1978; Scheid, 1982). At this location, the receptors are exposed to a rather low P_{CO_2} where their sensitivity curve is steep. Reversal of flow, on the other hand, would raise the P_{CO_2} in their microenvironment and would thereby bring the receptors into an unfavorable sensitivity range.

D. Crosscurrent Gas Exchange in the Parabronchi: A Series Inhomogeneity

To understand the principle of gas exchange in the avian parabronchial lung, it is essential to appreciate the anatomical relationship between airflow and blood flow in the parabronchus. The pulmonary artery branches into capillaries, and each blood capillary contacts the parabronchial air capillaries at only a very small fraction of the total parabronchial length.

Figure 6 represents a functional model to account for these anatomical features. This model has been termed "serial multicapillary," or crosscurrent, since airflow and blood flow in the region of gas exchange cross each other (Scheid and Piiper, 1970a). Scheid and Piiper (1970a) have used this model for quantitative analysis of gas exchange in avian parabronchial lungs. The result of this analysis is qualitatively shown for O_2 in Figure 6, where air with O_2 partial pressure P_I enters the parabronchus, and the P_{O_2} in mixed venous blood, entering all capillaries, is $P_{\bar{v}}$. Conversely, for CO_2, $P_{\bar{v}}$ is the highest and P_I is the lowest partial pressure value. The following features deserve attention:

1. The air, which flows through the parabronchus, gives off O_2 to, and accepts CO_2 from, all blood capillaries. Thus P_{O_2} and P_{CO_2} change continually along the parabronchus. The lowest levels of P_{O_2}, and

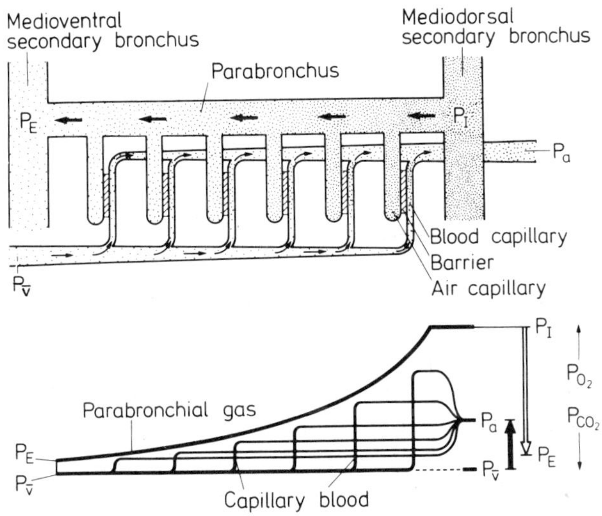

Figure 6 Top: Crosscurrent system for analysis of parabronchial gas exchange in birds. Bottom: Profiles of PO_2 or PCO_2 in parabronchial gas and capillary blood. For details, see the text. (Modified from Scheid, 1979.)

the highest of P_{CO_2}, in parabronchial gas are those at the end of the parabronchus, P_E.

2. The degree of arterialization in capillary blood decreases along the parabronchial axis, the arterial blood being a mixture from all capillaries. This feature, and feature 1 also, enable P_{O_2} in end-parabronchial gas to fall below the arterial level, and P_{CO_2} in end-parabronchial gas to exceed the value in arterial blood (Fig. 6).
3. The amount of gas exchanged per unit of parabronchial length is highest at the gas inflow end and diminishes continuously in the direction of gas flow, as the driving blood-gas partial pressure difference diminishes.

A remarkable intrinsic property of the parabronchial crosscurrent system is the independence of its gas exchange efficiency of gas flow direction. In fact, reversal of airflow would reverse the sequence in which the blood capillaries attain contact with the gas flowing through the parabronchus. But since arterial blood constitutes a mixture of blood from all capillaries, their sequence is immaterial. Reversal of gas or blood flow would retain the flow directions of both media relative to each other, and thus retain the crosscurrent system.

In search for the functional significance of unidirectional airflow (see above), a countercurrent model has been proposed for parabronchial gas exchange (Schmidt–Nielsen, 1971). In fact, reversal of the relative flow directions in the countercurrent model would turn that system into a cocurrent system and would thus seriously interfere with the gas exchange efficiency. Scheid and Piiper (1972) have experimentally reversed gas flow direction through the parabronchial lung of ducks, and have concluded that the crosscurrent rather than the countercurrent system is the more accurate model of parabronchial gas exchange.

The high gas exchange efficiency of the parabronchial system is reflected in the (potential) crossover of partial pressures in parabronchial gas and blood. As shown in Figure 6, arterial P_{O_2} (P_a) may exceed the expired level (P_E), which is impossible in the alveolar lung (negative alveolar-arterial P_{O_2} difference), and vice versa for CO_2. This crossover is, in fact, observed under physiologic conditions, particularly for CO_2 (Fig. 7). Thus for identical metabolic rate, ventilation, perfusion, diffusing capacity, and blood gas properties, the parabronchial system will reach a higher arterial P_{O_2} than the alveolar system (Piiper and Scheid, 1975). In parabronchial transfer of CO_2, the gas exchange efficiency of the crosscurrent system can be even further enhanced, by action of the Haldane effect, to such a degree that expired P_{CO_2} exceeds mixed venous P_{CO_2} (Meyer et al., 1976; Scheid, 1979).

Concentration gradients for respiratory gases along the parabronchus are typical for the crosscurrent system and occur even in the absence of any functional heterogeneity. In alveolar lungs, these concentration gradients within the gas exchanging airways are commonly referred to as "stratification." Although disagreement exists in the literature as to the significance of stratification as limiting gas exchange in humans under normal conditions, it can be shown that its presence would reduce alveolar gas exchange by imposing positive AaD_{O_2} and aAD_{CO_2} (gaps between gas and blood partial pressures; Scheid and Piiper, 1980). Stratification along the parabronchial axis, on the other hand, consequent upon the structural arrangement, is the decisive feature for the comparatively high gas exchange efficiency of this system. In fact, if mixing processes (e.g., provided by mechanical agitation of lung tissue by the heart or by diffusion along the parabronchial axis) attenuated the concentration gradients in the gas, the crosscurrent would approach the alveolar system with ensuing reduction in gas exchange efficiency. The essential difference between the effects of stratification in the alveolar and parabronchial systems resides in the mode in which both systems are ventilated: reciprocal in alveolar lungs; serial in avian lungs (Piiper and Scheid, 1978; Scheid and Piiper, 1980). It may thus be concluded that

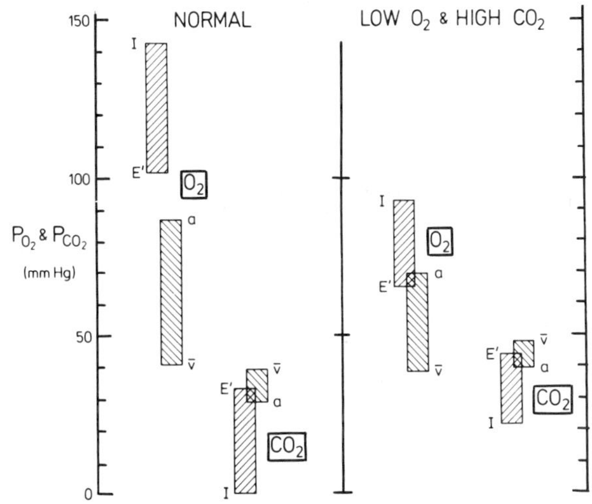

Figure 7 Measurement in the unanesthetized, spontaneously breathing hen of partial pressures for O_2 and CO_2 in inspired (I) and end-expired gas (E′) and in arterial (a) and mixed venous blood ($\bar{v}$). Left: air breathing; right: breathing a hypoxic-hypercapnic mixture. (Modified from Piiper and Scheid, 1973.)

stratification, in alveolar lungs a disadvantageous deviation from the ideal system, occurs even in the ideal parabronchial lung and reflects there the particularly high gas exchange efficiency of the system.

E. Diffusion Limitation in Air Capillaries: Another Series Inhomogeneity

The role of diffusion in the air capillaries of avian lungs in limiting gas exchange was first analyzed by Zeuthen (1942) and Hazelhoff (1943). An improved model which accounts for the microanatomy of the periparabronchial tissue (see above) has been used by Scheid (1978b). It consists of an air capillary in contact, all along its length, with a blood capillary in which blood flows from the peripheral end toward the entrance end of the air capillary (Fig. 8).

A particular feature of this system is that gases traverse the blood-gas separating tissue barrier all along the air capillary. This has two implications. First, not all gas molecules are subjected to the total diffusional resistance of air capillary gas, so that the peculiar arrangement of blood flow to the air capillary partially compensates the "stratified" resistance (Scheid and Piiper,

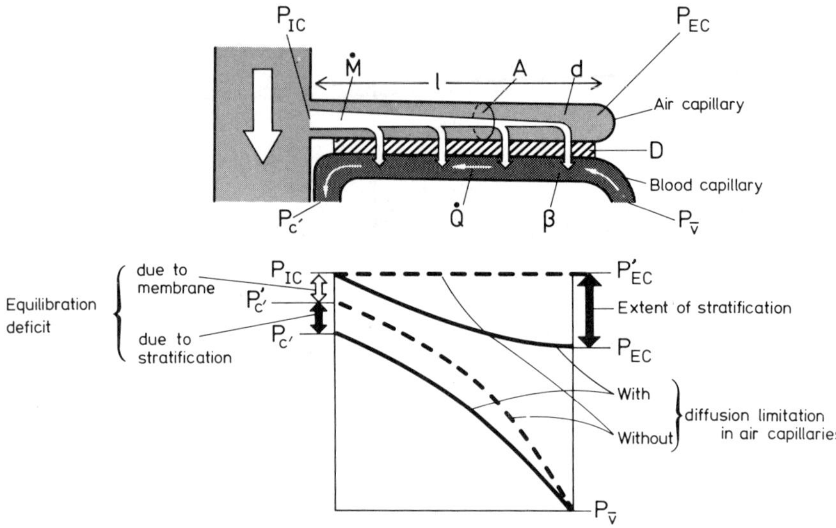

Figure 8 Top: Model for analysis of gas exchange between air capillaries and blood capillaries in avian parabronchial lungs. Air capillary, of length l and cross-sectional area A with flux ($\dot{M}$) (e.g., of O_2) (open arrow), due to diffusion alone (diffusivity d). Transport across gas-blood separating membrane (diffusing capacity D) into blood (flow rate $\dot{Q}$; effective solubility β). Bottom: Calculated PO_2 profiles along the air capillary, from initial-capillary (PIC) to end-capillary value (PEC), and in blood, from mixed-venous ($P\bar{v}$) to end-capillary value (Pc′). Solid lines calculated for finite diffusivity along the air capillary (finite stratification); dashed line indicates infinite diffusivity. (Modified from Scheid, 1979.)

1980). Second, the concentration gradient along the air capillary is not directly related to, and cannot be used to estimate, the diffusional resistance offered, as was shown by Zeuthen (1942) and by Hazelhoff (1943). In fact, if the blood-gas membrane were of infinite conductance, all gas would be taken up into blood at the entrance of the air capillary and the diffusive resistance of its gas phase would thus be immaterial; yet the partial pressure gradient along the air capillary in this case would be the highest possible, as the gas in the distal parts of the air capillary would equilibrate with mixed venous blood. A more reliable measure for the limitation to gas exchange offered by diffusion within the air capillaries is the increase in the degree of arterialization of end-capillary blood when diffusion resistance of the air capillary is reduced to zero.

This is shown schematically in Figure 8 by the partial pressure profiles in blood and gas along the air capillaries. The continuous lines are calculated for a finite value of diffusional resistance in air capillary gas, while for the dashed curves this diffusional resistance was assumed to be zero, in which case gas P values would be identical throughout the air capillary. The difference, at the end of the air capillary, in P values between the continuous (P_{EC}) and the dashed curves (P'_{EC}) corresponds to the extent of stratification, which appears to be marked in this case. However, removal of diffusion resistance in air capillaries results in an only small increase in end-capillary blood partial pressure (compare $P'c'$ with Pc').

Calculations suggest that under resting conditions the air capillaries impose no significant resistance to parabronchial gas exchange (Scheid, 1978b) and this is confirmed by measurement of O_2 and CO_2 exchange when diffusivities of these gases in the gas phase are increased about 2.5-fold by replacing air N_2 by He (Burger et al., 1979). However, under conditions of elevated gas exchange rates (e.g., exercise) the diffusion resistance in air capillaries may contribute significantly to the gas exchange resistance. There is substantial uncertainty in these estimates, as the morphometric information needed for the calculations is incomplete.

Recently, Crank and Gallagher (1978) have performed similar calculations with similar results. They have also considered diffusion of gases in axial direction within the parabronchus and found it to contribute significantly to longitudinal gas transport only at extremely low parabronchial flow rates.

Scheid (1978b) has termed the model for gas exchange between air capillaries and blood capillaries "countercurrentlike" since the partial pressure profiles in gas and blood phases resemble those of a countercurrent system. It should be noted, however, that there is convective flow only in the blood capillary, which makes this system distinct from a true countercurrent system. It sould also be noted that this model is not a substitute for the crosscurrent system, as the former describes gas exchange within the air capillary while the latter considers gas exchange between the bulk of parabronchial gas and capillary blood.

The countercurrentlike system takes account of the microscopic structure of the periparabronchial tissue observed by Duncker (1974). Other authors (Abdalla and King, 1975; Akester, 1971) have proposed slightly different structural relations among air capillaries and blood capillaries which lend themselves to different models for gas exchange. Scheid (1978b) has investigated these alternatives as well and found them to be inferior to the countercurrentlike system. It may thus be concluded that stratification may occur along the air capillaries but that the adverse effects on gas exchange are partially offset by the structural arrangement of blood flow, constituting a countercurrentlike system.

F. Parallel Inhomogeneity

Aside from the structural arrangement that gives rise to the series inhomogeneities of gas composition within the parabronchus, there may exist a heterogeneity of functional parameters, (e.g., perfusion, ventilation, diffusing capacity) which, as in the mammalian lung, impairs gas exchange efficiency in the avian lung. Two types of functional heterogeneity may be discerned: (1) along a given parabronchus (series inhomogeneity) and (2) between different parabronchi (parallel inhomogeneity; see Scheid, 1979).

It has been shown experimentally, using radioactive microspheres, that blood flow per unit of parabronchial length is higher at the caudal (gas inflow) end than at the cranial (gas outflow) end (Holle et al., 1978). This series heterogeneity results in impaired gas exchange efficiency only if the distribution of the diffusing capacity, D, along the parabronchus is not matched to the blood flow; in particular for infinite diffusing capacity, this series inhomogeneity is without effect (Holle et al., 1978).

Parallel inhomogeneity may result both from unequal ventilation/perfusion ratios or unequal diffusing capacity/perfusion ratios between parabronchi. They would give rise to differences in gas composition at corresponding sites in different parabronchi, and would thus be directly comparable to parallel inhomogeneity in alveolar lungs. Burger et al. (1979) have estimated parallel inhomogeneity on the basis of O_2 and CO_2 exchange. Recently, Powell and Wagner (1982a,b) have adopted the multiple inert gas technique, developed for analysis of $\dot{V}_A/\dot{Q}$ inhomogeneity in alveolar lungs (Wagner and West, 1980), for the goose lung. Both studies suggest that parallel heterogeneity exists in bird lungs but that its significance for gas exchange is limited.

III. Fish

A. Anatomy

The gas exchange apparatus of teleost fish gills is illustrated schematically in Figure 9. The gill arches (generally four) are covered by an operculum. They bear a double row of gill filaments which support on both sides a row of microscopic (secondary) lamellae. The secondary lamellae, with the filaments, form functionally a siev for the respiratory water current. Gas exchange occurs in this siev between interlammelar water and lacunar blood, across the lamellar epithelium. The lamellae contain blood lacunae which are perfused with venous blood from the ventral aorta, via afferent branchial arteries. After arterialization in the lamellae, blood is collected by efferent branchial arteries into the dorsal aorta and systemic arteries. It follows from the anatomical arrangement that, at the site of gas exchange, blood and water currents flow in opposite directions; the resulting countercurrent system is characterized by a particularly high gas transfer efficiency (see below).

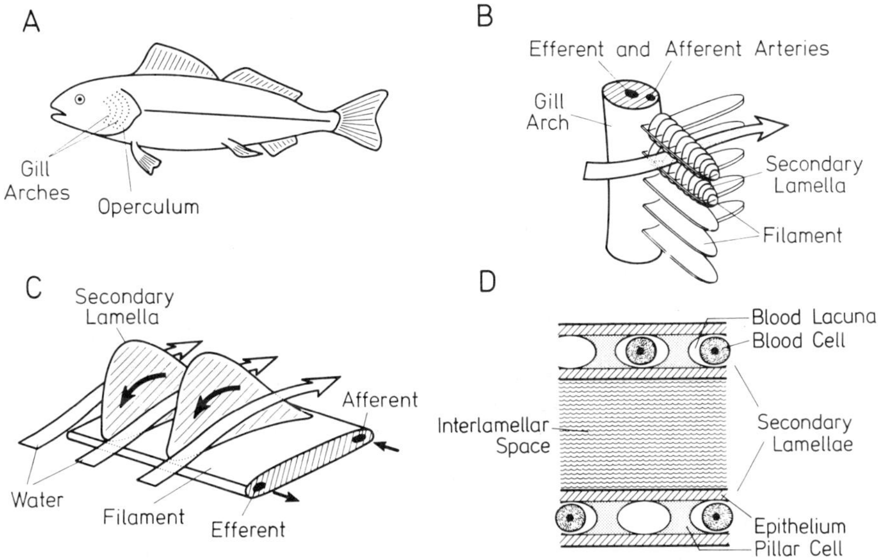

Figure 9 Anatomy of the respiratory system in teleost fishes. (A) Location of gill arches behind the operculum. (B) Section of one gill arch carrying a double row of gill filaments which, in turn, carry secondary lamellae. (C) Section of a gill filament with two secondary lamellae with blood flow in them and water flow between them, arranged in opposite directions. (D) Section of two neighboring secondary lamellae with epithelium and supporting pillar cells, leaving blood lacunae for blood perfusion. Water flow through interlammelar space.

In elasmobranch fish (dogfish, sharks, skates, rays), there is no operculum or, more correctly, each gill slit functionally has its own operculum, which is formed by the extension of the gill septum, whereby expired water exits (usually) from five gill slits on each side (Fig. 10). The arrangement of the filaments, lamellae, and of the blood flow is similar to that of teleost fish. Thus elasmobranch fish also appear to possess a countercurrent gas exchange system in their gills.

B. Respiratory Water Flow

The respiratory water flow is produced by the action of two pumps which are arranged in series and work at a phase difference: the "buccal pump" and the "opercular pump." Both pumps are capable of creating pressure and suction, produced by a complex set of muscles in combination with elastic recoil. Important for their action is the presence of two sets of valves, the

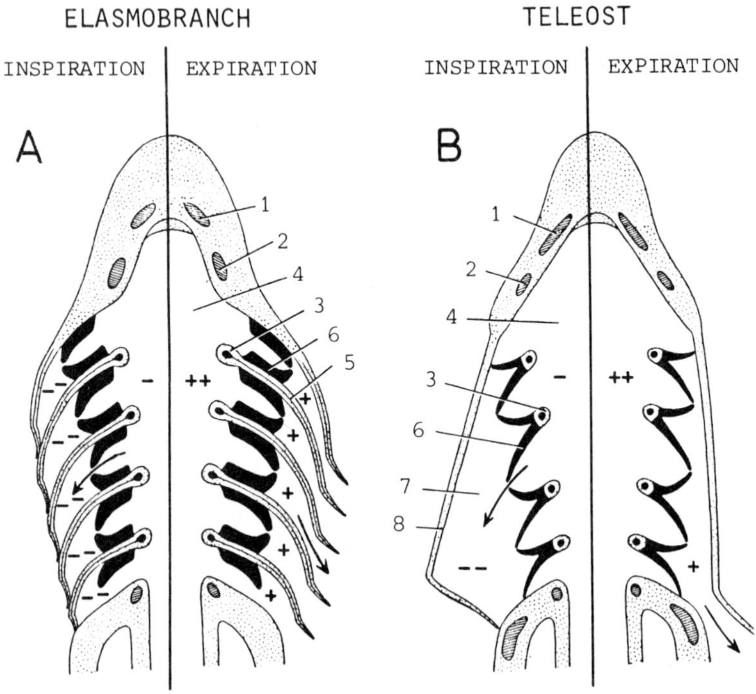

Figure 10 Schema of horizontal section through head region to show respiratory apparatus in elasmobranch (A) and teleost fish (B). 1, Mandibular arch; 2, hyoid arch; 3, gill arch; 4, buccal cavity; 5, interbranchial septum with gill rays; 6, gill filaments with secondary lamellae; 7, opercular cavity; 8, operculum. Signs + and – refer to direction of pressures (relative to ambient), and number of signs, to their amplitudes. (Modified from Portmann, 1965.)

mouth valve and the opercular valve, closing the buccal and opercular cavities, respectively. When the pressure inside the buccal cavity is negative, relative to the environment, the mouth valve opens; in contrast, the opercular valves open with positive pressure in the opercular cavity.

The four phases of a respiratory cycle according to Hughes (1963) are shown in Figure 11. They are defined with regard to the state of the two valves, which open and close with phase differences. In phase I, the pressure in both cavities is negative; the mouth valve is thus open, the opercular valve closed. Since opercular pressure is more negative than buccal prrssure, water flows from the buccal to the opercular chambers. In phase II, buccal pressure is positive and opercular pressure negative; both valves are closed, and

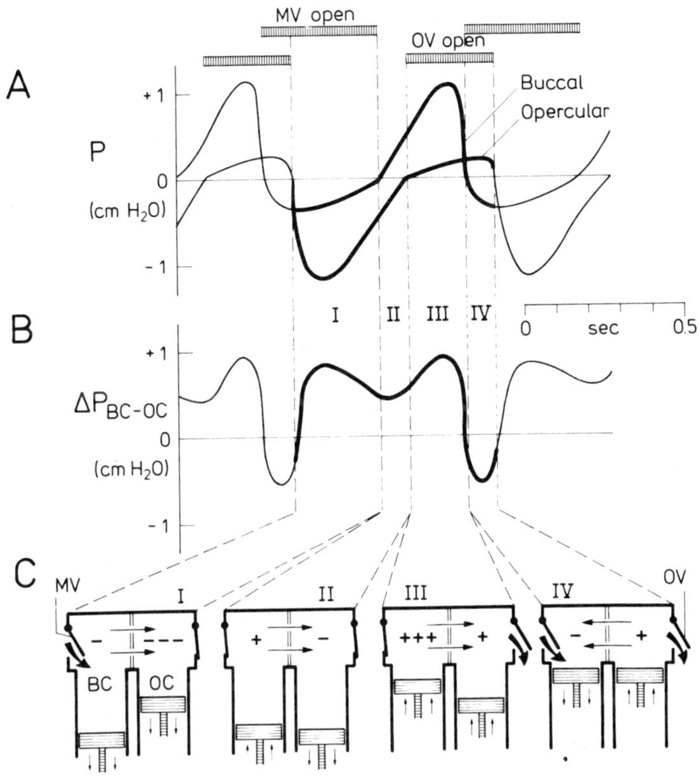

Figure 11 Variations of buccal and opercular pressures in the respiratory cycle (A) and of their difference [$\Delta P_{BC\text{-}OC}$ (B)]. Four phases (I-IV) defined by the time when one of the pressures becomes zero. (C) Schematic representation of the action in the four phases of the buccal and opercular cavities and the mouth valve (MV) and opercular valve (OV). BC, OC: buccal and opercular cavities. (Modified from Hughes, 1973.)

water flow keeps the direction of phase I. In phase III, both pressures are positive; the opercular valve opens and water flows across the gills and leaves the opercular chamber. Finally, in phase IV, buccal pressure becomes negative and water enters the buccal cavity both through the mouth and across the gills, from the opercular cavity.

Essential for gas exchange is the fact that water flow through the gill sieve occurs during the largest part of the respiratory cycle in the direction from the buccal to the opercular cavity, there being a reflux of water in the opposite direction only during a short period (phase IV of Fig. 11). However, the pattern of flow, which is probably similar to that of the differential pressure between the buccal and opercular cavities (Fig. 11), is thus far from constant.

Many fishes, particularly steady and constant swimmers, open their mouth during swimming and suppress respiratory movements, thereby obtaining a passive water flow through the gills (called ram-jet ventilation). In this case, the work of ventilation is performed by the locomotory muscles. This is probably energetically economical because the respiratory water flow is rather steady (no acceleration-deceleration work required). Moreover, steady water flow is also economical for gas exchange (see below).

The flow in the interlamellar spaces appears to be laminar since the Reynolds number is far below the critical value at which turbulence occurs (Hughes and Shelton, 1962). But in the buccal and opercular cavities, and across the mouth and opercular valves, the flow is expected to be turbulent.

The cost of breathing is expected to be higher in water than in air due to differences in the physical properties of both media. Thus the viscosity of water is much higher than that of air (high frictional resistance), and so is the density (acceleration-deceleration work); the O_2 solubility, on the other hand, is much lower in water than in air (high ventilation required) and so is the diffusivity for gases (high diffusion resistance). Estimates of the cost of breathing in fish span a wide range (reviewed by Holeton, 1980).

These unfavorable conditions are counterbalanced by a particularly effective gas exchange system (countercurrent system, see below) and probably by a high efficiency of respiratory muscles and low flow resistance of the gill apparatus (main resistance in the gill sieve, little resistance in the "conducting waterways," in contrast to mammalian lungs).

C. Countercurrent Gas Exchange in the Gills: A Series Inhomogeneity

Opposite directions of interlamellar water flow and lacunar blood flow are the basis for countercurrent gas exchange in fish gills. The simplified model of the countercurrent system in Figure 12A shows schematically that partial pressures in both respiratory water and blood change along the gill slit as gases are exchanged across the lamellar membrane. Due to the countercurrent arrangement, arterial partial pressures may equilibrate closely to inspired partial pressures, whereby a substantial water-blood overlap in partial pressures is produced. This is the basis for the particularly high gas exchange efficiency of the countercurrent system. Reversal of either flow (Fig. 12B), which converts the countercurrent into a cocurrent system, abolishes this overlap and thus impairs the efficiency.

The high gas transfer efficiency of the countercurrent system is bound

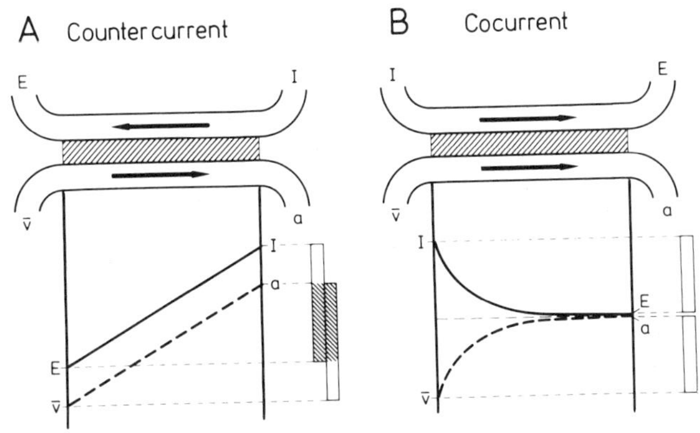

Figure 12 Countercurrent and cocurrent systems and representative partial pressure profiles. For details, see the text.

to a number of conditions (reviewed by Piiper and Scheid, 1982, 1984): (1) the ventilation/perfusion conductance ratio must be close to unity, and (2) there must be only a small extent of diffusion limitation, including diffusion in the medium and in blood, and chemical reaction kinetics of O_2 and CO_2.

If PO_2 and PCO_2 gradients in series (longitudinal) direction within the gas exchange area are considered as "stratified inhomogeneity," there is a pronounced stratified inhomogeneity in fish gills. But in contrast to the stratified inhomogeneity in mammalian lung models, this stratification enhances gas exchange in fish gills (see Sec. IV). Thus the situation is comparable to the series inhomogeneity of gas composition along the parabronchial gas phase of avian lungs (Sec. II.D).

D. Diffusion Limitation in Interlamellar Water: Another Series Inhomogeneity

Since the width of the interlamellar spaces (20-100 μm) is much greater than the thickness of the water-blood tissue barrier (0.2-10 μm; see Piiper, 1971), a sizable, possibly major part of the total diffusive resistance to water-blood gas transfer should reside in the interlamellar water. The role of diffusion in interlamellar water in limiting branchial gas transfer has been studied by Scheid and Piiper (1971b) using a highly simplified gill model (Fig. 13). This model represents an interlamellar space bounded by two lamellae of trapezoidal shape, the length at the edge being a fraction λ (<1) of the length at the base (ℓ_0). The slit width is b_0 and the lamellar height, h_0.

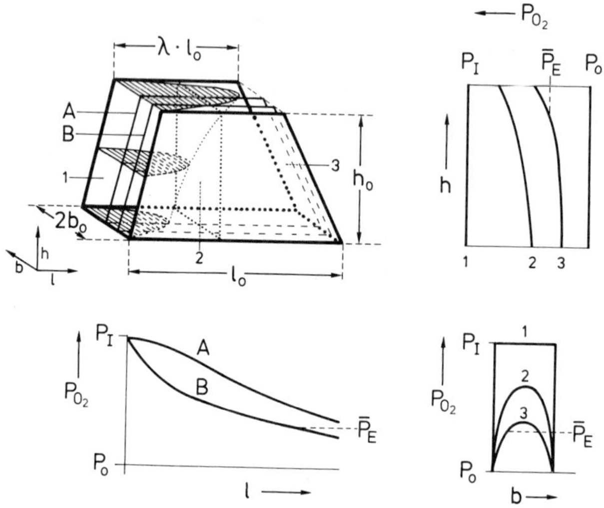

Figure 13 Model for analysis of diffusion limitation in interlamellar water. For details, see the text. (From Piiper and Scheid, 1984.)

The O_2 partial pressure in water at the lamellar surface is assumed to be constant at P_0 throughout the lamella (in reality, this PO_2 decreases from the water inflow to its outflow end). Water flow is assumed to be laminar (with parabolic velocity profile) and inversely proportional to slit length, which decreases linearly from the base to the free edge due to the trapezoidal shape of the lamella. Thus there are velocity gradients in both the b and h directions (see Fig. 13). Oxygen is assumed to diffuse in the b direction only (i.e., perpendicularly to the lamellar surface).

The resulting PO_2 profiles, shown schematically in Figure 13, display PO_2 gradients in all three space dimensions:

1. $\partial P/\partial \ell$, reflecting the progressive O_2 depletion
2. $\partial P/\partial b$, due to resistance to diffusion
3. $\partial P/\partial h$, due to the base-to-apex velocity gradient

Because of gradients 2 and 3, PO_2 in outflowing water (P_E) varies across the cross section. The decisive variable for the overall O_2 uptake is the PO_2 in the mixed expired water ($\bar{P}_E$) obtained by (flow-weighted) double integration of P_E with respect to b and h.

The inefficiency of O_2 equilibration may be expressed by the inefficiency parameter, $\epsilon = (\bar{P}_E - P_0)/(P_I - P_0)$. Since, in the absence of diffusion limitation in water, $\bar{P}_E$ must equal P_0, ϵ constitutes an equivalent shunt which may be termed the "water diffusion shunt" to distinguish it from the "diffusion shunt" due to membrane diffusion (Piiper and Scheid, 1984).

It can be shown (Scheid and Piiper, 1971b) that ϵ is determined by the tapering factor λ and by a dimensionless parameter $\phi = (b^2{}_0\bar{v})/(\ell_0 d)$. The parameter ϕ contains two geometric variables (the half-width of the interlamellar space, b_0, and its base length, ℓ_0); the mean water velocity, $\bar{v}$; and the diffusion coefficient of O_2 in water, d. ϕ is proportional to the mean water velocity, $\bar{v}$, and thereby to the water flow rate, $\dot{V}_W$.

Figure 14 shows, for the model of Figure 13, theoretical curves for ϵ as a function of ϕ at some values of λ. ϵ increases with increasing ϕ and with decreasing λ. Estimates using experimental values for ventilation and morphometric data yield ϕ values ranging from about 0.02 to about 10 (Scheid and Piiper, 1971b). The corresponding ϵ values range from close to zero to about 80%. Typical ϵ values for basal resting conditions are 0-5%; and for increased ventilation due to hypoxia or activity, 10-15%.

Since the mechanism involved is diffusion limitation, it is appropriate to transform the inefficiency parameter, ϵ, into an equivalent or apparent diffusing capacity, D_{app}, defined as the diffusing capacity in an equivalent model in which diffusion limitation is offered by a stagnant water layer of appropriate thickness bordering on the interlamellar surface, water in the

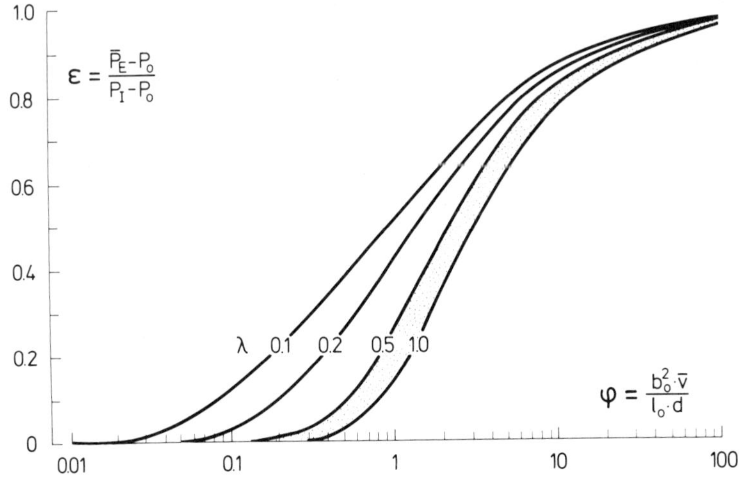

Figure 14 Inefficiency ϵ of interlamellar partial pressure equilibration due to finite diffusivity in interlamellar water in the model of Figure 13. For details, see the text. (From Piiper and Scheid, 1984.)

central portions of the interlamellar space being well mixed in both the b and h directions (Fig. 13). Remarkably, D_{app} increases considerably with increasing ϕ and thus with increasing mean water flow velocity, $\bar{v}$, or increasing ventilation, $\dot{V}_w$. This feature may be important for facilitating O_2 uptake in conditions of increased O_2 requirement (swimming, hypoxia).

Since the lamellar surface PO_2 was assumed to be constant (at P_0) in the simplified model of Figure 13, diffusion resistance offered by water was artificially isolated from other resistances to gas transfer, notably from those due to membrane diffusion and blood perfusion. If it is assumed that water diffusion and membrane diffusion resistances may be considered to be arranged in series, D_{app} can be compared with membrane D in an attempt to estimate their relative magnitudes. This has been done by Scheid and Piiper (1971b, 1976). Both D values were found to be of comparable magnitude in the dogfish.

Recently, a more comprehensive model has been investigated in which diffusion both across a tissue barrier and in flowing water are considered simultaneously and blood perfusion is finite (J. Piiper, C. Hook, and P. Scheid, unpublished). According to preliminary results of calculations, the effects of diffusion limitation in interlamellar water are slightly less than calculated for the simplified model because their water and membrane diffusion resistances are functionally not strictly in series (or additive) in the comprehensive model. However, the simplified model seems to yield sufficiently good estimates of the order of magnitude for diffusion limitation in interlamellar water.

It may be concluded that series inhomogeneities in interlamellar water, both across the lamellar slit and along its height, result from finite diffusion coefficients. These inhomogeneities are qualitatively comparable with stratified inhomogeneity in the alveolar lung in that they impose a resistance to gas exchange and thus reduce the gas transfer efficiency. The extent of this effect, however, depends on the structure of the gas exchange system and is thus expected to be different in gills and in alveolar lungs.

E. Parallel Inhomogeneity

The effects of unequal ventilation-perfusion distribution in fish gills are, in principle, similar to those in mammalian or avian lungs. They may occur on different scales: in individual interlamellar spaces/lamellae, in entire gill slits/branchial arches, or at any intermediate level.

The effects of $\dot{V}/\dot{Q}$ inequalities may be described in terms of water shunt, equaling parallel dead space ventilation, and of blood shunt, equaling venous admixture (see Piiper and Scheid, 1984). But "true water shunts" are also likely to occur, as water may flow outside the interlamellar spaces between departed lamellar rows. In fact, given the anatomically unstable gill sieve, it is astonishing that the water shunts are rather small according to measurements on resting fish.

IV. Mammals versus Birds and Fish: Search for Similarities

It was shown in the preceding sections that structural elements in the gas exchange system lead to particularly high gas exchange efficiency (Secs. II.D and III.C) and may minimize detrimental effects of mixing impairment (Sec. II.E). In this section we shall investigate whether some of these elements can be applied to the mammalian lung as well.

A. "Countercurrentlike" Element

There appears to be considerable stratification in the air capillaries of avian lungs but, due to the peripheral-to-central capillary blood flow in the parabronchial unit, this "stratification" has no or little effect on blood arterialization (see Sec. II.E). It is conceivable that in mammalian lungs, capillary blood flow is preferentially directed from distal to proximal alveolar ducts, as has been envisaged by West et al. (1969). A simplified model for this situation is shown in Fig. 15B, where the alveolar duct is represented by two serially arranged compartments with blood contacting these elements in a countercurrentlike fashion. The partial pressures in blood and gas phases, as well as in expired and arterial blood, are indicated. It is evident that arterial blood (Pa) can equilibrate to expired gas (PE). Hence, as in the avian air capillary, serial concentration gradients (stratification) exist, but their effects on gas exchange are minimized. In fact, with blood contact to the distal compartment only, positive AaD_{O_2} and aAD_{CO_2} due to stratification would exist.

On the other hand, the gas transfer efficiency of this countercurrentlike element is inferior to that of the countercurrent system (Fig. 15A), as it cannot create negative AaD_{O_2} and aAD_{CO_2} values. It should be noted, however, that there is no anatomical or physiological basis for countercurrentlike blood flow arrangement in the alveolar lung.

B. "Crosscurrentlike" Element

The alveolar ducts of mammalian lungs are relatively elongated structures surrounded by the blood capillary network along their length, and are thereby comparable to avian parabronchi (the ramification, extensive in mammalian lungs but practically absent in avian lungs, is not an essential difference for this consideration). Hence a crosscurrentlike arrangement, as shown in Figure

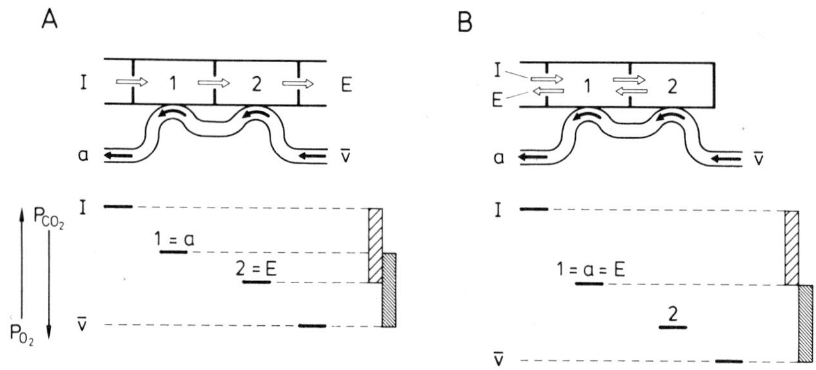

Figure 15 Simplified model to compare countercurrent system (A) and countercurrentlike system (B). For details, see the text.

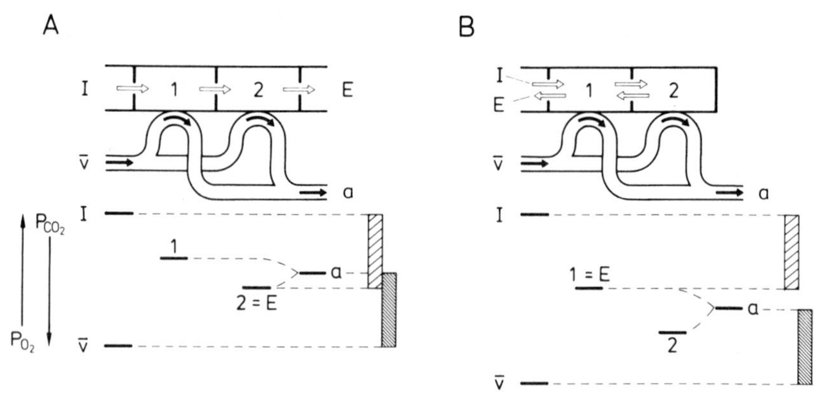

Figure 16 Simplified model to compare crosscurrent system (A) with crosscurrentlike system (B). For details, see the text.

16, may exist in the acinus, which has recently been considered by Weibel et al. (1981).

It was shown above (Sec. II.D) that the crosscurrent arrangement of gas and blood flows in avian lungs is decisively beneficial, increasing gas exchange efficiency beyond that attained by simple alveolar lung models. Could this be true for mammalian lungs as well? The essential difference between both systems resides in the circumstance that the avian parabronchi are open at both ends and are thus ventilated in a flow-through manner, whereas the alveolar ducts constitute a dead-end alley which must be ventilated in a to-and-fro fashion. As shown in Figure 16, in the parabronchial (A) as in the alveolar duct system (B), arterial P_{O_2} derives as a mixture from the serially arranged capillaries. However, expired gas P_{O_2} (P_E) represents the lowest P_{O_2}, being below Pa, in the parabronchial lung, while for the alveolar duct it constitutes the highest P_{O_2}, above Pa (normal, positive AaD_{O_2}). Hence compared with the true crosscurrent system, the crosscurrentlike element of the alveolar duct does not show the high intrinsic efficiency.

However, the gas exchange efficiency of this system exceeds that of an alveolar duct model in which perfusion is restricted to the distal compartment (no perfusion in the capillary to compartment 1 in Fig. 16B). This has been shown by Scheid (1978b), who analyzed the crosscurrentlike element for gas exchange in the avian air capillary and showed that this system is superior to the "alveolarlike" model in which blood flow is only at the dead end of the air capillary.

C. Conclusion: Elements for Minimizing Effects of Stratified Inhomogeneity in Alveolar Lungs

Figure 17 is a summary of the various systems considered in this chapter and of the concentration gradients in their gas exchange regions. In the countercurrent (A) and crosscurrent systems (B) these gradients are closely linked to the high gas exchange efficiency. In the alveolar pool model (C), in which alveolar gas mixing is complete, the gas exchange efficiency is inferior to that of the counter- or crosscurrent systems.

The models of Figure 17D-F constitute the elements for considering imperfect mixing (i.e., stratification in its strict sense) in alveolar ducts. They also apply, however, to imperfect mixing in other systems (e.g., countercurrentlike element for avian air capillaries). The "dead-end contact" system (Fig. 17F), which imposes a series stratificational resistance, results in positive stratificational AaD_{O_2} and aAD_{CO_2} when compared with the mixed pool system (Fig. 17C). Part of this stratificational resistance can be eliminated when the blood flow arrangement creates a crosscurrentlike system (Fig. 17E). The countercurrentlike element (Fig. 17D) can (ideally) remove entirely the effect of stratification on gas exchange, thus removing the AaD_{O_2} and aAD_{CO_2}.

It thus appears that the alveolar lung, due to its to-and-fro ventilation, is particularly prone to series stratificational resistances. Elements of structural arrangement of blood flow may minimize the effects of stratification on gas exchange. The anatomical basis, however, and the physiologic effectiveness of these structural elements, remain to be demonstrated.

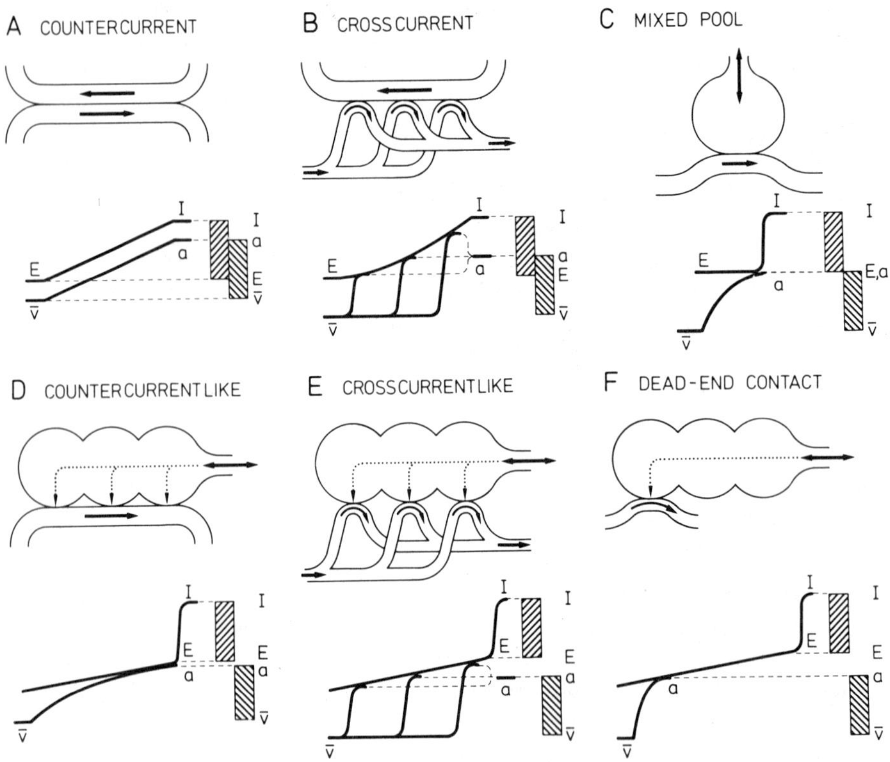

Figure 17 Potential models for gas exchange in the acinus of alveolar lungs in the presence of stratified inhomogeneity (D-F) and comparison with gas exchange in the basic models for fish gills (A), avian lungs (B), and ideal alveolar lungs (C). For explanations, see the text.

References

Abdalla, M. A., and King, A. S. (1975). The functional anatomy of the pulmonary circulation of the domestic fowl. *Respir. Physiol.*, **23**:267-290.

Akester, A. R. (1971). The blood vascular system. In *Physiology and Biochemistry of the Domestic Fowl*, Vol. 2. Edited by D. J. Bell and B. M. Freeman. London, Academic Press, pp. 783-839.

Bouverot, P. (1978). Control of breathing in birds compared with mammals. *Physiol. Rev.*, **58**:604-655.

Bouverot, P., and Dejours, P. (1971). Pathway of respired gas in the air sacs-lung apparatus of fowl and ducks. *Respir. Physiol.*, **13**:330-342.

Brackenbury, J. H. (1971). Airflow dynamics in the avian lung as determined by direct and indirect methods. *Respir. Physiol.,* **13**:319-329.

Brackenbury, J. H. (1972). Physical determinants of air flow pattern within the avian lung. *Respir. Physiol.,* **15**:384-397.

Bretz, W. L., and Schmidt-Nielsen, K. (1970). Patterns of air flow in the duck lung. *Fed. Proc.,* **29**:662.

Bretz, W. L., and Schmidt-Nielsen, K. (1971). Bird respiration: flow patterns in the duck lung. *J. Exp. Biol.,* **54**:103-118.

Bretz, W. L., and Schmidt-Nielsen, K. (1972). The movement of gas in the respiratory system of the duck. *J. Exp. Biol.,* **56**:57-65.

Burger, R. E., Meyer, M., Graf, W., and Scheid, P. (1979). Gas exchange in the parabronchial lung of birds: experiments in unidirectionally ventilated ducks. *Respir. Physiol.,* **36**:19-37.

Burggren, W. W., Glass, M. L., and Johansen, K. (1978). Intrapulmonary variation of gas partial pressures and ventilation inequalities in chelonian reptiles. *J. Comp. Physiol.,* **126**:203-209.

Crank, W. D., and Gallagher, R. R. (1978). Theory of gas exchange in the avian parabronchus. *Respir. Physiol.,* **35**:9-25.

Donnelly, P., and Woolcock, A. (1978). Stratification of inspired air in the elongated lungs of the carpet python, *Morelia spilotes variegata. Respir. Physiol.,* **35**:301-315.

Duncker, H.-R. (1971). The lung air sac system of birds. *Ergeb. Anat. Entwicklungsgesch.,* **45**(6):1-171.

Duncker, H.-R. (1972). Structure of avian lungs. *Respir. Physiol.,* **14**:44-63.

Duncker, H.-R. (1974). Structure of the avian respiratory tract. *Respir. Physiol.,* **22**:1-19.

Fedde, M. R. (1976). Respiration. In *Avian Physiology,* 3rd ed. Edited by P. D. Sturkie. New York, Springer-Verlag, pp. 122-145.

Gratz, R. K., Ar, A., and Geiser, J. (1981). Gas tension profile of the lung of the viper, *Vipera xanthina palestinae. Respir. Physiol.,* **44**:165-176.

Hazelhoff, E. H. (1943). Bouw en functie van de vogellong. *Versl. Gewone Vergad. Afd. Natuurk. Kon. Ned. Akad. Wet.,* **52**:391-400. English translation (1951): Structure and function of the lungs of birds. *Poult. Sci.,* **30**:3-10.

Holeton, G. F. (1980). Oxygen as an environmental factor of fishes. In *Environmental Physiology of Fishes.* Edited by M. A. Ali. New York, Plenum Press, pp. 7-32.

Holle, J. P., Heisler, N., and Scheid, P. (1978). Blood flow distribution in the duck lung and its control by respiratory gases. *Am. J. Physiol.,* **234**:R146-R154.

Hughes, G. M. (1963). *Comparative Physiology of Vertebrate Respiration.* London, William Heinemann.

Hughes, G. M. (1973). Comparative vertebrate ventilation and heterogeneity. In *Comparative Physiology: Locomotion, Respiration, Transport and Blood.* Edited by L. Bolis, K. Schmidt-Nielsen, and S. H. P. Maddrell. Amsterdam, North-Holland, pp. 187-220.

Hughes, G. M., and Shelton, G. A. (1962). Respiratory mechanisms and their nervous control in fish. *Adv. Comp. Physiol. Biochem.,* **1**:275-364.

King, A. S., and Payne, D. C. (1960). Does the air circulate in the avian lung? *Anat. Rec.,* **136**:223.

Macklem, P. T., Bouverot, P., and Scheid, P. (1979). Measurement of the distensibility of parabronchi in duck lungs. *Respir. Physiol.,* **38**:23-35.

Magnussen, H., Willmer, H., and Scheid, P. (1976). Gas exchange in air sacs: contribution to respiratory gas exchange in ducks. *Respir. Physiol.,* **26**: 129-146.

Meyer, M., Worth, H., and Scheid, P. (1976). Gas-blood CO_2 equilibration in parabronchial lungs of birds. *J. Appl. Physiol.,* **41**:302-309.

Moalli, R., Meyers, R. S., Jackson, D. C., and Millard, R. W. (1980). Skin circulation in the frog, *Rana catesbeiana:* distribution and dynamics. *Respir. Physiol.,* **40**:137-148.

Molony, V., Graf, W., and Scheid, P. (1976). Effects of CO_2 on pulmonary air flow resistance in the duck. *Respir. Physiol.,* **26**:333-349.

Piiper, J. (1971). Gill surface area: fishes. In *Handbook of Respiration and Circulation.* Edited by P. L. Altman and D. S. Dittmer. Bethesda, Md., Federation of American Societies for Experimental Biology, pp. 119-121.

Piiper, J., and Scheid, P. (1973). Gas exchange in avian lungs: models and experimental evidence. In *Comparative Physiology.* Edited by L. Bolis, K. Schmidt-Nielsen, and S. H. P. Maddrell. Amsterdam, North-Holland, pp. 161-185.

Piiper, J., and Scheid, P. (1975). Gas transport efficacy of gills, lungs and skin: theory and experimental data. *Respir. Physiol.,* **23**:209-221.

Piiper, J., and Scheid, P. (1978). Series ventilation and stratified inhomogeneity in avian vs. mammalian lungs. *Physiologist,* **21**:92.

Piiper, J., and Scheid, P. (1981). Oxygen exchange in the metazoa. In *Oxygen and Living Processes.* Edited by D. L. Gilbert. New York, Springer-Verlag, pp. 150-176.

Piiper, J., and Scheid, P. (1982). Physical principles of respiratory gas exchange in fish gills. In *Gills.* Edited by D. F. Houlihan, J. C. Rankin, and T. J. Shuttleworth. Cambridge, Cambridge University Press, pp. 45-61.

Piiper, J., and Scheid, P. (1984). Model analysis of gas transfer in fish gills. In *Fish Physiology,* Vol. X. *Gills,* Part A. Edited by W. S. Hoar and D. J. Randall. New York, Academic Press, pp. 229-262.

Portmann, A. (1965). *Einführung in die vergleichende Morphologie der Wirbeltiere.* Basel, Schwabe.

Powell, F. L., and Wagner, P. D. (1982a). Measurement of continuous distributions of ventilation-perfusion in nonalveolar lungs. *Respir. Physiol.,* **48**:219-232.

Powell, F. L., and Wagner, P. D. (1982b). Ventilation-perfusion inequality in avian lungs. *Respir. Physiol.,* **48**:233-241.

Powell, F. L., Geiser, J., Gratz, R. K., and Scheid, P. (1981). Airflow in the avian respiratory tract: variations of O_2 and CO_2 concentrations in the bronchi of the duck. *Respir. Physiol.,* **44**:195-213.

Read, J., and Donnelly, D. M. (1972). Stratification of blood flow in the elongated lungs of the carpet python. *J. Appl. Physiol.,* **32**:842-846.

Scheid, P. (1978a). Estimation of effective parabronchial gas volume during intermittent ventilatory flow: theory and application in the duck. *Respir. Physiol.,* **32**:1-14.

Scheid, P. (1978b). Analysis of gas exchange between air capillaries and blood capillaries in avian lungs. *Respir. Physiol.,* **32**:27-49.

Scheid, P. (1979). Mechanisms of gas exchange in bird lungs. *Rev. Physiol. Biochem. Pharmacol.,* **86**:137-186.

Scheid, P. (1982). Respiration and control of breathing. In *Avian Biology,* Vol. VI. Edited by D. S. Farner and J. R. King. New York, Academic Press, pp. 405-453.

Scheid, P., and Piiper, J. (1969). Volume, ventilation and compliance of the respiratory system in the domestic fowl. *Respir. Physiol.,* **6**:298-308.

Scheid, P., and Piiper, J. (1970a). Analysis of gas exchange in the avian lung: theory and experiments in the domestic fowl. *Respir. Physiol.,* **9**:246-262.

Scheid, P., and Piiper, J. (1970b). Direkte Messung der Strömungsrichtung der Atemluft in der Entenlunge. *Pfluegers Arch. Gesamte Physiol.,* **319**:R59.

Scheid, P., and Piiper, J. (1971a). Direct measurement of the pathway of respired gas in duck lungs. *Respir. Physiol.,* **11**:308-314.

Scheid, P., and Piiper, J. (1971b). Theoretical analysis of respiratory gas equilibration in water passing through fish gills. *Respir. Physiol.,* **13**:305-318.

Scheid, P., and Piiper, J. (1972). Cross-current gas exchange in avian lungs: effects of reversed parabronchial air flow in ducks. *Respir. Physiol.,* **16**:304-312.

Scheid, P., and Piiper, J. (1976). Quantitative functional analysis of branchial gas transfer: theory and application to *Scyliorhinus stellaris* (Elasmobranchii). In *Respiration of Amphibious Vertrebrates.* Edited by G. M. Hughes. London, Academic Press, pp. 17-38.

Scheid, P., and Piiper, J. (1980). Intrapulmonary gas mixing and stratification. In *Pulmonary Gas Exchange,* Vol. I. Edited by J. B. West. San Francisco, Academic Press, pp. 87-130.

Scheid, P., Slama, H., and Piiper, J. (1972). Mechanisms of unidirectional flow in parabronchi of avian lungs: measurements in duck lung preparations. *Respir. Physiol.,* **14**:83-95.

Scheid, P., Slama, H., Gatz, R. N., and Fedde, M. R. (1974a). Intrapulmonary CO_2 receptors in the duck: III. Functional localization. *Respir. Physiol.,* **22**:123-136.

Scheid, P., Slama, H., and Willmer, H. (1974b). Volume and ventilation of air sacs in ducks studied by inert gas wash-out. *Respir. Physiol.,* **21**: 19-36.

Scheid, P., Worth, H., Holle, J. P., and Meyer, M. (1977). Effects of oscillating and intermittent ventilatory flow on efficacy of pulmonary O_2 transfer in the duck. *Respir. Physiol.,* **31**:251-258.

Schmidt-Nielsen, K. (1971). How birds breathe. *Sci. Am.,* **225**(6):72-79.

Schmidt-Nielsen, K., Kanwisher, J., Lasiewski, R. C., Cohn, J. E., and Bretz, W. L. (1969). Temperature regulation and respiration in the ostrich. *Condor,* **71**:341-352.

Spragg, R. G., Ackerman, R., and White, F. N. (1980). Distribution of ventilation in the turtle *Pseudemys scripta. Respir. Physiol.,* **42**:73-86.

Torre-Bueno, J. R., Geiser, J., and Scheid, P. (1980). Incomplete gas mixing in air sacs of the duck. *Respir. Physiol.,* **42**:109-122.

Wagner, P. D., and West, J. B. (1980). Ventilation-perfusion relationships. In *Pulmonary Gas Exchange,* Vol. I. Edited by J. B. West. San Francisco, Academic Press, pp. 219-262.

Warncke, G., and Stork, H. J. (1977). Biostatische und thermoregulatorische Funktion der Sandwich- Strukturen in der Schädeldecke der Vögel. *Zool. Anz.,* **199**:251-257.

Weibel, E. R., Taylor, C. R., Gehr, P., Hoppeler, H., Mathieu, O., and Maloiy, G. M. O. (1981). Design of the mammalian respiratory system: IX. Functional and structural limits for oxygen flow. *Respir. Physiol.,* **44**: 151-164.

West, J. B., Glazier, J. B., Hughes, J. M. B., and Maloney, J. E. (1969). Pulmonary capillary flow, diffusion, ventilation and gas exchange. In

Circulatory and Respiratory Mass Transport. Edited by G. E. W. Wolstenholme and J. Knight. London, J. & A. Churchill, pp. 256-272.

Zeuthen, E. (1942). The ventilation of the respiratory tract in birds. *K. Dan. Vidensk. Selsk. Biol. Medd.*, **17**:1-50.

Concluding Remarks

LUDWIG A. ENGEL

Westmead Hospital
Sydney, New South Wales, Australia

MANUEL PAIVA

Institute of Interdisciplinary Research
and Respiratory Research Unit
Free University of Brussels
Brussels, Belgium

The eight chapters provided by our contributors represent a comprehensive review of our present understanding of gas mixing and ventilation distribution in the lung. Rather than summarize the different chapters, we shall attempt to identify some of the areas that require further intense investigation, and venture to predict those in which advances may be expected in the foreseeable future.

Although the anatomy of the bronchial tree has been rigorously studied and the patterns of branching quantitatively described, the details of the structure of a lung acinus are poorly understood. Yet, recent model analyses have illustrated the sensitivity of gas distribution to local acinar anatomy. Since most of the mixing in the lung takes place within the acinus, an outstanding problem is the accurate definition of the anatomy of the acinus and its range of variation. Subsequently, a better description of the changes in structure occurring in various diseases will be required. The methods of serial section used in the past have been extraordinarily time-consuming and tedious, so that the shortage of this type of data is understandable. However, the application of computerized histological imaging techniques and three-dimensional reconstructions now available could make the task much less odious.

Hopefully, these techniques will be applied to lung morphometry in the near future.

It is curious that the mechanisms underlying the sloping alveolar plateau, an old friend of physiologists working in the field of gas mixing, still elude our understanding. Although theories of diffusion-dependent inhomogeneity date back to the beginning of this century, it is only in recent years that mathematical techniques for analyzing the mixing of gases within complicated structures have been capable of putting these theories to a rigorous test. The results have been illuminating but give rise to further questions. Multibranch-point models clearly point to the presence of intraacinar inhomogeneities of gas concentration and a diffusion-dependent pattern of emptying. However, the alveolar plateaus thus generated are always curvilinear. They therefore differ qualitatively from the linear slopes frequently observed experimentally. What is the basis for these slopes? Because it is difficult to conceive of a systematic distribution of mechanical properties within a single acinus, most model simulations assume a uniform and synchronous convective filling and emptying pattern. However, a mechanical basis for nonreversibility exists in the form of surface tension, and the surfactant lining of the lung introduces a hysteresis to the pattern of volume change. What is the effect of this nonuniformity? We do not know. Is it possible that the mechanical hysteresis and the gaseous convection-diffusion interaction combine to determine both the temporal and spatial distribution of inspired gases as well as the expired pattern of gas concentration? Further research is urgently needed to answer these questions.

At a macroscopic level, sequential emptying of unequally ventilated units has long been proposed as an explanation for the intraregional component of the sloping alveolar plateau. Yet, experimental data in support of this hypothesis are not available. Recently, new imaging techniques using small metallic markers in excised lung lobes have begun to provide some experimental evidence in support of the concept of unequal compliances among small portions of the lung parenchyma. Whether these units fill and empty sequentially is not yet clear. Further developments in this approach and its application to studies of gas distribution offer a fertile ground for many an investigator.

The study of alveolar ventilation at high frequencies using tidal volumes smaller than the anatomic deadspace (HFV) is a new and rapidly moving field. Much additional material will probably be available by the time this volume is published. The basic mechanisms of gas transport during HFV are currently being worked out, but precisely how these mechanisms are translated into gas exchange is still unclear. A major direction for future research will be to determine methods of quantitatively predicting (theoretically) and assessing (experimentally) the distribution of gas transport during HFV. These results will provide the basis for predicting the ventilation/perfusion distribution in the lung, and hence the critical factors determining oxygenation during HFV. The elucidation of the mechanisms underlying HFV will be as satisfying to the physiologist as a definition of the role of HFV in clinical practice will be to the clinician. Both these developments are likely in the near future and we look forward to them with great interest.

Ventilation distribution among topographically distributed lung regions is related to lung weight, gravity-induced chest wall deformation, and gradients in lung expansion. Sophisticated imaging techniques have succeeded in describing with increasing accuracy the regional inequality of lung expansion and inspired gas distribution. We can expect that improved tomographic imaging methods will further refine the resolution with which we shall be able to trace the distribution of inspired tracer gases into the different lobes, segments, and even subsegments of the lung. However, the most exciting prospect in the immediate future is the likelihood of identifying the contribution that gravity makes to the distribution of ventilation. By comparing measurements made during weightlessness in space with those obtained on the Earth's surface, we shall be able to partition the inequality of regional ventilation distribution into that due to gravity and that due to differences in regional mechanical properties of the lung. Experiments designed to address this question are in the making and will be performed in Spacelab 4, scheduled to fly in January 1986. Indeed, experiments planned for this and subsequent ventures into space will open new horizons for the study of pulmonary function during weightlessness and should provide exciting information on the behavior of the lung even on the Earth's surface.

In this volume we have set out to provide a comprehensive summary of what is known of gas mixing and ventilation distribution in the lung. The summary is intended not as a definitive and final statement but as an incentive to further research. It is clear that application of new and powerful computer technology will enable progress to be made in areas hitherto considered impossibly difficult. It is equally clear that this progress will depend on the dedicated collaboration among investigators from a variety of different disciplines. If this volume succeeds in stimulating some young scientists to work in this area and enter into such a collaboration it will have served its purpose.

AUTHOR INDEX

Italic numbers give the page on which the complete reference is listed.

C

D

E

F

I

J

K

L

M

N

O

S

T

SUBJECT INDEX

B

C

D

V

W